The Provider's Guide to Hospital-Based Psychiatric Services

Edited by
Allen H. Collins, M.D., M.P.H.
Lenox Hill Hospital and
New York Medical College
New York

Herbert H. Krauss, Ph.D.
Lenox Hill Hospital and Hunter College
New York

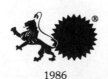

AN ASPEN PUBLICATION®
Aspen Systems Corporation

1986

Rockville, Maryland
Royal Tunbridge Wells

Library of Congress Cataloging in Publication Data

The Provider's guide to hospital-based psychiatric services.

"An Aspen publication."
Includes bibliographies and index.
1. Psychiatric hospitals—Administration. 2. Psychiatric hospital care. I. Collins, Allen
H. II. Krauss, Herbert, 1940-   . [DNLM: 1. Psychiatric Department, Hospital—
organization & administration. WM 27.1 P969]
RC439.P815   1985   362.2'1'068   85-15706
ISBN: 0-87189-232-4

Editorial Services: Jane Coyle

Library of Congress Catalog Card Number: 85-15706
ISBN: 0-87189-232-4

Printed in the United States of America

1 2 3 4 5

To our wives and children

for their patience and endurance
in the writing of this book.

Table of Contents

Contributors

Lisa Aiken, Chief Psychologist, Lenox Hill Hospital, New York; and Clinical Instructor in Psychiatry, New York Medical College, Valhalla, New York

Roger Barker, Vice President for Research and Evaluation, Brownlee, Dolan, Stein Associates, New York

Karen Ann Burns, Patient Care Coordinator, Medical-Surgical Intensive Care Unit, Department of Nursing, Lenox Hill Hospital, New York

Murry J. Cohen, Associate Attending Psychiatrist, Chief of Psychiatric Outpatient Services, and Psychiatric Consultant to the Methadone Maintenance Treatment Program, Lenox Hill Hospital, New York; and Assistant Professor of Psychiatry, Mount Sinai School of Medicine, New York; formerly Medical Director, Drug Rehabilitation Center, Mount Sinai Hospital and Medical Center, New York

Allen H. Collins, Attending Psychiatrist and Acting Director, Department of Psychiatry, Lenox Hill Hospital, New York; and Clinical Associate Professor of Psychiatry, New York Medical College, Valhalla, New York; and Psychiatric Consultant, Region II Office of the National Institute of Mental Health, New York

Joel Gonchar, Associate Attending Psychiatrist and Psychiatric Consultant to the Nephrology Service, Lenox Hill Hospital, New York; Assistant in Psychiatry at Columbia University, College of Physicians and Surgeons, New York; and Assistant Attending Psychiatrist at St. Luke's-Roosevelt Hospital Center, New York

Larry S. Goldblatt, Attending Psychiatrist and Chief of Psychiatric Consultation-Liaison Services, Department of Psychiatry, Lenox Hill Hospital, New York; and Clinical Assistant Professor, Department of Psychiatry, New York Medical College, Valhalla, New York

Martin H. Greenstein, Counselor, Employment Assistance Program Consortium, New York; Clinical Instructor in Psychiatry, New York Medical College, Valhalla, New York; formerly Coordinator, Psychiatric Outpatient Clinic, Department of Psychiatry, Lenox Hill Hospital, New York

Jerald Grobman, Adjunct Attending Psychiatrist and Psychiatric Consultant to the Cardiovascular Surgical Service, Lenox Hill Hospital, New York; formerly Associate Clinical Professor, Tufts University School of Medicine, Boston; and Assistant Psychiatrist and Director of Group Psychotherapy Training, Tufts-New England Medical Center Hospital, Department of Psychiatry, Boston

Ira R. Hoffman, Associate Director, Department of Medicine, Lenox Hill Hospital, New York; and Clinical Professor of Medicine, New York Medical College, Valhalla, New York

Natalie Jacobson, Psychiatric Social Worker, Psychiatric Outpatient Clinic, Lenox Hill Hospital, New York

Alice Keating, Mental Health Nurse Clinician to the Psychiatric Outpatient Clinic and Psychiatric-Psychosocial Emergency Program, Department of Nursing, Lenox Hill Hospital, New York

Beatrice J. Krauss, Assistant Professor of Psychology, College of New Rochelle, New Rochelle, New York

Herbert H. Krauss, Affiliate Psychologist, Lenox Hill Hospital, New York; Professor of Psychology, Hunter College, New York; Supervising Psychologist, International Center for the Disabled, New York; Clinical Associate Professor of Psychiatry (Psychology), Cornell University College of Medicine, New York; and Associate Attending Psychologist, New York Hospital and Payne Whitney Clinic, New York

Leo Kron, Adjunct Attending Psychiatrist, Departments of Psychiatry and Pediatrics, Lenox Hill Hospital, New York; Assistant Clinical Professor of Psychiatry, Columbia University College of Physicians and Surgeons, New York; and Instructor in Psychiatry, New York Medical College, Valhalla, New York

Charles Mazzone, Vice President, Patient Accounting and Records, Lenox Hill Hospital, New York

Marlene Nadler-Moodie, nursing consultant, educator, and clinician in private practice, Carlsbad, California; formerly Mental Health Nurse Specialist, Psychiatric Inpatient Scatter-Bed Program, Department of Nursing, Lenox Hill Hospital, New York

Richard Rosner, Associate Attending Psychiatrist, Department of Psychiatry, Lenox Hill Hospital, New York; Clinical Associate Professor of

Psychiatry, New York University, New York; Visiting Associate Professor of Psychiatry, Albert Einstein College of Medicine, Bronx, New York; and Adjunct Clinical Associate Professor, New York Medical College, Valhalla, New York

Thomas Sedlock, Adjunct Attending Psychiatrist and Psychiatric Consultant to the Medical-Surgical Intensive Care Unit, Department of Psychiatry, Lenox Hill Hospital, New York

Loren Skeist, Associate Attending Psychiatrist and Coordinator of Psychiatric Education, Department of Psychiatry, Lenox Hill Hospital, New York; Assistant Professor of Psychiatry, New York Medical College, Valhalla, New York; and Lecturer, Mount Sinai School of Medicine, New York

Eugene Wallsh, Chief of Cardiovascular Surgery, Department of Surgery, Lenox Hill Hospital, New York

Sheldon Zimberg, Adjunct Attending Psychiatrist, Department of Psychiatry, Lenox Hill Hospital, New York; Director of Psychiatry, North General Hospital, New York; and Associate Professor of Psychiatry, Mount Sinai School of Medicine, New York

Foreword

It is a pleasure for me to write a brief introduction to this highly informative book on hospital-based psychiatric services. As a director of medicine in a moderate-sized, acute care general hospital, I have had the rather unique experience of being administratively responsible for a Section of Psychiatry. By virtue of this organizational structure, the chief ("attending-in-charge") of this section has reported to me for the past two decades. This has permitted me, as an administrator and clinician of a different medical specialty, to maintain a bird's eye view of the day-to-day operations, as well as the longer-range evolution of the Psychiatry Service.

In actual fact, I inherited the administrative responsibility for the Psychiatry Service with my appointment as director of the Department of Medicine in 1966. The intervening 20 years can be roughly divided into two periods with respect to psychiatry. The first, 1966–1976, was one marked by repetitive programmatic and clinical difficulties. These are rather well-detailed in several chapters in the book (Chapters 1, 2, 3, 5, and 7). The principal problem came down to that of providing proper administrative leadership *within* the section. The intrinsic lack of familiarity that even a competent medical director has of the psychiatric specialty limits the director's ability to provide the leadership necessary for the growth and development of a general hospital psychiatric service. Indeed, many attempts were made to recruit able psychiatrists who were thought to represent potentially good leaders for this service. The fact that many fine clinicians were not able to accomplish the mandate to build the service attests to intrinsic differences between administrative and clinical skills. The complexities that exist in managing hospital clinical departments require considerable talents from the few physicians who are motivated and capable of meeting the challenges. Our experiences are one more example of the fact that accomplished clinicians do not necessarily make able administrators.

The second period, 1976–1984, was one of significant growth, development, and maturation of the Psychiatry Service. I am proud to have participated in this process. Many of the clinical services and training programs that were initiated are documented in the pages of this text. A major thread can be seen to run through virtually all of the descriptions of these programs: the relevance of psychiatry to, and its close coordination with, other medical-surgical services. I believe that this has been an extremely important byproduct of the anomaly in the organizational relationship between medicine and psychiatry. The fine working relationship that has evolved between the two disciplines has been reinforced by the new brand of psychiatrist that has arrived on the hospital scene—one who is medically adept, comfortable in the hospital setting, and able to provide specialty care that can be integrated into that of other medical-surgical specialists. Non-psychiatric physicians of all specialties have responded with enthusiasm to the extremely helpful participation of their psychiatric colleagues in jointly rendering care to patients. Moreover, the new psychiatric leadership has been welcomed into the wider arena of hospital administration, joining with their medical-surgical colleagues and lay managers in providing direction for the hospital as a whole.

From my vantage point, the present book is unusual in at least two other respects: First, the realistic perspective that it maintains—that of elucidating the provision of clinical care within the organizational matrix of the general hospital—is not very often seen in the professional literature. Consequently, the book is both practically informative and refreshing. Second, the program developments that form the substance of most of the chapters bear a striking resemblance to the actual realities as they unfolded. Many of us in organizational medicine, clinical medical practice, and academia are quite familiar with the fact that considerable discrepancies often exist between the manner in which a subject is treated in an article or chapter and the actual nature of the experience. This book is an exception in that regard.

In summary, the *Provider's Guide to Psychiatric Services in the General Hospital* offers a well-written, comprehensive, and practically oriented approach to professionals who devote themselves to caring for patients with emotional difficulties in the hospital environment. It provides useful guidelines for administrators in developing medically relevant mental health programs and valuable information for clinicians who choose to affiliate with general hospitals so that they can care for their patients more effectively. Indeed, as medicine becomes more sophisticated and complex, there are few alternatives to providing the necessary integration of biologically based medical services and psychosocially based care in hospital settings.

Michael S. Bruno, M.D.
Director, Department of Medicine
Lenox Hill Hospital, New York
Associate Dean and Professor of Medicine
New Yrok Medical College
Valhalla, New York

Preface

In the years following World War II, the role played by general hospitals in providing mental health services to communities has expanded greatly. Once of secondary importance, general hospitals have now assumed a central position in mental health care.[1] The era of community mental health centers, which saw its heyday in the 1960s and early 1970s, has yielded to the present epoch of "remedicalization" of those services. Mental health services have found their way back to the general hospital. Under the organizational aegis of clinical departments of psychiatry, mental health care has become increasingly coordinated with the other specialty health care services provided in this setting.

The evidence for the striking expansion of general hospital psychiatry over the past four decades is documented by the following:

- the increase in psychiatric patient care episodes[2,3]
- the growth of psychiatric inpatient units[4]
- the increased utilization of psychiatric clinics[5]

Furthermore, individuals seeking treatment for alcoholism[6] and substance abuse[7,8] and those requiring emergency psychiatric intervention[9,10] now frequently turn to their community general hospital for help. Psychiatric consultation-liaison services have become almost standard fare on medical surgical wards, bringing mental health support to medical patients and to nonpsychiatric physicians, nurses, and other health professionals.[11]

There are many fine general psychiatric texts and other specialized volumes that are concerned with the provision of psychiatric care in various settings, including that of the general hospital. By and large, these volumes emphasize purely clinical phenomenology, that is, the characteristics of patients that fulfill diagnostic criteria and the related treatment approaches to the disorders.[12-14] Other texts proceed one step further in providing practical illustrations of provider-patient interpersonal transactions and stressing the importance of considering hospital milieu factors that play a vital part in clinical care.[15-17] Only one reasonably current text consistently depicts the influence that organizational structures of the general hospital have upon clinical care, while also emphasizing the more purely "clinical" considerations.[18] An older text provides an excellent model of how to weave milieu-clinical interfaces into a variety of institutional program case examples.[19] However, considerable time has elapsed since its publication and major changes have occurred in the psychiatric field. Consequently, it is now dated. One recent book provides a similar case-study perspective.[20] It lacks more general application, however, by virtue of its focus on the provision of psychiatric services in smaller general hospitals, its brief survey design, and its omission of detailed descriptions of clinical care.

In sum, few psychiatric textbooks have integrated the specific organizational elements of the general hospital into their descriptions of how mental health clinical care is achieved in that setting. They describe clinical transactions as if they occur between provider and patient in an organizational vacuum. The physical, funding, legal, and marketing factors and the role of other health care personnel in rendering these services within the framework of the general hospital environment are largely omitted. Consequently, mental health professionals who want to affiliate with a general hospital in clinical, administrative, teaching, or other supportive role do not have a single text to which they can refer as a comprehensive resource. It is for this specific purpose that the present volume has been written.

The text offers a comprehensive view of mental health, alcoholism, and substance abuse services that are provided within the organizational matrix of the general hospital. Each chapter strives for a careful balance between clinical considerations, that is, the actual care provided to patients, and the milieu factors that impact on that care. The chapter authors are mental health professionals from various disciplines who have been involved for many years as program managers, clinicians, and teachers in the general hospital setting. Their focus is on the interface elements between clinical care/teaching and the milieu. Who are the professionals who provide these services? In which programmatic settings, and to which patient groups? What are the characteristics of the physical and health care personnel environment in which such services are delivered? And, most importantly, what are the relationships between the mental health providers/services and the wider hospital and community milieus?

With two exceptions, all of the chapters are written by members of the health care professional staff of Lenox Hill Hospital in New York City. Several of the authors have utilized their experiences in mental health programs of other general hospitals (Mt. Sinai Hospital and Medical Center, St. Luke's/Roosevelt Hospital Medical Center, North General Hospital—all in New York City) as reference points in their discussions. Consistent with the overall emphasis of the text, specific institutional milieu factors are described whenever applicable so that the organizational context can be appreciated. Also, wherever possible, the authors have utilized particular community, organizational, and programmatic contexts to illuminate general principles and recommendations for improving clinical practice in other general hospitals with similar missions.

The initial series of chapters focuses on the development and operation of several discrete clinical and teaching programs often found in general hospitals. These chapters (1 through 6) on psychiatric administration, innovative inpatient services, consultation-liaison services, outpatient services, emergency care, and teaching follow a traditional program format.

These are followed by a discussion of psychiatric services from the internist's perspective (Chapter 7), which offers a nonpsychiatric view of the programs described in the previous chapters. The author considers the availability of general hospital psychiatric services in the wider context of the concerns of medicine.

Subsequently, six chapters (8 through 13) focus on the provision of mental health services to specific patient populations and medical services—the child-adolescent psychiatry service, the intensive care unit, the cardiac surgery service, the renal dialysis unit, and services for alcoholism and substance abuse. These chapters provide the flavor of their specialized service milieus and patients, each with its own clinical challenges. They also address the ways in which the mental health providers who participate in the programs adapt to meet the unique clinical needs that are encountered.

The next three chapters (14 through 16) consider the roles of nonmedical mental health professionals—psychiatric nurses, psychologists, and social workers—in the medical environment of the general hospital. These disciplines are assuming increased importance in the delivery of mental health care in the acute care institutional setting. In spite of the parochial and often senseless national debates that drag on between the professional societies representing the various mental health disciplines, these professionals can work together in a collaborative manner in the medical hospital setting.

The last series of chapters deals with the increasingly important legal, financial, and marketing aspects of hospital-based mental health services. These have become vitally important in the 1980s as all health care delivery services have become concerned with the seemingly contradictory requirements of providing a high quality of care while containing health care costs. Caught in the crunch of such conflicting demands, mental health professionals who bear the responsibility for hospital-based services must become thoroughly familiar with the knowledge and skills offered in the legal, financial, and marketing areas.

The closing chapter on the future of mental health services presents some extrapolations from current trends in the context of historical realities.

We believe that professionals engaged in the administration, clinical practice, and teaching of mental health services will profit from this text, whether their primary organizational frame of reference is the general hospital or some other site. The realities of working within the structures and operational procedures of the general hospital can often be frustrating and dismaying. However, for those clinicians who regard the general hospital as a useful vehicle for providing up-to-date clinical care to patients, the setting has great creative potential.

REFERENCES

1. H.C. Schulberg, *The Treatment of Psychiatric Patients in General Hospital: A Research Agenda and Annotated Bibliography,* Mental Health Service System Reports, Series DN no. 4, Publication no. (ADM) 84–1294 (Washington, D.C.: U.S. Department of Health and Human Services, National Institute of Mental Health, 1984).

2. R. Redick, M. Witkin, and H. Bethel, *N.I.M.H. Mental Health Statistical Note No. 167,* Publication no. (ADM) 84–158 (Washington, D.C.: U.S. Department of Health and Human Services, 1984).

3. R. Redick and M. Witkin, *Separate Psychiatric Settings in Non-Federal General Hospitals, United States 1977–78,* Series CN no. 4, Publication no. (ADM) 82–1140 (Washington, D.C.: U.S. Department of Health and Human Services, National Institute of Mental Health).

4. R. Glasscote, J. Gudeman, and A. Beigel, *The Uses of Psychiatry in Smaller General Hospitals* (Washington, D.C.: Joint Information Service, 1983).

5. D. Regier and C. Taube, "The Delivery of Mental Health Services," in *The American Handbook of Psychiatry,* 2nd ed., vol. 7, ed. S. Arieti and H.K. Brodie (New York: Basic Books, 1981).

6. M. Galanter and J. Sperber, "General Hospitals in the Alcoholism Treatment System," in *Encyclopedic Handbook of Alcoholism,* ed. E.M. Pattison and E. Kaufman (New York: Gardner Press, 1982).

7. F.S. Tenant, C.M. Day, and J.T. Ungelerder, "Screening for Drugs and Alcohol Abuse in the General Medical Population," *Journal of the American Medical Association* 242(1979):533–535.

8. M.E. Perkins, "Psychiatric Management and the Future System of Care in Drug Abuse," in *Drug Abuse, Current Concepts and Research,* ed. N. Keup (Springfield, Mass.: Charles C. Thomas, 1972), pp. 452–458.

9. E. Bassuk and S. Schoonover, "The Private General Hospital's Psychiatric Emergency Service in a Decade of Transition," *Hospital and Community Psychiatry* 32(1981):181–185.

10. E. Bassuk and S. Gerson, "Into the Breach, Emergency Psychiatry in the General Hospital," *General Hospital Psychiatry* 1(1979):31–45.

11. M. Greenhill, "Liaison Psychiatry," in *American Handbook of Psychiatry*, 2nd ed., vol. 7, ed. S. Arieti and H. K. Brodie (New York: Basic Books, 1981), pp. 672–702.

12. H. Kaplan and B. Sadock, eds., *Comprehensive Textbook of Psychiatry/IV* (Baltimore, Md.: Williams & Wilkins, 1985).

13. L.C. Kolb and H.K. Brodie, *Modern Clinical Psychiatry,* 10th ed. (New York: W. B. Saunders, 1982).

14. A. Nicholi, ed., *The Harvard Guide to Modern Psychiatry* (Cambridge, Mass.: Belknap Press of Harvard University Press, 1978).

15. L. Sederer, *Inpatient Psychiatry Diagnosis and Treatment* (Baltimore, Md.: Williams & Wilkins, 1983).

16. S. Dubovsky and M. Weissberg, *Clinical Psychiatry in Primary Care,* 2nd ed. (Baltimore, Md.: Williams & Wilkins, 1982).

17. H.J. Lane, *Practical Problems of Emotional Disorders in Medicine* (New York: Raven Press, 1982).

18. T.P. Hackett and N.E. Cassem, eds., *The Massachusetts General Hospital Handbook of General Hospital Psychiatry* (St. Louis, Mo.: C. V. Mosby, 1978).

19. L. Linn, ed., *Frontiers of General Hospital Psychiatry* (New York: International Universities Press, 1961).

20. Glasscote, Gudeman, and Beigel, *The Uses of Psychiatry.*

Chapter 1

Psychiatric Administration: Organizational Structures, Operational Processes, and Essential Services

Allen H. Collins, M.D., M.P.H.

INTRODUCTION AND BACKGROUND

The term *psychiatric administration,* is used to describe the management principles, practices, structures, and processes utilized by individuals in leadership positions in mental health systems. Fifty years ago, these systems were limited to state mental hospitals, mental hygiene and other outpatient psychiatric clinics, several "psychopathic" hospitals, and a few general hospital psychiatric units. Today, such systems can be found in:

- state psychiatric hospitals
- Veterans Administration and other federal psychiatric hospitals
- county and municipal psychiatric institutions
- private (proprietary) psychiatric hospitals
- general hospital psychiatric services (including outpatient clinics, emergency services, inpatient units and scatter-bed programs, partial hospital services, alcoholism and substance abuse treatment programs, consultation-liaison services, and crisis intervention services)
- community mental health centers
- free standing psychiatric clinics
- free standing alcoholism and drug abuse residential treatment centers
- transitional and other residential treatment facilities
- medical school departments of psychiatry
- psychoanalytic and other training institutes
- psychiatric research institutes
- prison mental health services and other forensic psychiatric programs
- a myriad of governmental, quasigovernmental, and private mental health bureaucracies

The American Psychiatric Association (APA) was founded in 1844 (originally called the Association of Medical Superintendents of American Institutions for the Insane) by a group of 13 psychiatric administrators: "Six were in charge of state institutions, five directed incorporated hospitals, and two were the proprietors of private hospitals."[1] Their collective goal was to further research, improve patient care, and stimulate the development of organizational structures and systems within which the medical discipline of psychiatry would advance. The emphasis on administration reflected the belief that the quality of patient care was inextricably woven into the fabric of the organization in which it was provided.

In the years since the founding of the APA, the revolutionary changes that have occurred in clinical psychiatry have emphasized the direct, one-to-one physician-patient relationship. However, progress has been significantly slower in the related area of mental health administration. The profoundly increased complexity of organizational structures and available clinical services has placed a great strain on the ability of mental health administrative leaders to meet the needs and challenges of their tasks. As Saul Feldman, one of the leaders in the field of mental health administration, notes, "this new complexity has not been matched by increased administrative sophistication."[2] In fact, until the past two decades, "psychiatric administration has been very slow coming of age."[3] "Middle and top management echelons of our mental health organizations are occupied largely by professionals who are minimally equipped by education, and often by interest, to understand and cope creatively with their managerial responsibilities."[4] This situation is in marked contrast to that in the American business establishment, in which quality management practices have long been recognized as essential to organizational success.

For all intents and purposes, the considerable literature and expertise that have accumulated over the past several decades in the field of business administration have been all but neglected by most psychiatric administrators. It was expected that clinical psychiatry's knowledge of human psychology and behavior, individual and group dynamics, and psychopathology could be applied with relative ease to administrative-management tasks. The fact that this has not occurred has fostered an overdue reexamination of the problems involved and renewed exploration of the possible solutions.

"Administration is strongly modified by the nature of the environment in which it is performed."[5] This is especially true in the mental health field in which "the organizational ethos we ordinarily call the milieu is a very strong factor in treatment."[6] In order to understand the administrative structures and processes that have evolved, it is therefore necessary to become familiar with the nature of the psychiatric programs that have developed in general hospitals.

There has in fact been an explosive development of general hospital psychiatric services since World War II. The number of psychiatric beds increased almost 50 percent from 1963 to 1971,[7] then doubled again between 1971 and 1975.[8] This trend has continued in the 1980s. Increasing numbers of psychiatric administrators are working in general hospital settings.

CASE STUDIES: LENOX HILL HOSPITAL PSYCHIATRIC SERVICES

In each of the following administrative case studies, the case description is followed by a discussion of the relevant administrative issues involved in developing psychiatric services at Lenox Hill Hospital:

* organizational structures and processes
* obstacles to program development and operational management
* the management skills required to overcome these obstacles
* the range of solutions to resolve the difficulties

Background

Lenox Hill Hospital is a 698-bed general hospital located in the upper eastside of the borough of Manhattan in New York City. It was founded in 1854 as the German Dispensary and Hospital and, over the next 90 years, grew slowly in size and stature. Since World War II, however, the hospital has changed dramatically. These changes are highlighted by the statistics shown in Table 1-1.

Postgraduate intern and residency training programs also burgeoned during the 1946-1983 period. In 1946, there were 41 house staff positions in the 5 specialties of medicine, surgery, orthopedics, pediatrics, and thoracic surgery. By 1983, there were 165 house staff. Training programs are now well-established in 14 medical specialties, including psychiatry. Patient care

Table 1-1 Lenox Hill Hospital Growth Statistics

Characteristic	1946	1983	Percent Change
Total bed complement	552	698	+ 26.4%
Percentage of beds ward service	65%	15%	− 50.0%
Number of patients admitted	13,060	24,533	+ 87.8%
Number of patient days	176,277	229,447	+ 30.0%
Average length of stay (LOS)	17.9 days	9.3 days	− 48.0%

services became more intensive and acute-care oriented. In virtually all aspects of diagnostic, therapeutic, and support services, modern medical technology replaced obsolescent equipment.

Along with these changes in direct patient care activities and teaching services, the hospital has developed a wide range of community relations, public affairs, patient relations, planning, management information systems, ambulance, and other supportive services. Indeed, the leisurely paced, relatively nonacute-illness-oriented, and administratively modest attributes that once characterized the institution have now been replaced by medical care services that are high-powered, fast-paced, and technologically sophisticated. These services are supported and integrated by an administrative network that is streamlined, comprehensive, and efficient.

In 1978, an affiliation agreement with the New York Medical College (based in Valhalla, Westchester County, New York) capped a ten-year informal relationship that has transformed the hospital into a university teaching institution. This has resulted in greatly increased involvement in the training of undergraduate medical students. In short, the Lenox Hill Hospital of today would probably be unrecognizable to someone who knew it a mere quarter century ago.

Pre-1974 History

An anachronistic feature of Lenox Hill Hospital as late as the beginning years of the 1970s was the relatively primitive and undeveloped state of its psychiatric services, despite the fact that it was located in the heart of New York City and known for the quality of its medical-surgical patient care. From 1931 through 1959, psychiatry at Lenox Hill had grown and prospered in "neuropsychiatric" form. An outpatient clinic had operated for decades; inhospital consultation services were just becoming established; child and adolescent clinical and training programs were active and enjoyed a fine local reputation; and an acute care inpatient unit was on the verge of becoming a reality in a newly completed wing of the hospital. The untimely death of the charismatic director of the Department of Psychiatry and Neurology led abruptly to the transformation of the psychiatric unit into a neurology ward. The profound disappointment and anger of the psychiatric leadership and voluntary attending staff resulted in the resignations of two key leaders, the attending-in-charge of psychiatry and the chief of child psychiatry. The Psychiatry Service was subsequently reassigned as a section within the Department of Medicine, where it has remained up to the present time. Thus, in the span of a six-year period, there was a precipitous decline in the organizational status of psychiatry and in the viability of its clinical services. The specialty then entered a destructive cycle characterized by:

- an ineffective and unsupported leadership that was unable to muster the necessary strength to reverse the chain of events
- repetitive resignations of psychiatrists from the voluntary attending staff and difficulties in replacing them with those of comparable quality
- a decline in the quality of clinical services and an inability to meet the mental health intervention needs of the hospital patient population and professional staff
- criticisms of psychiatric services by other clinical departments and the hospital administration, resulting in the eventual depiction of the Psychiatry Service as an inept and embarrassing medical discipline
- a loss of professional self-esteem and morale by those psychiatric attendings who remained on the voluntary staff through the period of decline
- repeated reluctance of the hospital medical and lay leadership to make the necessary decisions to recruit new psychiatric leadership and fund new program development

Indeed, just when major developments were transforming psychiatry as a medical specialty—developments like diagnostic conceptual clarifications, revolutionary psychopharmacologic advances, psychotherapeutic refinements, major expansions of clinical programs especially suited to the general hospital in the new era of community mental health, and the availability of governmental funding for general and specialized psychiatric training—Lenox Hill psychiatry took giant steps backward into the pre-World War II era.

These difficulties persisted for eight years (1966–1974), despite repeated attempts by the recently (1966) appointed director and associate director of the Department of Medicine to attract young, energetic, and well-trained psychiatrists to the institution. All that remained of psychiatric services during this time was a very modest, analytically oriented outpatient clinic that was administered and staffed principally by social workers. An informal psychiatric consultation network barely operated; it involved a few members of the voluntary psychiatric attending staff who performed emergency and acute consultations for inpatients upon the request of attending and house staff medical-surgical physicians.

Case Study 1: Establishment of Quality Clinical Services and Training Programs

Developing a Program Proposal

The preceding historical background of Lenox Hill Hospital and its Psychiatry Service provides the organizational context in which the author inadvertently found himself when he joined the hospital's voluntary attending staff in May 1973. It was his primary intention to become involved in consultation-liaison activities on the various medical-surgical wards. During the first year, he became acquainted with the kinds of patients who were admitted to these "service" areas, their medical problems, and their needs for psychiatric care. He came to know many house staff and attending nonpsychiatric physicians who were concerned about their patients' health and welfare and desperately wanted responsive psychiatric involvement that was relevant to their needs.

The author was surprised to discover the nature of the "system" by which consultation-liaison services were provided to the medical wards. This amounted to an unreliable, catch-as-catch-can network in which the Psychiatric Clinic's clerical staff, upon receiving a consultation request, telephoned various members of the psychiatric attending staff until a professional was found to perform the service. A consequence of this process was that psychiatric evaluations were provided in only the most emergent situations, for example, for suicide attempts, acutely psychotic "medical" patients, and acutely agitated, uncooperative patients who were unmanageable for the medical-nursing staff. Members of the attending staff who were interested in consultation-liaison psychiatry provided these services on an uncoordinated, individual basis. Emergency, on-call coverage existed only on a nominal basis. Attending participation in the outpatient services of the Psychiatric Clinic was minimal; it involved the provision of some individual psychotherapy and medication and an occasional initial patient evaluation. Training programs in psychiatry were essentially nonexistent.

These discoveries led the author to consider what could be done to improve the situation. The first line of approach seemed to be to join with other interested members of the attending staff to discuss the perceptions of needs for psychiatric services in the hospital and the problems involved in providing these services within the existing structures. Fortunately, there was a cadre of dedicated and consistently involved attendings who desired constructive change and were willing to work to accomplish it. What seemed to be lacking was an individual who could coalesce these individuals into a working, task-oriented group.

A proposal to develop a formal psychiatric consultation-liaison service provided the requisite impetus. The author's experience as a grantsman and program consultant at the National Institute of Mental Health gave him the necessary expertise and authority within the group to provide leadership. Some senior members of the staff seemed to resent this leadership by a new junior attending and intermittently manifested obstructive and hypercritical behavior toward the group's work. This was overcome by the absence of a combative response and the intense desire of the group to accomplish its tasks.

Over a period of four months, the group developed and implemented a plan by which the proposal for a formal psychiatric consultation-liaison service would be generated. Committee members were assigned specific tasks. These involved the collection of available data on potential and actual requests for psychiatric consultations by the medical-surgical wards, on the numbers and quality of consultations that were provided, on the psychiatric attendings who were interested in providing such services, and on the clinical (and legal) problems that had resulted from the inadequacies of the existing network.

From these data, a narrative was developed, covering the following seven areas of program operations:

1. delineation of clinical services to be provided; their policies and procedures
2. specific voluntary attending staffing of the program
3. administrative organization with clearly delineated lines of responsibility and accountability
4. expected impact on existing psychiatric services
5. ramifications for training of medical-surgical house staff and future teaching programs for psychiatric residents and undergraduate medical students
6. ramifications for clinical research
7. funding specifications

A formal proposal for consultation-liaison services was completed and approved by the group and then presented to the entire voluntary psychiatric attending staff in a special meeting called for the purpose. A lively discussion was followed by unanimous endorsement, with the recommendation that the proposal be sent to the director of the Department of Medicine for approval and presentation to the medical board. The director and the medical board both responded with encouragement and support, much to the surprise of many older members of the psychiatric attending staff. Indeed, the nonpsychiatric physicians and administrators seemed relieved and hopeful that relevant psychiatric services for the hospital would result from this process. In July 1974, with the initiation of operations of the Psychiatric Consultation-Liaison Service, a new era of psychiatric programs was launched at Lenox Hill Hospital.

Discussion: Administrative Skills Necessary in Program Development and Operations

Several observations concerning the administrative process in a general hospital are relevant to an understanding of the above developments at Lenox Hill Hospital. First and foremost is the need to become familiar with the historical and current hospital milieu in which psychiatric programs are provided. This includes:

- organizational structures and idiosyncracies
- personality attributes of the principal clinical departmental and lay administrators
- strengths and weaknesses of the existing clinical services (including unmet needs) provided by each department
- perceptions held by various hospital personnel regarding each specialty and department
- the specific administrative processes and procedures by which proposals for programmatic changes are accomplished.

The more one knows about these variables, the better one can plan workable strategy and tactics. This saves a great deal of time and avoids unnecessary mistakes.

The second observation is that it is important to be aware of the realities of each person's professional position relative to those of other members of the specialty group and to the larger hospital setting. Does the person have a formal position of authority and responsibility for program services, or is the person acting alone or on behalf of a group that wants to change the status quo? Also, it is important to know how the person is perceived by colleagues and others relative to seniority, age, attending rank, and clinical and administrative experience and skills; these are all important factors in determining the degree to which the person is accepted and effective in the leadership role. On the other hand, insofar as a person actively and openly participates in an undertaking that seeks to effect a significant change in the status quo, regardless of how constructive such a change is felt to be, some measure of anxiety, resentment, envy, or jealousy will probably be felt by other members of the hospital community.

The third observation concerns the importance of working with available professional staff who may be highly motivated, experienced, and knowledgeable regarding the new project. All too frequently, newly arrived leaders on the general hospital scene confuse the sad state of existing programs with the quality and dedication of the psychiatric staff.

The fourth observation focuses on the importance of developing in the leadership role the capacity to facilitate small group cohesion. In this connection, it is useful to become acquainted with the task-oriented group literature, particularly, the Tavistock model and the techniques of Wilfred Bion,[9] A.K. Rice,[10] and R. Newton and D. Levinson.[11] A leader's attention to the sentient needs of group members within boundaries that are consistent with the tasks and goals of the group frequently makes the difference between focused success and chaotic failure.

Apart from the above qualities, the ability to document needs and problem areas, to specify the services to be provided (by which staff, by what procedures), to delineate the positive consequences of program implementation for other services of the hospital, to outline clearly the administration and operational management of the program, and to determine the necessary funding, space, and other support necessary for the program's operations is essential in translating existing deficiencies and needs into operational solutions in any proposal for a new clinical service. The managerial skills required to develop a program proposal are in fact different from those needed to see that it becomes implemented. In the latter process, interpersonal skills—involving promotion, salesmanship, and political sensitivity— are important assets. Above all, persistence in the face of obstacles and negative receptions is required. The professional knowledge and expertise learned in medical school and postgraduate training does not adequately prepare a person to deal with such challenges. The practical cognitive and interpersonal skills involved are largely intuitive, acquired in one's family or neighborhood. They may, however, also be gleaned from postgraduate training in public health, public administration, or business administration by those few mental health administrators who have the requisite motivation and persistence.

By the same token, the administrative skills needed to facilitate initial program implementation are not the same as the leadership attributes that are tapped in the ongoing operation of a mental health program. Such operational management requires:

- attention to detail, including the development of data management systems that maintain records, statistics, and other program operations data; the writing of periodic reports, correspondence, and memoranda; and the preparation of other documentation required for program review and evaluation
- a focus on the important issues that relate to the program and an avoidance of matters that are peripheral
- careful time management (there is always more to do than one has time for)

- assumption of responsibility for program services
- expertise in the mental health services being provided and the ability to provide them in situations of emergency and clinical overload
- ability to work well with other professionals and supporting staff to maximize motivation and efficiency (especially relevant when relying on voluntary (nonsalaried) psychiatric staff whose interests and gratifications must be encouraged)
- ability to plan phased goals in a strategic way, taking into account manpower, financial, spatial, and political constraints

Case Study 2: The Psychiatric Consultation-Liaison Service

The Crisis in Staffing

The Psychiatric Consultation-Liaison Service at Lenox Hills Hospital achieved important clinical goals relatively early (in the first two years) in its development. As expected, the assignment of able psychiatric clinicians to specific inpatient medical-surgical units prompted their utilization by attending and house staff physicians. The psychiatric clinicians were asked to see patients who had significant psychopathology as a consequence of or independently of the somatic disease processes. These consultations stimulated more active case finding, resulting in earlier detection of and intervention for emotional disorders. Liaison support and the education of medical-nursing staff developed slowly but surely in the wake of the patient-oriented consultations. Many outside psychiatrists who were well-trained and clinically adept heard about the new service and applied for hospital privileges. This enabled the author, as part-time attending-in-charge, to recruit with relative ease nonsalaried psychiatrists for the rapidly growing program.

For a time, these new attendings performed their clinical assignments on the various medical-surgical units in a consistent and responsible manner. However, after the initial 2–3 year period, a significant number became disenchanted with the affiliation. Many expected referrals of private patients to occur with considerably greater frequency than actually developed. Some were disappointed with the level of academic stimulation they encountered, since at the time there was no academically oriented training or medical school affiliation in psychiatry. Others had hoped that the hospital would serve as an acute care facility to which they could admit private patients. The admission status of patients with primary psychiatric diagnoses was unclear at the time.

These disappointments with the deficiencies of psychiatry at the hospital resulted in a disturbing number of resignations from the attending staff.

This, in turn, caused concern and criticism of psychiatry in the medical board and the board of trustees, both of which were involved in the administrative review of all applications to and resignations from the voluntary medical attending staff. The director of medicine, who was administratively responsible for the Section of Psychiatry, was the major recipient of this criticism and, in turn, transmitted them to the author. Attempts to explain the resignations in terms of the chronic problems psychiatry had experienced in the institution and the current efforts to alleviate them had a limited impact on the hard-pressed director. "The bottom line is to see to it that this does not happen any longer. Attendings cannot continue to come and go."[12] Thus, it was the author's clearly delineated task to stem, if not stop entirely, the loss by whatever creative mechanisms he could develop. The solutions had to be found in the existing organizational structure, with all its programmatic, financial, academic, and private practice referral constraints. The task seemed impossible. Given that structural context, it was all too clear why so many able and talented psychiatrists had left the hospital over the previous ten years, after brief attempts to alter the status quo.

Discussion: Administrative Problem-Solving Skills

The development of a new clinical service, training program, or research endeavor invariably involves many obstacles and frustrations. The tasks involved in breaking new ground are in fact quite different from those required in directing a pre-existing psychiatric program with developed structures, processes, and internal and external relationships. A central task of creative administration is to discover solutions to seemingly insoluble organizational problems.

The problems that developed following the initial attempts to provide voluntary professional staffing for the Lenox Hill Consultation-Liaison Service were unanticipated. The basic task was to consider the controllable variables in the management of the Psychiatric Service and to change them in the direction of positive outcome. Here, the natural reflective qualities that psychiatric training develops in its residents and young specialists can prove of great value in the administrative setting.

Thus, through an introspective process, the author came to realize that his management of the attending staff application interview process needed considerable improvement. The failure to explore sufficiently certain motivational, personality, logistical, and subspecialty factors in the applicants was found to have led to errors in judgment in selecting new members of the psychiatric attending staff. Also, the failure to orient the applicants to the realities of practice in the hospital milieu inadvertently reinforced their erroneous expectations and led to further disappointments and frustrations when they began their work in the institution.

Clearly, mechanisms had to be developed to improve the evaluation of new applicants to the voluntary psychiatric attending staff. These mechanisms, based on the lessons gleaned from past mistakes and problems, were incorporated in a new applicant evaluation process. An improved set of criteria for applicant attributes was developed, making it easier to predict how prospective attendings would fare at the hospital. The criteria included the following:

- What were the physician's reasons for joining the hospital and participating in the existing (or planned) psychiatric clinical programs? How did the applicant imagine involvement in these programs? Here, it was important that identifiable areas of program need be matched with the applicant's clinical interests, special training, and professional experience.
- What were the applicant's existing professional time allocations? How would the new hospital affiliation meld into these commitments?
- Which members of the medical attending staff were professionally known to the applicant, and how did these relationships affect mutual referrals of patients?
- What was the extent of the applicant's involvement with (and desired development of) the private practice of psychiatry?
- What were the medical-model (versus social, psychoanalytic, or other) orientation and experience of the applicant?
- What were the applicant's personality characteristics as they related to the ability to take initiatives; to engage in adaptational (rather than passive) activity, and to develop social skills?
- Would the applicant be able to tolerate a minimal programmatic structure and provide active, constructive input into the development of new structures and processes?

As noted earlier, it was also necessary to address the erroneous expectations that prospective attendings had in joining the voluntary staff. A special orientation was developed and included in the evaluation interview to correct the expectational distortions. The following areas were addressed:

- The *quid-pro-quo* referral of private patients as a "natural" result of diligently performing one's service assignment was ruled out, and the ways referral networks actually operated at the hospital were discussed. It was stressed that referrals were ultimately dependent on the development of positive interpersonal relationships with other members of the medical attending staff. While the author could facilitate the introduction of new attendings on his staff to other hospital physicians, it was the responsibility of the attendings to develop their own referral relationships.

- It was necessary to document clearly the extent of medical school affiliations in psychiatry and other training programs. Many prospective attendings assumed mistakenly that a New York City acute care general hospital would have many such opportunities available.
- Attendings were required to provide a minimum of three hours per week of voluntary clinical service to nonreferred patients and medical-nursing staff in order to maintain an active attending affiliation with the hospital.
- Attendings were required to provide on-call emergency psychiatric coverage to the ER and inpatient wards for one week periods on a rotational basis with other members of the attending staff. This amounted to a total of two on-call periods per year. The specific procedures and service demands of this emergency system were discussed with each applicant.
- The applicant's clinical needs for admitting privileges for acute care hospitalization of private patients were determined. The existing hospital policy, which did not provide for such psychiatric admissions, was discussed with the applicant; and how this policy impacted on the applicant's motivation to join the staff was explored.

In the orientation process, it was important that applicants understood all of these limitations. If applicants then still appeared well-motivated to join the staff, they were asked to make a nonbinding commitment to remain affiliated with the hospital for at least two years. The reasons for this—the serious political problems precipitated by repetitive new appointments and resignations from the attending staff—were explained in a direct and serious manner.

Of course, not all of the application interview was so negatively focused. If there seemed to be the realistic possibility of a mutually beneficial collaboration between the Psychiatry Service and the applicant, the considerable assets of the hospital were then discussed, for example, the quality of the medical-surgical attending staff; the opportunity to join a young and expanding psychiatric staff at an early stage in its development; the mutually respectful and cooperative relationships between the voluntary psychiatric attendings and the service leadership, and the advocacy of the private attendings by the leadership throughout the hospital; the considerable opportunities for private practice referrals, provided certain conditions were met; and the active involvement and participation of the attending staff in the planning and implementation of future clinical services and training programs.

The author as attending-in-charge was actively involved in facilitating the smooth integration of new attendings into the medical staff (introductions to other physicians) and the hospital system (the clinical program area in which the prospective attendings would be involved). Further, a commitment was made to provide assistance in the area of referrals of private patients (if this was a significant reason for joining the hospital staff) after the new attending demonstrated the expected level of clinical performance.

After all these issues and problem areas became clarified in the initial evaluation interview as a basis for proceeding with the application process, the number of new psychiatric attendings who came on staff, only to resign within a short period of time (less than 3 years), significantly declined. Thus, the reevaluation of the interviewing process for new applicants to the voluntary psychiatric attending staff succeeded in resolving the staffing crisis. The Psychiatric Consultation-Liaison Service was able to continue its growth and development and to serve as the basis for the creation of a new psychiatry service at Lenox Hill Hospital.

Case Study 3: Expanding Psychiatric Programs
An Attempt to Initiate an Inpatient Service

It was clear, even in the early years of the Psychiatric Consultation-Liaison Service, that a major limitation in the development of more comprehensive psychiatric programs stemmed from the lack of a psychiatric inpatient service and the absence of admitting privileges for attending psychiatrists. Indeed, the psychiatric clinicians who were found to be the most desirable applicants for the attending staff were those who had active and acute care private practices that required hospitalization resources for their patients. In this area, existing hospital policy regarding psychiatric admissions was, at best, unclear. A few older members of the "neuropsychiatric" staff continued to admit selected private patients (largely depressives) to the neurology ward. And, although no formal, organized psychiatric inpatient service existed, these patients received psychotropic medication, individual psychotherapy, and electroconvulsive therapy (ECT) at the bedside on the ward. Not infrequently, as in many community general hospitals, patients with primary psychiatric diagnoses were admitted to the general care units; such patients had somatic symptoms, neurasthenic complaints, and sometimes frank psychological presentations. This practice seemed to be tolerated, provided no serious management problems arose; however, the numbers of such admissions remained limited.

In 1976, the author and a colleague on the Lenox Hill attending staff wrote a proposal for a 25-bed acute care psychiatric inpatient unit. The proposal had the support of the hospital "in principle" and was thus submitted to the lengthy community and public mental health agency review process for consideration. It was, however, severely criticized in the initial community board meetings by a much larger, local general hospital and was subsequently rejected. The recommendation of the local review groups was that the hospital's existing mental health service elements (outpatient, consultation-liaison, and emergency) utilize other community inpatient facilities in a collaborative system. Unfortunately, the promised collaboration by the local general hospital that had opposed the development of the Lenox Hill inpatient unit failed to materialize, and the serious service deficiencies for patients and providers of Lenox Hill Hospital have persisted.

Discussion: Working Within the Review Process in a Political Environment

There are several important administrative lessons to be learned from the above case study. First, it is essential to understand thoroughly every step of the program review process. Which groups do the review and in what sequence? What are the perspectives and concerns of these groups? What are the specific review functions of each group (advisory, approval/veto, and so on)? What institutions and agencies are represented on the groups, and who are their designated individual representatives? Finally, what are the overt and covert agendas of these representatives?

Second, it is necessary to have an intimate appreciation of the general health care political climate of the community, city, and state. This appreciation should encompass the political perceptions of the need for specific clinical programs; of the need for certain patient populations to be served; of the adequacy or inadequacy of existing acute care, intermediate care, long-term care, and residential treatment beds in the catchment area, borough, city, and region; and of the need for additional inpatient programs.

Third, it is important to engage in a dialogue with the various community institutions, providers, and consumer and patient advocate groups prior to formal program presentation at the reviewing bodies. This facilitates understanding of the issues cited above and permits the incorporation of the needs and concerns of the review groups in the program proposal. It also fosters the development of the necessary relationships with those individuals, groups, and institutions that will play important roles in the subsequent formal review process. At the same time, interinstitutional service networks can be developed to influence the documentation of the need (or lack of need) of the requested service. Sometimes, institutional "deals" are made through such networks with politically influential city and state officials, thereby circumventing normal relationships, but such arrangements are usually short-sighted and ultimately more disruptive than helpful in the review process.

Fourth, it is vital to develop a firm foundation of support within one's own institution before proceeding to outside groups. This foundation requires the development of clinical services and training programs that are viewed as strong, credible structures by the other administrative-clinical departments of the hospital. This will minimize the chance of internal institutional ambivalence or reservation in the review process. It will also help to demonstrate the need for the proposed new program in the light of existing clinical and training facilities.

Fifth, the process of developing a new inpatient service is a lengthy one, entailing community and public mental health agency consultation, review, approval, and implementation. It requires considerable patience, tact, openness, and flexibility to program effectively the input from all of these extrainstitutional groups.

Case Study 4: The Evolution of Management

The Transition to Group Leadership

In the years 1977–1980, a major expansion occurred in the clinical services and training programs of the Psychiatry Section at Lenox Hill. This resulted in a radical restructuring of the administration of the section. A small group of salaried mental health professionals were appointed to provide executive leadership for designated programs. The author's role as an independently functioning clinician-executive was transformed to one in which he functioned as the leader of a group of clinician-administrators. The entrepreneurial model had to be supplanted by a group model.

In May 1978, the author was promoted from his position as chief of psychiatric inpatient services (which included responsibility for the consultation-liaison program) to attending-in-charge of psychiatry (both half-time positions); in the new position, he was responsible to the director of the Department of Medicine. The new administrative arrangement replaced the transitional administrative structure of the Psychiatry Service, in which leadership was shared between an attending-in-charge of inpatient psychiatry and an attending-in-charge of outpatient psychiatry. In the new arrangement, the latter position was made subordinate to the former.

In the years 1977–1978, the conceptual bases and procedural elements of a psychiatric inpatient scatter-bed program were formulated (see Chapter 2).

The new program started operating in June 1978. A full-time chief of Psychiatric Inpatient Services was appointed to assume the administrative direction of the program, responsible to the attending-in-charge. A full-time inpatient mental health nurse specialist was in charge of the nursing staff for the new program and also provided consultation-education support for the nursing staff of the medical-surgical units.

In 1978, following several years of negotiation, an affiliation agreement was concluded on a preliminary basis between Lenox Hill Hospital and the New York Medical College. As part of this process, agreement was reached between the Department of Psychiatry of the medical school and the Department of Medicine, Section of Psychiatry, of the hospital to develop clinically based training programs for undergraduate medical students and rotating PGY 2-3 psychiatric residents. Provision was made for the joint selection and appointment of a full-time coordinator of psychiatric education, a process completed in December 1978. Psychiatric training programs were formally initiated at the hospital in April 1979.

During the first year of his tenure as attending-in-charge, the author reviewed the administrative and clinical operations of the Psychiatry Service. These reviews focused on (1) performance levels of existing staff program chiefs, other administrative personnel, and clinicians; (2) the status of coordination between the various programs; (3) the responses of staff to suggestions for programmatic changes to increase effectiveness and collaboration; (4) the levels of agreement on future program development to address areas of deficiency or unmet needs; and (5) the utilization of resources (personnel, financial, space) to achieve maximum program impact.

These reviews resulted in decisions to alter certain administrative structures: (1) the half-time position of attending-in-charge of psychiatric outpatient services was eliminated. (2) The position of full-time clinical coordinator of the Psychiatric Outpatient Clinic was upgraded to that of coordinator, with overall program authority and responsibility for the clinic. (3) An additional position of half-time chief of Psychiatric Consultation-Liaison Services was established to assume the administrative leadership of those services. These changes were implemented over a six-month period and were completed in September 1979. The successive structural changes are summarized graphically in Figures 1-1 through 1-4.

The reviews also indicated a need to change the existing psychiatric emergency on-call system, which was functioning poorly (see below and Chapter 5). However, a "moonlighting" proposal was rejected by the hospital administration as too costly, and no other solution was immediately available.

A certification review of the Psychiatric Outpatient Clinic was conducted in the Spring of 1979 by the New York State Office of Mental Health

Figure 1–1 Organizational Structure of the Psychiatry Service of Lenox Hill Hospital: 1970

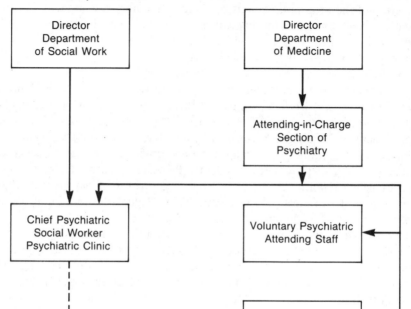

(OMH). The clinic was found to be not in compliance with newly promulgated, minimal professional salaried staffing requirements. To receive the recertification by OMH that would be necessary to operate legally as a mental health facility, the hospital decided to hire the requisite number of mental health professionals for the clinic. The specific mental health disciplines of the new staff were determined by the attending-in-charge and the clinic coordinator, based on the kinds of clinical services required to fulfill unmet needs, the desire to keep the cost of new staff to an acceptable level, and the need for other programs related to the clinic's services (ER, other outpatient clinics, and so on). The addition of a full-time outpatient mental health nurse specialist, two part-time psychiatrists, and a clinical psychologist provided considerable opportunities for the development of limited psychotherapy, crisis intervention, and emergency programs by the end of 1979.

Figure 1–2 Organizational Structure of the Psychiatry Service of Lenox Hill Hospital: 1974

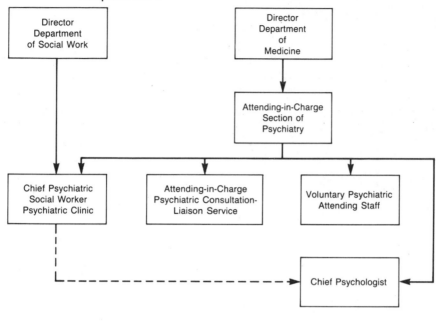

A reexamination of the psychiatric emergency on-call system was made in the light of the above clinic staffing changes. Discussions revealed that a concurrent system of ER "psychosocial" consultations was being provided by the Social Work Department. Thus, a new system was devised, combining the two existing programs with joint staffing. The outpatient mental health nurse specialist was designated the program director of the new service, answering to the attending-in-charge of psychiatry.

The development of these new clinical service and training programs and the hiring of several clinician-executives to provide administrative leadership profoundly altered the structure of the Psychiatry Service. Mechanisms had to be developed to coordinate the various programs, review program operations, develop data management systems, plan future programs, and devise the overall strategy and tactics to continue the service's growth and development. The old model, in which the author operated as a single administrator, with little consultation and few joint planning activities with other individuals, was clearly unworkable in the new context. The practice of recruiting assertive, independently minded professionals as program directors was at variance with a pyramidal administrative system. More-

Figure 1–3 Organizational Structure of the Psychiatry Service of Lenox Hill
Hospital: 1976

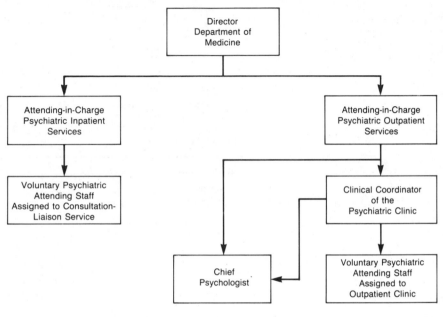

over, such an authoritarian (pyramidal) system would overly tax the time
and personal resources of the author in managing the new, more complex
organizational structure. Substantive delegation of authority and responsibility was obviously required.

A new administrative vehicle grew out of a two-year experience (1978–
1979) with informal, irregularly held meetings with the chiefs of the inpatient and outpatient services and the coordinator of education. The poorly
structured, aperiodic character of these meetings had resulted in an inadequate group process and low task output and failed to meet the administrative demands for coordination and planning. The succeeding group,
designated the Executive Committee of the Psychiatry Service, began meeting in October 1979. Its membership was determined on the basis that each
member have authority and responsibility for a distinct clinical service or
training program. There were initially six members in the group: (1) the
attending-in-charge (chairman), (2) the chief of Psychiatric Inpatient Services, (3) the chief of the Psychiatric Consultation-Liaison Service, (4) the
coordinator of the Psychiatric Outpatient Clinic, (5) the coordinator of
psychiatric education, and (6) the inpatient mental health nurse specialist.

Figure 1–4 Organizational Chart of the Lenox Hill Hospital Psychiatry Service: 1980

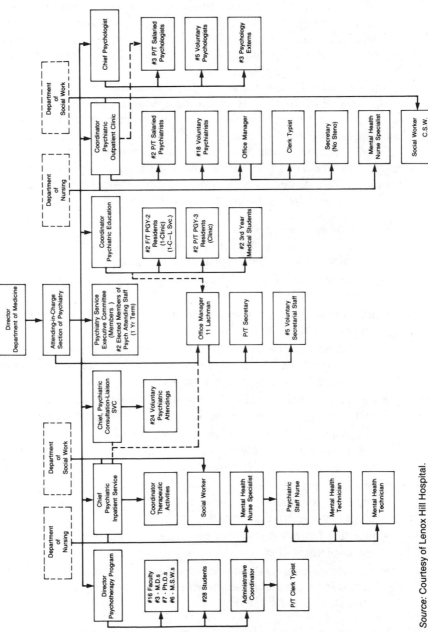

Source: Courtesy of Lenox Hill Hospital.

Over the next four years, five additional members were appointed to the Executive Committee: (1) an outpatient-emergency mental health nurse specialist, (2) a chief psychologist, (3) a director of the postgraduate psychotherapy training program, (4) an elected representative from the senior voluntary psychiatric attending staff, and (5) an elected representative from the junior voluntary psychiatric attending staff.

The Executive Committee meetings are conducted weekly for a period of 90 minutes. Each meeting is structured around a formal agenda, the items of which are determined in advance by the group members. The chairman encourages open and free discussion of all issues brought to the committee. The only constraints on discussion are relevance to the work setting, respectful relatedness, time limitations, and the indications for closure on an issue. As the content and process of the committee's meetings have evolved, its tasks have evolved to include the following:

- evaluating ongoing clinical service and training programs to ensure quality, appropriate utilization, and adequate coordination with other Psychiatry Service and hospital programs
- modifying, adding, or eliminating operating programs in accordance with the results of evaluations
- formalizing program policies and procedures and developing orientation and operating manuals
- evaluating compliance with Psychiatry Service policies and procedures and the quality of the clinical/teaching performance of members of the salaried and voluntary professional staff
- discussing recommendations for new appointments, reappointments, and nonreappointments to the voluntary attending staff
- discussing the status of the relationships of the Psychiatry Service with other hospital departments and community agencies, and recommending strategies as needed to improve them
- planning for the hospital's annual capital and operating budgetary process, coordinating requested budgetary items, and reviewing the programmatic issues involved
- planning future directions of programs, including the phasing of tactics and implementation
- improving members' interpersonal relations and their sensitivities to each other's emotional needs with respect to their professional responsibilities in the work setting

The Executive Committee has become the embodiment of the style in which the Psychiatry Service is managed. It is conducted as a task-oriented, peer work group that takes into account the sentient needs of its members. The member program directors have a wide latitude of responsibility in the direction and operation of their individual programs. They are expected to provide assertive representation and advocacy for their programs in the committee. There is little sense of hierarchy in the group. The authority of the attending-in-charge is largely a passive presence; it has been employed only in those few instances when irreconcilable member differences impeded necessary discussion or decision making. It has also been used on the rare occasion when the majority of the committee wished to pursue a course of action that the attending-in-charge felt strongly would be detrimental to the service. Overall, the Executive Committee has become very adept at airing and resolving interpersonal and interprogram problems and differences and at coordinating operations and planning.

Discussion: Clinician-Executive versus Group Leader

It is impractical to try to maintain the entrepreneurial clinician-executive administrative model in a climate of expanding and more complex structures of clinical/teaching services. In the latter setting, the recruitment of additional administrative staff and the delegation of authority and responsibility for program planning and operation are essential. This, of necessity, produces a cadre of managers who must learn to work together in a collaborative manner to achieve maximal program effectiveness. The clinician-executive often has blind spots with regard to planning, evaluation, operations, and interpersonal relations. Administrative vehicles like the Lenox Hill Psychiatry Service Executive Committee can act as invaluable quality control mechanisms for the elimination of such blind spots. In addition, this type of finely honed task-oriented group can tap unexpected resources to stimulate managerial creativity.

In the more complex administrative structure, a peer group (collegial) model, exemplified by the Executive Committee, is recommended. Unlike more authoritarian vehicles, it stresses mutual respect, preserves individual autonomy and responsibility, and fosters collaboration between members. This type of small, task-oriented group model is certainly not the easiest to establish and maintain. It requires restricting the easy use of the leader's formal authority to close discussions prematurely and to dictate the course of action. Kernberg warns against the administrator's temptation toward such exercises of authority, relating it to difficulties in controlling aggressive urges.[13] Leadership in the peer group model requires attention to the emotional states of being and the affectual needs of the supporting administrative staff; and it requires nurturing that staff, when necessary.[14]

Rioch has observed that "the formation of a human group seriously and consistently dedicated to a serious task without fanaticism or illusion is an

extremely difficult process and a relatively rare occurrence."[15] She describes
the powerful forces within the group that operate to keep its members
childishly dependent on a leader. Wilfred Bion,[16] together with the later
Tavistock group theorists (A.K. Rice, A.D. Coleman, W.H. Bexton, E.J.
Miller, and P.M. Turquet) have drawn conceptual distinctions between
"basic assumption groups," that is, groups driven by largely unconscious,
irrational, nontask-oriented factors, and "work groups." However, "neither
the work group nor the basic assumption group exists in pure culture for
very long. What one sees in reality is a work group which is suffused by,
intruded into, and supported by the basic assumption groups."[17] It is useful
to review briefly at this point the characteristics common to all work
groups. The processes of such work groups can be evaluated by the following seven criteria:

1. The primary task of the group is defined as that which must be
   performed in order for the group to survive.
2. The group's activity is engaged in consciously and cooperatively by
   the members.
3. The group activity draws on the specific training, experience, and
   talents of the members who act rationally.
4. The members retain their sense of selfhood and separateness from
   each other.
5. The members desire to acquire all relevant knowledge and information.
6. The group's activity is related to reality, that is, to the outside environment, and hence the group is concerned with group boundary regulations.
7. The leadership function of the group is a boundary function that
   controls transactions between the members and the outside.

Burns notes that the leader is an agent of the group, in defining and
maintaining the group's primary task, and is also the center of group
communication.[18] Turquet adds that the leader is the agent of executive
action in decision making and implementation and is a facilitator of the
members' skills, of changes in leadership in accordance with the appearance
of new and different facets of the primary task, and of the assessment
process related to the use of members' skills in primary task implementation.[19]

These functions of the work group leader will be aided or inhibited by
certain attributes the leader has or lacks:

- degree of formal authority ("Hierarchy in the work group ordinarily corresponds to the hierarchy in the larger institution.")[20]
- competence as related to the tasks and goals group members value
- ability to fulfill the members sentient expectations
- ability to tolerate anxiety and doubt when making executive decisions with incomplete knowledge and uncertainty about outcome

The last of the above four attributes actually pertains to every member of a peer-oriented, small work group, not only to the group leader. Group support and collaboration can work to either highlight or obscure the personality assets and deficiencies of the leader. Managerial uncertainties can thereby either be realistically confronted or be denied. The path taken by the group process, at any given time, indicates either its healthy, adaptive functioning or its psychopathology.

From these considerations, one can see that a major aspect of the role of clinician-executive is the ability to participate in and lead small, task-oriented work groups.[21] "However, to conduct group business without regard for group processes and the feelings that lie beneath the surface is to invite resistance and possible failure through subtle sabotage."[22]

Many of the developmental phases and related leadership tasks in small, task-oriented groups are cited by Collins and Grobman in their discussion of psychiatric liaison groups.[23] The leader must be sensitive to the members' anxiety levels, to the phase-specific needs for group structure, and to the need to control disruptive interpersonal transactions and facilitate discussions of personal difficulties. The leader must be aware that a task-oriented work group is not a therapy group; psychodynamic interpretations are inappropriate. There is clearly a distinction, albeit subtle at times, between the leader's awareness of the needs of the members and attempts to deal with those needs as therapeutic issues. If the leader engages in "therapeutic" leadership, the significant limitations of applying the clinical model to the administrative setting will quickly become apparent.

ADMINISTRATIVE ISSUES

Walter Barton, the dean of American administrative psychiatry, has noted that "the issue of highest priority, at the moment, is the containment of health care costs."[24] Prospective payment plans like the diagnosis related group (DRG) system, increasing competition among health care institutions for consumer utilization, aggressive marketing and pricing strategies, and better and better informed consumers are major elements in current efforts to contain health care costs. The impact of these factors on the quality of care of mental health delivery systems has yet to be fully measured and assessed.

Against this backdrop, twenty years after the first calls for relevant training in mental health administration, Barton points out that, in order to increase the number of psychiatrists and mental health professionals in the field, formal training for leadership posts is required.[25] In this connection, it is often suggested that the knowledge base of clinical psychiatry is easily applicable to training programs in mental health administration. Indeed, there is a considerable amount of information concerning human developmental psychology, psychodynamics, psychopathology, interpersonal relationships, and group dynamics that can be applied in the day-to-day work of the mental health administrator. But, if administrators attempt to use such knowledge as if they were in the clinical setting, the results are often quite different from what they might expect. As Patteson notes, "it is tempting to suggest that the clinician need only extrapolate from his psychodynamic clinical experience to the problems and issues of administration. [But] . . . the well-qualified clinician cannot necessarily move successfully into administration on the basis of demonstrated clinical skills; indeed, just the reverse may apply."[26] Indeed, application of the adage, "treat one's fellow administrator as your patient," may lead to failure as an executive/manager.

By and large, the general propensities for clinicians to be passive, introspective, nonaction oriented, comfortable with their clinical control without unnecessary risks, and not clearly goal-oriented are at variance with the requirements of administrative processes, structures, and goals. In fact, psychiatric clinician-executives are at some initial disadvantage with their colleagues in their general wariness of being "psychoanalyzed." Only after consistent demonstrations to the contrary—by acting spontaneously and straightforwardly and displaying a detailed knowledge of administrative matters—do such suspicions disappear. In short, clinical knowledge may be quite helpful in aiding the clinician-executive to think about an interpersonal problem with a colleague, or in formulating a strategy to overcome transactional obstacles. But it is not helpful as the basis for role playing by the psychiatric clinician in the administrative setting.

A critical attribute of any executive, manager, or administrator is the ability to develop positive interpersonal relationships in the organizational setting. A colleague once expressed the opinion that "all so-called 'political' issues can be reduced to the underlying nature of the interpersonal relationships that are operating between the interested parties."[27] This may not be true in all circumstances; individuals who represent different organizations, or groups within the same organization, may have irreconcilable policy differences in the context of positive interpersonal relationships. Still, with respect to a substantial number of organizational interactions that fall into the gray zone of cooperation-conflict, the nature of the interpersonal relationships between the principals will certainly play a major role in the determination of events.

A great majority of the acute care, community general hospitals in the United States are or have been in situations similar to that of Lenox Hill Hospital in the development of psychiatric clinical services and training programs. The author's experience is that one learns most about mental health administration from reviewing specific events and their contexts. Thus, current teaching about mental health organizations should be "heavily oriented toward the real-life situations in which administrators work, and the real-life problems with which they must cope."[28] As Feldman notes, "it is the shape and substance of mental health services that determines the nature of the administrator's job."[29]

REFERENCES

1. Nolan D.C. Lewis, "American Psychiatry from Its Beginnings to World War II," *American Handbook of Psychiatry,* 2nd ed., ed. Silvan Arieti (New York: Basic Books, 1974), p. 33.

2. S. Feldman, "Administration in Mental Health: Issues, Problems and Prospects," *Bulletin of the Pan American Health Organization* 9 (1975): 212.

3. M. Greenblatt, "Administrative Psychiatry," *American Journal of Psychiatry* 129 (October 1972): 33.

4. D.I. Levinson and G.L. Klerman, "The Clinician-Executive Revisited," *Administration in Mental Health* 1 (1973): 64.

5. S. Feldman, "Perspectives on Mental Health Administration," *Hospital and Community Psychiatry* 29 (June 1978) 389.

6. Ibid., 390.

7. C. Kanno et al., "Psychiatric Treatment in the Community," *Joint Information Service* (1974): V9.

8. M. Greenblatt, "Special Problems Facing the Psychiatrist Administrator," *Hospital and Community Psychiatry* 30 (November 1979): 761.

9. W.J. Bion, *Experiences in Groups* (New York: Basic Books, 1959).

10. A.K. Rice, *Learning for Leadership: Interpersonal and Intergroup Relations* (London: Tavistock Publications, 1965).

11. R.M. Newton and D.J. Levinson, "The Work Group within the Organization: A Sociopsychological Approach," *Psychiatry* 36 (1973): 115–142.

12. Personal communication, M.S. Bruno, 1977.

13. O.F. Kernberg, "Leadership and Organization: Functional Organizational Regression," *International Journal of Group Psychotherapy* 28 (January 1978): 3–25.

14. E.L. Miller, *Task and Organization* (New York: John Wiley, and Sons, 1976).

15. M.L. Rioch, "Group Relations, Rationale and Techniques," *International Journal of Group Psychotherapy* 20 (1970): 347.

16. Bion, *Experiences in Groups.*

17. M.L. Rioch, "The Work of Wilfred Bion on Groups," *Psychiatry* 33 (1970): 62.

18. J.M. Burns, *Leadership* (New York: Harper & Row, 1978).

19. P.M. Turquet, "Leadership: The Individual and the Group," in *Analysis of Groups,* ed. G.S. Gribbard, J.J. Hartmen, and R.D. Mann (San Francisco: Jossey-Bass, 1974), pp. 337–371.

20. Newton and Levinson, "The Work Group," 117.

21. D.J. Levinson and G.L. Klerman, "The Clinician-Executive: Some Problematic Issues for the Psychiatrist in Mental Health Organizations," *Psychiatry* 30 (1967): 3–15.

22. J. Racy, "Psychiatrists as Administrators: Problems of Leadership and the Exercise of Power," *Hospital and Community Psychiatry* 26 (August 1975): 529.

23. A.H. Collins and J. Grobman, "Group Methods in the General Hospital Setting," in *Comprehensive Textbook of Group Psychotherapy,* ed. B. Sadock and H. Kaplan (Baltimore, Md.: Williams and Wilkins, 1982), pp. 289–293.

24. W.E. Barton, "Current Issues and Trends in Administrative Psychiatry," *Psychiatric Annals* 14 (1984): 837.

25. Ibid., 838.

26. E.M. Patteson, "Young Psychiatrist Administrators," *American Journal of Psychiatry* 131 (February 1974): 157.

27. E. Witenberg, personal communication, 1980.

28. Feldman, "Administration in Mental Health," 215.

29. Ibid., 219.

Chapter 2

Innovative Psychiatric Inpatient Services: Psychiatric Units and Scatter-Bed Programs

Allen H. Collins, M.D., M.P.H., and Loren Skeist, M.D.

INTRODUCTION

In 1752, 30 years after the first general hospital psychiatric inpatient unit was established at Guy's Hospital in London, England, Benjamin Rush founded the first American unit at the Pennsylvania Hospital. Over the next 200 years, there was little growth in the number of such general hospital units in the United States. In 1933, however, the Rockefeller Foundation initiated the funding of psychiatric units in major medical teaching hospitals, and by 1942 there were 39 such units throughout the country. This development inaugurated the major role that general hospitals have increasingly played in the provision of psychiatric hospitalization care. The evolution of this role has been insightfully considered in several articles.[1-6] Thus, only certain highlights concerning the further growth of these units over the past 50 years will be considered here. In this context, the role of such units in the acute psychiatric hospitalization of patients and their relation to scatter-bed inpatient services will be the major focus.

The experiences of psychiatrists in the military during World War II demonstrated that it was possible to treat large numbers of emotionally dysfunctional soldiers, provided there was prompt accessibility to these patients at the site of "breakdown." The large numbers of newly trained psychiatrists who returned from the war with these successes stimulated the development of new acute care psychiatric inpatient units in large community general hospitals. By 1950, the number of such units had almost doubled; and, by 1958, a total of 164 units had been established.

Action for Mental Health, the 1961 report of the Joint Commission on Mental Illness and Health, specifically recommended that, in order to be regarded as providing comprehensive care, community general hospitals of 100 or more beds should accept mental patients for short-term hospitaliza-

Figure 2-1 The Development of Segregated Psychiatric Units in
Short-Term General Hospitals

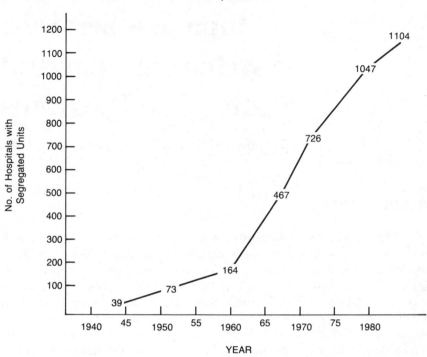

tion and therefore provide a psychiatric unit or psychiatric beds.[7] The community mental health movement resulting from these deliberations led to the development of several hundred more such inpatient units, many in affiliation with federally funded community mental health centers (CMHCs). By 1971, 726 psychiatric units were established in community general hospitals. Figure 2–1 shows that the rate of increase of "segregated" units was greatest from 1963 to 1976, following the report of the joint commission.

The following factors contributed significantly to the growth of the role of nonfederal general hospitals in the provision of psychiatric care:[8]

- clinical factors—early diagnosis, continuity of care, availability of psychopharmacologic agents, brief hospitalization, avoidance of institutionalization
- economic factors—third party insurance coverage for short-term psychiatric hospitalization

- legal factors—restrictions on long-term hospitalization
- social-psychological factors—changes in public attitudes toward psychiatric illness and treatment and the resulting enlightened consumerism

An additional factor of great importance was the desire of state governments to reduce their budgets by lowering their state hospital censuses.

Since 1976, fewer psychiatric units have been opened. One reason for this can be seen in Figure 2–2. By 1981, more than 80 percent of general hospitals with 500 or more beds had already established psychiatric units. These institutions were the ones most likely to possess the necessary

Figure 2–2 Percentage of General Hospitals Reporting Having a Segregated Psychiatric Unit in 1981, by Size of Hospital

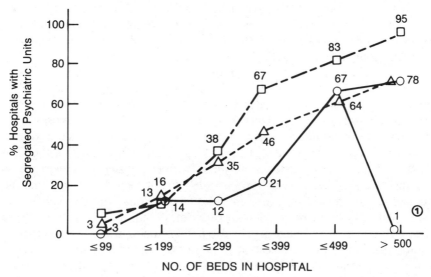

Source: Hospital Statistics, 1981 edition, Copyright 1981 by the American Hospital Association.

resources to set aside beds exclusively for psychiatric admissions. Smaller hospitals have more difficulty in generating sufficient numbers of psychiatric admissions to justify the maintenance of segregated units. This suggests that discrete psychiatric units are not as practical for smaller general hospitals as they are for hospitals with bed complements in excess of 500 beds. It also raises the possibility that the development of alternative models providing appropriate services for the acute inpatient care of psychiatric patients in smaller facilities is necessary. In fact, alternative approaches to psychiatric admissions to general hospitals have already been developed, namely, the informal admission of psychiatric patients on open medical-surgical floors and the more formally designed scatter-bed programs.

For many years, the National Institute of Mental Health (NIMH) has carefully tabulated the statistics of psychiatric admissions to hospitals. In spite of the great increase in the number of segregated psychiatric inpatient units between 1965 (467) and 1979 (844), the number of "inpatient psychiatric episodes"* appears to have increased only slightly over this period, from 519,000 to 572,000. This has led Klerman to note that "the number of inpatient care episodes per 100,000 population has remained relatively stable at about 800 since 1955."[9]

A major reanalysis of the data reflecting inpatient psychiatric episodes was made by Kiesler and Sibulkin.[10,11] They utilized hospital discharge data (rather than patient care episodes as defined by NIMH) to obtain the total number of discharges of patients with primary psychiatric diagnoses from all hospitals, including those general hospitals without segregated psychiatric units. Their findings were quite striking. They confirmed that the total number of inpatient episodes in hospitals with segregated psychiatric units minimally increased between 1965 and 1979. But they discovered that the number of psychiatric inpatient episodes in hospitals without such segregated units increased by more than 6½ times! Indeed, as of 1979, there were twice as many primary psychiatric patients being treated by alternative approaches on general medical-surgical floors (1,203,000) than on segregated psychiatric units (592,000). The relevant data are shown in Figure 2–3.

These data are especially remarkable in light of the fact that very little is known about psychiatric patients who are admitted to nonsegregated general hospital medical beds, that is, scatter-beds. Kiesler and Sibulkin have summarized the few observations that have been documented about such admissions: The patients involved have a shorter length of stay (7.9 days)

---

*"Inpatient psychiatric episodes" are defined as the number of residents in inpatient facilities at the beginning of the year plus the total admissions to these facilities during the year.

Figure 2–3 Number of Inpatient Psychiatric Episodes in General Hospitals: 1965–79

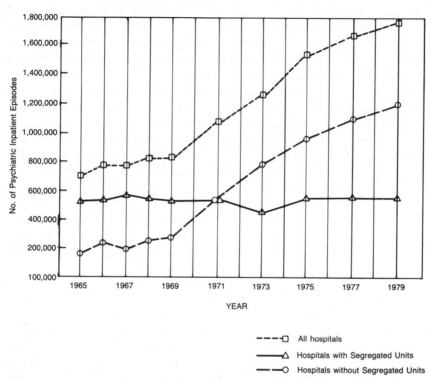

YEAR

----☐ All hospitals

———△ Hospitals with Segregated Units

— —○ Hospitals without Segregated Units

Source: American Journal of Psychiatry, Vol. 141, No. 1, p. 46, January 1984.

---

than patients admitted to segregated units (17 days); they have more frequent diagnoses of alcoholism and neuroses, in contrast to diagnoses of schizophrenia and personality disorder in units; and they tend to be older, with a higher percentage of men, than patients admitted to units.[12]

The paucity of information available on the psychiatric patients admitted to medical-surgical beds in general hospitals extends as well to the nature of the in-hospital psychiatric programs and resources provided to them during their hospitalizations. The assumption one makes is that, by and large, the great majority of hospitals that admit psychiatric patients to open medical-surgical floors have not specifically delineated and developed programs for these patients. In other words, these psychiatric patients are treated in roughly the same manner, with the same physical and personnel resources, as are medical patients. It is not even clear, at this point, what percentage of these patients receive their care from psychiatric (or other mental health) specialists as opposed to nonpsychiatric primary care physicians. (In the following discussion, where no specifically designed in-hospital psychiatric program has been developed to address the diagnostic and treatment needs of psychiatric patients, the situation is referred to as "informal admissions to medical beds"; where specific programs have been developed, they are referred to as "psychiatric scatter-bed programs.")

Over the past 20 years, there have been relatively few articles in the literature on the development of scatter-bed programs designed to address the clinical needs of psychiatric patients admitted to open medical-surgical (general care) floors. The first such program appears in a report by Castelnuovo-Tedesco that describes the treatment of female psychiatric patients on a medical ward at the 5005th USAF Hospital.[13] There was apparently no other facility available for hospitalizing these patients, but "the arrangement has proven to be a happy one and devoid of any significant drawbacks."[14] Castelnuovo-Tedesco cautioned against admitting too high a proportion of psychiatric patients, or those whose behavior was too severely disruptive. He further suggested that steps be taken to dispel the negative attitude toward psychiatric patients by nurses.

In a report on his experiences at the Franklin Square Hospital in Baltimore, Ayd emphasized the importance of rapid tranquilization of patients and of training nursing staff to ensure that medications were taken.[15] He claimed positive benefits from placing psychiatric patients on medical wards, for example, decreased stigma, early treatment, reduced cost, better liaison for medical care, training for house staff and nursing staff, and decreased fear and misinformation about psychiatric illness. He gave only a brief description of the program itself, but it apparently did not include the services of an occupational therapist.

Dale and Wright described a three-year experience at Greenwich Hospital in Connecticut, where patients were admitted to medical floors and followed by their private physicians or medical house staff.[16] They noted problems involving a lack of beds during winter months, inadequate space for therapy, limited activity during the day, and difficulty in modifying the rigid schedules of psychiatrists in private practice. However, overall, their experience demonstrated that a wide variety of psychiatric disorders could be treated on beds scattered throughout the hospital. It is instructive to compare their original experience with a later one, as described in 1970.[17] By that time, they had hired a psychiatric liaison nurse and dismissed a psychiatrist-administrator. These personnel changes still allowed them to continue and expand (which underscores the crucial importance of liaison with medical-nursing staff), but they felt limited in their ability to provide emergency service and to manage patients who were unaware they were ill.

An important and innovative program was described by Reding and Maguire.[18] In the program, psychiatric emergencies were admitted to medical floors, but remained for the most part under the direct supervision of their primary care physicians. Of particular interest is the authors' detailed description of how they tried to overcome a generally hostile attitude toward psychiatric patients on the part of nursing and medical staff. They emphasized that, to manage psychiatric emergencies, close monitoring and rapid use of parenteral medications were essential. Physical restraints and ECT were not used. A mental health nurse, psychiatric social worker, and drug-abuse coordinator were added. They felt their program demonstrated that acute psychiatric episodes could and should be treated on the nonpsychiatric wards of general hospitals.

In response to the Reding and Maguire article, several interesting letters were published describing similar programs. The most negative, by Mutty, cautioned against (1) a medical setting that forced the acceptance of the sick role, (2) overmedication to control disruptive patient behavior, and (3) failure to provide sufficient opportunities to patients to engage in meaningful activity.[19] Mutty's experience apparently was in hospitals that did not provide psychiatric support staff and organized programs. Anderson described his experience at a naval hospital in which psychiatric patients were managed easily on an open medical ward.[20]

Werner, Knorr, and Stack described a ten-bed psychiatric service with beds scattered throughout the hospital.[21] The rural setting of the hospital did not provide sufficient resources for a segregated unit, and the only alternative to a scatter-bed program was transfer to a distant state hospital. Primary care physicians were trained and participated extensively, in most cases maintaining primary responsibility for the care of their patients.

Radman and Davidson reported the use of an open emergency medical ward for rapid evaluation and disposition following suicide attempts.[22] They felt this provided both preparation for longer-term treatment of serious psychopathology and short-term intensive interventions for acute situational disorders.

Finally, Smith reported on the development of a nonsegregated system of care in a rural, 59-bed county general hospital (Howard County General Hospital in Columbia, Maryland) to which private attending psychiatrists admitted their patients.[23] In over three years, 455 patients were admitted to the program, with an average length of stay of 7.3 days. The inpatient program included psychiatric nursing care, group, and activities therapy components.

In summary, the authors found in the literature only seven reports of psychiatric scatter-bed programs designed to provide comprehensive in-hospital care to selected, acutely ill, psychiatric patients. None of these reports included a detailed account of the process by which the scatter-bed program was conceptualized and implemented. Few operational features were described. Moreover, there was no information provided on the specific policies and procedures that were proven useful and those that were problematic.

CONCEPTS AND DEFINITIONS

It is clear from the above observations that, though a great majority of mental health professionals are familiar with the acute hospitalization care resources offered by short-term segregated psychiatric units of general hospitals, few are aware of how psychiatric inpatient management can be provided on open, medical-surgical units. This is remarkable in the context of the statistics comparing "nonsegregated" admissions with those to psychiatric units. Consequently, before discussing the kind of scatter-bed system developed at Lenox Hill Hospital, some definitions of terms are in order.

Psychiatric inpatient units are synonymous with the terms *mental health unit, division for mental and nervous diseases, neuropsychiatric ward,* and *segregated inpatient services, units,* or *beds.* All of these terms denote a contiguous group of beds in a designated floor, wing, or complex of buildings for the in-hospital treatment of psychiatric patients. These unit areas are physically distinct and separate from "medical-surgical" or "general care" beds or units. Most importantly, their beds are specifically reserved for the admission of patients with primary psychiatric diagnoses. By definition, they exclude patients with "medical" illnesses. In most units, this exclusion pertains both to patients with primary medical diagnoses and to those with secondary medical disorders that require substantial medical management. The unit areas are staffed by a multidisciplinary mental health team, which includes psychiatrists (attendings and residents), medical students, psychologists (graduates and interns), psychiatric nurses, psychiatric social workers, occupational and recreational therapists, and mental health technicians (aides, paraprofessionals). Generally, this staff has had specialized training or experience in the in-hospital treatment of psychiatric patients. By and large, they feel ill-equipped to care for medical patients on the unit or in other areas of the hospital. The in-hospital milieus of psychiatric inpatient units have evolved a specialized ethos that is quite different from that found on medical-surgical floors. In fact, "therapeutic community" techniques and various offshoots of such approaches have become standard fare on such segregated inpatient units.

Psychiatric inpatient scatter-bed programs or, as they are sometimes called, nonsegregated psychiatric admissions, denote general hospital psychiatric hospitalization services without physically separate facilities. In these scatter-bed programs, patients with primary psychiatric disorders are admitted to medical-surgical beds on open general care units. The admission of psychiatric patients to these beds is done in the same manner as that for patients with any acute medical illness. The beds are not segregated exclusively for psychiatric patients, hence the term *nonsegregated*. By definition, these beds and the care areas in which they are located are not separate and distinct from medical areas.

The staffing of scatter-bed programs is quite variable. Many have no specialized psychiatric professional personnel exclusively assigned to them. Others employ a special multidisciplinary mental health team. The scant literature on these programs is especially deficient in describing their staffing patterns. The in-hospital management of patients admitted to scatter-bed programs is also quite variable, ranging from limited bedside general nursing care, with individual psychotherapy and psychoactive medication provided by the patient's private general physician or psychiatrist, to more comprehensive therapeutic milieu programs. Once again, there is a paucity of descriptions of these clinical management arrangements in the available literature.

A CASE STUDY: THE DEVELOPMENT OF A PSYCHIATRIC INPATIENT SCATTER-BED PROGRAM AT LENOX HILL HOSPITAL

Pre-1977 Conditions

The period of years during which limited numbers of patients with primary psychiatric diagnoses were informally admitted to general care beds on open medical-surgical wards at Lenox Hill Hospital is difficult to document. The best indications are that it continued over several decades. In this period, generally prior to 1977, such admissions could be subdivided into the following three categories:

1. Patients who were openly admitted with primary psychiatric diagnoses by members of the "neuropsychiatric" attending staff. These admissions were openly accepted and managed by the attending physicians, medical house staff, floor nursing staff, admitting office, and business office.
2. Psychiatric patients who were admitted with spurious nonpsychiatric diagnoses with the probable knowledge of the attending physician. In

most cases, the true nature of the patient's disorder became quickly known to the floor medical and nursing staff because of the nature of the diagnostic and therapeutic services rendered. The true diagnostic status of the patient may or may not have become known to the admitting and business offices. Primary discharge diagnoses of these patients included both psychiatric and nonpsychiatric categories.

3. Patients who were hospitalized with nonpsychiatric medical diagnoses without the attending physician being aware of the psychiatric nature of the condition at the time of admission. The lack of awareness of the patient's primary emotional disorder was variably maintained as the medical work-up proceeded with negative findings. Until 1974, the absence of formal psychiatric consultation-liaison at Lenox Hill reinforced this clinical shortsightedness. Some of the patients were treated with psychoactive medication and other psychiatric therapies. For the purposes of the present discussion, this category of patients does not include those "psychosomatic" conditions—such as ulcerative colitis, gastric and duodenal ulcer disease, migraine headaches, asthma, and neurodermatitis—all of which have well-delineated somatic components. The question of the psychological contribution to the etiologies of these conditions was (and still is) in dispute.

Patients in the second and third categories were admitted by many members of the medical attending staff, including neuropsychiatrists. In the absence of a segregated psychiatric inpatient unit and given the lack of a supporting inpatient psychiatric medical-nursing staff, the in-hospital management of patients with primary psychiatric diagnoses was tolerated, as long as (1) their numbers remained small, or were so perceived; (2) the patients did not pose significant management problems for the floor nursing staff or other patients on the ward; and (3) their presence was not overly visible to the clinical service (medical) directors and chiefs or to the lay administration.

Lenox Hill Hospital's formal policy regarding the admission of patients with primary psychiatric diagnoses was at best ambiguous. It was clear, however, that the hospital's operating certificate from New York State Department of Health did not include a specific proviso for the admission of such a patient population.

As documented in the preceding chapter, the failure to establish a discrete psychiatric inpatient unit in 1959 was a significant blow to the members of the voluntary psychiatric attending staff. Many of these attendings maintained practices that required hospitalization facilities. Most of them had developed other hospital affiliations and used the psychiatric inpatient units of those institutions for their acute hospitalization needs. A few, however, hospitalized their private patients at Lenox Hill on general care units or on the neurology ward. This amounted to an informal scatter-bed system.

As noted in Chapter 1, significant problems were encountered from 1975 to 1977 in recruiting and retaining voluntary attending psychiatrists. One of the principal reasons for this was the absence of a psychiatric inpatient service at the hospital. Several of the newly recruited attending psychiatrists had great need for hospitalization resources. In the absence of a clear hospital policy regarding such admissions, they began hospitalizing patients in general care beds with increasing frequency.

This development disrupted the existing fragile equilibrium at Lenox Hill. Medical-surgical floor nurses became increasingly anxious about providing bedside care to the "psych" patients, and they complained about being unprepared for and unsupported in these tasks. The hospital administration became concerned about the ambiguity in the hospital's operating certificate with respect to the institution's legal status in treating these patients. Finally, the hospital's Department of Medicine, to which the Section of Psychiatry organizationally reported, and other clinical departments became progressively more alarmed about these admissions. Objections to the admission of psychiatric patients were based on assertions that (1) the hospital was not equipped to treat such patients; (2) such admissions would jeopardize the care of medical-surgical patients insofar as the latter would be anxious about the presence of "emotionally disturbed" individuals on the units; and (3) such admissions took up valuable general care beds, which made it even more difficult for the nonpsychiatric physicians to admit their patients to the hospital. The latter claim reflected the very high occupancy rate of the institution.

The concerns and objections of various hospital personnel to the admission of psychiatric patients to general care beds resulted in a decision to declare a moratorium on such admissions, pending the outcome of a study of the problem by the chief of Psychiatric Inpatient Services and the director of the Department of Medicine.

1977–1978 Developments

In the light of the earlier (1975) unsuccessful effort to obtain the approval of the city and state mental health and health departments for a new segregated psychiatric inpatient unit at Lenox Hill Hospital, a completely different approach had to be found to break the impasse. During a two-year period, 1977–1978, the study by the chief of Psychiatric Inpatient Services and the director of the Department of Medicine blossomed into a concerted effort to formulate a new program; the result was a proposal for a psychiatric inpatient scatter-bed program. The process of developing the proposal focused on formulating programmatic policies and procedures that would both meet the needs of the hospital and the psychiatric attending staff and overcome the many concerns that had been raised on the issue of psychiatric admissions. The mandate to study the situation proceeded along two separate, but very much related, tracks: (1) intrainstitutional and (2) extrainstitutional.

The Intrainstitutional Track

The process of intrainstitutional program development included discussions with the members of voluntary psychiatric attending staff, the professional staff of the Psychiatric Outpatient Clinic, the clinical departmental directors and service chiefs, the professional leadership and staff of the Nursing Department, the professional leadership and staff of the Department of Social Work, the professional staff of the emergency room, members of the executive staff of the Administration, the staff of the Business Office, and the staff of the Admitting Office. In the course of these discussions, the particular concerns of the various groups were elaborated. For example, none of the other clinical departments were prepared to give up beds to the Psychiatry Service. The general care bed occupancy rate exceeded 95 percent, which meant that members of the voluntary medical attending staff had considerable difficulty in getting their patients admitted to the hospital, especially in emergency and acute situations. In addition, there were no psychiatric house staff available to provide care to psychiatric patients (there was no psychiatric residency program at the time). The issues of who would provide admission histories, physical examinations, and initial work-up orders for these patients and who would cover medical/ psychiatric emergencies that might arise during hospitalization had to be clarified.

Medical-surgical floor nurses who would provide most of the bedside care for the psychiatric patients and who were considerably apprehensive about their clinical adequacy with regard to "psych cases" had to be educated and supported in the new endeavors. In that context, the quality of care and the lengths of stay for psychiatric inpatients had to be closely monitored and controlled. The concern with lengths of stay reflected the generally held impression that most psychiatric patients required hospitalizations in excess of 30 days, thereby occupying acute care medical beds for unacceptably long periods of time.

Apart from these staffing and resource concerns, the health insurance reimbursement status of the psychiatric patients had to be clarified. Third party payers had to approve the scatter-bed program before the hospital administration would approve it.

A coverage system involving on-site psychiatric physicians and/or nurses was needed to back up private psychiatric attendings in emergency situations involving in-hospital patients. In such problem situations, psychiatric residents were not available to the floor medical-surgical physician and nursing staff, and there were reservations about the telephone accessibility of psychiatric attendings once they left the hospital for their private offices. In this situation, answering machines and services were not deemed to be adequate response vehicles.

Finally, the admission of "clinically inappropriate" patients to general care beds had to be addressed. Which categories of psychiatric patients were appropriate for in-hospital management on open medical wards in semiprivate rooms occupied by "medical" patients? The answer involved such variables as the nature of the presenting problem, the diagnosis, the treatment requirements, the anticipated length of stay, and other factors. All of these admitting criteria had to be incorporated in a clinical admission screening mechanism to prevent problems before they arose.

The Extrainstitutional Track

The extrainstitutional process involved meetings with the New York State Office of Mental Health regarding the regulations and procedures that governed the establishment and operation of psychiatric scatter-bed services. Preliminary inquiries revealed that, in fact, there were no existing regulations that appeared to apply to such programs. The certification regulations applied only to segregated inpatient units. Since scatter-bed services did not fall under any existing guidelines, they were ruled to be outside the purview of the certification procedures of the state agency. Similarly, there were no guidelines regarding the maximum census of patients that such a scatter-bed program could have. The rough figures of 15–20 patients were arbitrarily cited as an upper limit.

It was clear from these inquiries that the public mental health agencies were confused about their positions regarding scatter-bed programs. In the end, in the absence of clear and pertinent regulations, they absolved themselves of involvement in reviewing, certifying, and monitoring such programs. This, paradoxically, offered important advantages, in that it was unnecessary to devote the considerable amount of administrative time and effort to satisfy the complex bureaucratic regulations involved in certification. But it also had the serious detrimental consequence of excluding such an inpatient service from the mainstream of hospitalization resources, mental health planning, and catchmenting.

In addition, this situation restricted the hospital's ability to admit all clinically appropriate Medicaid patients. This consequence devolved from the following regulatory logic: (1) In-hospital psychiatric treatment is approved for any Medicaid-eligible patient admitted to a facility that is certified as such by the State Office of Mental Health. (2) The regulations of the State Office of Mental Health concerning such certification pertained only to segregated psychiatric inpatient units, not to scatter-bed programs. Thus, Medicaid certification for the latter services was not possible. In effect, Medicaid did not approve the care of psychiatric patients in scatter-bed programs.

The proscription against providing psychiatric care to Medicaid patients by general hospital scatter-bed services included, of course, any reimbursement for such care. Beyond the financial issue, however, was the more imposing question of the institution's legal liability for providing care to this patient population. What would be the hospital's legal exposure stemming from untoward episodes that might occur during such hospitalizations?

Discussions with the New York City Department of Mental Health, Mental Retardation, and Alcoholism Services concerning the relation of the proposed scatter-bed program to the psychiatric hospitalization needs of the local Manhattan upper eastside community also revealed equating acute psychiatric inpatient services with certified segregated units. The net effect was to preclude the program from being considered in the borough and city-wide mental health planning process and to prohibit the catchmenting of its services in any way. In sum, the clinical restrictions on a scatter-bed service, which precluded its utilization by all diagnostic categories of patients and the Medicaid reimbursement restrictions served to reinforce the basic attitude of unfamiliarity and aloofness on the part of the city agency staff regarding scatter-bed services. The end result was to view such an inpatient service as "irrelevant to the needs of the community."[24]

Discussions were also held with representatives of Blue Cross/Blue Shield of Greater New York, Inc., and with other third party insurance payers. After reviewing the program protocol and interviewing the hospital-based clinical staff, these groups tentatively approved the Lenox Hill scatter-bed program for reimbursement.

Policies and Procedures

In order to provide some inpatient acute care psychiatric resources to members of the voluntary psychiatric attending staff and their patients, Lenox Hill Hospital initiated the psychiatric inpatient scatter-bed program in June 1978. As noted, the program was designed to meet the issues and concerns raised by the various interested individuals and groups. A detailed, formal program protocol was developed, which clearly specified all relevant policies and procedures.[25] The essential characteristics of the clinical care system of the program are described in this section.

The admission of patients with primary psychiatric diagnoses to nonsegregated medical-surgical beds on open general care wards is on an as-available basis. These admissions are, in effect, no different from those of any other diagnostic group of patients. Initially, ten general care nursing units were selected for the scatter-bed admissions. As the program evolved, these areas were expanded to include virtually every nonspecialized medical-surgical ward of the hospital. The "as-available" characteristic is an extremely important aspect of the program. It means that no beds or areas are specifically reserved for psychiatric patients. It also means that such admissions must compete with the general mix of medical patients placed on the list of the Admitting Department according to three categories of priority: emergency, urgent, and elective.

Patients with primary psychiatric diagnoses are admitted under the care of their private psychiatrist or nonpsychiatric physician. The scatter-bed program was designed as a private practice system because there was no psychiatric house staff (residents). It was considered important to permit all members of the attending medical staff to admit psychiatric patients under the auspices of the program. In fact, several internists and "neuropsychiatrists" (primarily neurologists) occasionally did admit such patients to the hospital. To avoid discriminating against these nonpsychiatric physicians, the program stipulated that they need not necessarily refer patients with primary psychiatric diagnoses upon admission to the care of psychiatric colleagues. In such cases, the quality of care provided by the nonpsychiatric physician could be reasonably maintained by the close, daily involvement of the inpatient mental health team, which could at any time recommend the inclusion of a psychiatric consultant on the case in an adjunctive capacity or, if that proved insufficient, in a primary care capacity.

The program's patients are given informal admission status. That is, patients with primary psychiatric diagnoses are admitted in the same manner as any other medical patient. In other hospitals, "voluntary" admission procedures are employed only for psychiatric patients, which entails administrative segregation. Furthermore, "involuntary" admissions for psychiatric patients were not sanctioned under the operating certificate of Lenox Hill Hospital (another consequence of the exclusion of the scatter-bed program from certification). It was also clear that a clinical program that utilized primarily semiprivate general care beds on open medical-surgical units would be inadequate for the in-hospital management of involuntary psychiatric patients who required a more secure and structured milieu.

The program stipulates the preadmission clinical screening of patients by a peer review panel of members of the psychiatric attending staff. A major concern of the Lenox Hill medical board and administration was that clinically "inappropriate" psychiatric patients, that is, patients who could not be managed on open medical floors, would be admitted to the hospital under the new program. It was unclear whether this concern was real or imaginary. In any case, if the new program was to have any chance of succeeding, caution had to be exercised in this very critical admission area. Senior clinicians of the voluntary psychiatric attending staff (and one member of the Department of Medicine) volunteered to provide this screening on a 24-hour/day, 7-day/week basis. Each patient referred for admission is evaluated on a case-by-case basis according to guidelines for clinical indications for hospitalization incorporated in the "Lenox Hill Hospital Psychiatric Physician Medical Care Criteria."[26] Relative exclusory criteria included the following factors:

- expectation of hospitalization in excess of 30 days
- acute manic symptomatology
- acute suicidal risk
- impulsive and acting-out behavior
- violent behavior

These factors must be considered in the context of the patient's overall clinical presentation, present and past psychiatric history, the clinical skills of the patient's admitting psychiatrist (especially in the area of providing acute inpatient care), family and other support systems, and so on.

The program includes *preadmission or immediate postadmission financial screening*. As with any privately admitted medical patient, credit office review of the patient's financial and insurance coverage is included as an important part of the admissions procedures (see Chapter 18).

Appropriately screened medical-surgical inpatients may be transferred to psychiatric status. Many medical-surgical patients admitted to the general and specialized care units fall into the clinical categories that lead to consideration for "conversion," that is, transfer to the Psychiatric Inpatient Program. Such conversions are possible in the case of mixed medical-psychiatric diagnoses, if and when the medical care of the patient comes to a successful conclusion or begins to take on secondary importance to psychiatric management, and continued in-hospital stay is justified on psychiatric clinical grounds. A conversion is also possible when the diagnostic work-up of a medical patient proves negative, psychogenic etiology becomes probable, and continued in-hospital management is clinically justified (provided psychiatric management is available). Both of these situations involve members of the Psychiatric Consultation-Liaison Service, who facilitate the determination of the psychiatric components of clinical presentation, the significance of the underlying psychiatric disorder, and the need for continued hospitalization on a psychiatric basis. The service members also function as the initial clinical screeners to determine suitability for conversion to the scatter-bed program. A patient who is judged clinically justified for such transfer must consent to the move, with the concurrence of the patient's medical physician and the attending psychiatrist, who agrees to provide further private in-hospital care. When conversion is effected, the patient remains on the same unit, in the same bed. The inpatient mental health team becomes involved in the patient's care, and the various therapeutic modalities of care provided by the program are ordered, as indicated.

A full-time, hospital-based, multidisciplinary inpatient mental health team is maintained. This team formally meets on a daily basis in clinical rounds to review new admissions and to discuss the progress of and develop discharge plans for previously admitted patients. The private attending physician of every scatter-bed admission is required to present the patient to the team in order to develop coordinated case management and a discharge planning strategy. Diagnostic and therapeutic orders are reviewed, including the specific orders for patient participation in group and activities therapies. In addition to the daily rounds, two teaching conferences and a "rap session" are held each week by the staff. Cohesiveness of the team and coordination of its members' individual efforts are considered vital for optimum program effectiveness. The members of the inpatient mental health team include:

- The chief of inpatient services (psychiatrist), who is responsible for the overall administrative direction and clinical coordination of the program. This includes admissions screening, clinical coordination and supervision, quality control, and modification of existing policies and procedures.
- An inpatient mental health nurse specialist, a master's level psychiatric nurse clinician/educator who is responsible for supervising the psychiatric nursing staff, providing education/support to medical-surgical floor nurses, and engaging in one-to-one and group clinical patient care.
- A psychiatric staff nurse, an RN with specialized training and experience in acute care hospital psychiatric nursing. This nurse provides one-to-one and group psychiatric nursing care and support for the administration of ECT.
- Two mental health technicians, mental health paraprofessionals who are responsible for assisting the psychiatric and medical-surgical nursing staffs in the management of scatter-bed patients.
- A coordinator of therapeutic activities, a mental health professional with training and experience in acute care in-hospital occupational or

activities therapy. This person is responsible for assessing the needs, capabilities, and interests of scatter-bed patients in relation to daily living, vocation, and recreation and for providing them with outlets of expression through art, music, drama, and so on.

- A psychiatric social worker, a master's level social worker with acute care psychiatric inpatient experience, preferably in a general hospital. This professional assesses the psychosocial needs of scatter-bed patients and provides diagnostic and therapeutic casework with their families.

All the above professional staff participate in patient progress conferences, discharge planning, and utilization review discussions on scatter-bed admissions.

The program operates in a centralized, inpatient mental health administrative-treatment area. The inpatient team is based on this centralized psychiatric administrative-treatment area; but emphasis is placed on its mobility to move throughout the hospital, especially to those general care nursing units to which the scatter-bed patients are admitted. This balance between centralized location and mobility enables the staff to provide many of the therapeutic activities of more traditional segregated psychiatric unit milieus as well as to maintain the ability to respond to the needs of patients, house staff, and nursing staff on the "scattered" medical-surgical floors.

The full range of in-hospital psychiatric diagnostic and treatment services are available to the program. These services include:

- Diagnostic psychiatric and medical work-ups under the direction of the patient's admitting psychiatric (or medical) attending physician. These work-ups encompass all historical, physiological, psychological (mental status examinations, psychological testing, neuropsychological assessment), and interpersonal studies conducted in order to establish clinical diagnoses and formulate treatment plans. Initial admission histories and physical examinations are performed by the medical house staff physician assigned to the general care floor. Nonpsychiatric specialty consultations are ordered, as clinically indicated, by the admitting physician.

- Individual psychotherapy on a daily basis, seven days per week, by the admitting physician or covering psychiatrist.

- Psychopharmacologic medications, as clinically indicated, under the medical direction of the admitting physician.

- Electroconvulsive therapy (ECT), as clinically indicated, administered by members of the psychiatric attending staff who are specifically authorized to render this care under established guidelines.[27] These guidelines stipulate procedures covering clinical indications, prior medical clearance, informed consent, locations of administration, anesthesia, post-ECT monitoring, supporting professional staff, necessary equipment, and records and charting.

- Psychological testing and neuropsychological assessment, as ordered by the admitting physician, as clinically indicated, and performed by a staff-affiliate clinical psychologist.

- Psychiatric nursing care, provided at the bedside and on the psychiatric inpatient treatment area by members of the scatter-bed nursing team.

- Group psychotherapy, as clinically indicated and ordered by the admitting physician. This therapy is provided on a three-times-per-week basis by members of the inpatient mental health team.

- A therapeutic activities program, as clinically indicated and ordered by the admitting physician. The program is provided on a daily basis under the direction of the coordinator of therapeutic activities by members of the inpatient mental health team.

- Psychosocial needs assessment, diagnostic and therapeutic family casework, and discharge planning, as clinically indicated. These services are performed by the psychiatric social worker in consultation with the admitting physician and members of the inpatient mental health team.

- Emergency coverage of psychiatric scatter-bed patients, as provided by the admitting physician or designated covering physician. The members of the inpatient mental health team provide back-up coverage during daytime shifts. The attending psychiatrist on emergency call provides back-up coverage during evenings and nights and on weekends and holidays.

A close working relationship is maintained with the Psychiatric Consultation-Liaison Service. The scatter-bed program of providing nonsegregated clinical care to patients with primary psychiatric diagnoses must collaborate closely with the Psychiatric Consultation-Liaison Service. Since 20 to 30 percent of all patients admitted to the scatter-bed program are converted from medical inpatient status, the two clinical programs must work closely together to determine the appropriateness of each transfer and the changes required in inpatient status between medicine and psychiatry. The principal clinical criterion used to determine the appropriate administrative status of a patient with mixed medical-psychiatric diagnoses is that of clinical management, that is, what are the principal diagnostic-therapeutic efforts being employed, and which problems are the most acute.

Operational Experience with the Psychiatric Inpatient Scatter-Bed Program: 1978–1983

At this writing, the psychiatric inpatient scatter-bed program has been providing clinical services at Lenox Hill Hospital for almost seven years. Members of the Lenox Hill Hospital professional community are pleased that the program has operated smoothly and without major clinical difficulty during this period. The success of the program is due to a great extent to the careful planning that was done prior to implementation. It is also due to the continuing open-mindedness and willingness to experiment shown by all the physicians, nurses, social workers, administrators, and support personnel who have contributed to the program. At the outset, these contributors were clearly conservative in determining admitting criteria, in defining management issues, and in discharge planning. However, as they became more familiar with the program's procedures, strengths, and limitations, and as they continued to address problems that needed correction, the scatter-bed program became increasingly popular, to the point where it is now fully accepted by virtually all groups. It is important to note that the individuals who are most enthusiastic about the program are the patients who have been admitted and their families. With few exceptions, patients with previous general hospital admissions to psychiatric units have reported to us that the Lenox Hill program of psychiatric hospitalization is more effective and less onerous to them.

Table 2–1 presents the admission statistics of the Lenox Hill Hospital psychiatric inpatient scatter-bed program in various categories for the six-year period, 1978 through 1983. As can be seen, the number of scatter-bed admissions reached an average level of 250 patients per year in the years 1980–1983. This reflected the relatively high medical-surgical occupancy rate (over 95 percent) during those years, which reduced the availability of general care beds for acute psychiatric admissions. A great majority of the patients for whom admission was requested could not wait the period (from two to ten days) it took to procure a bed. Their emergency or acute clinical status required a more responsive admission at another institution.

As noted earlier, state regulations did not permit Medicaid patients to be admitted to the program, and this also limited the number of admissions, especially from the Psychiatric Clinic, other outpatient department clinics, and the ER. Another factor which kept the census down was the political sensitivity of such admissions in organizational relationships with the Department of Medicine and other clinical departments in the hospital. The hospital had an extremely high occupancy rate, and the great majority of the attending medical staff regarded their ability to admit patients to the hospital as an important aspect of their practice of medicine. Since each psychiatric

Table 2-1 Psychiatric Inpatient Scatter-Bed Program Admissions at Lenox Hill Hospital: 1978–1983

	1978	1979	1980	1981	1982	1983
Total Admissions	92	196	268	245	257	230
Male	32	66	102	87	56	54
Female	60	130	166	158	201	176
White	75	163	225	198	221	193
Black	15	27	40	39	28	28
Other	2	6	3	7	8	9
Type of Admission						
Emergency	34	56	77	59	55	52
Urgent	30	83	82	89	86	100
Elective	28	57	109	97	116	78
Source of Admission						
Office	57	99	151	160	168	133
Transfer of med/surg pt.	19	54	82	57	54	66
Emergency rm.	14	36	32	26	33	27
Psych. clinic	1	4	2	1	1	1
Other hospital	1	3	1	1	3	3
Admitting Diagnoses						
Depression	36	86	138	119	156	132
Depression with suicide attempt	13	21	14	20	12	10
Agitated depression	4	10	9	22	15	9
Mania	8	11	15	4	11	16
Schizophrenia	7	17	12	21	16	10
Schizoaffective disorder	1	4	2	3	1	4
Other psychosis	9	23	48	31	14	13
Alcoholism	7	12	12	11	7	14
Substance abuse	3	5	13	11	13	13
Anorexia nervosa	1	0	1	2	2	7
Transient situational disorder	3	5	4	0	0	0
Psychosomatic disorders	0	2	0	0	0	2
Other	0	0	0	1	11	0
Average Length of Stay (Days)	17.1	17.6	14.9	15.3	18.3	14.7
Average Daily Census (Patients)	8.3	9.4	11.8	10.4	12.9	10.4
Insurance[a]						
Blue Cross/Blue Shield	44	80	87	115	122	125
Medicare	37	89	139	126	117	102

(continued)

Table 2–1 continued

	1978	1979	1980	1981	1982	1983
Commercial & government	7	14	14	28	2	13
Manhattan Health Plan	0	8	1	0	4	0
Self-pay	4	5	27	3	0	4
Unknown	0	0	0	0	12	0
Dispositions						
Home/outpatient treatment	65	151	245	203	213	193
Conversion to med/surg status	10	8	3	20	8	9
Nursing home	4	7	10	17	15	14
Transfer to psych. unit	7	10	5	2	5	3
Left A.M.A.	6	15	3	3	7	5
Alcohol rehab. unit	0	0	0	0	6	3
Physical rehab. unit	0	0	0	0	1	1
Expired	0	0	0	0	2	2
Other	0	5	2	0	0	0

[a]Some patients had multiple insurance.

admission represented one less medical patient admitted to the same bed, given the precarious developmental status of the section of psychiatry, the resulting organizational tensions had to be closely monitored.

It is also clear from the Table 2–1 statistics that the majority of patients (51–65 percent) were referred for admission from the offices of the psychiatric attending staff. Administrative transfers (conversions) of medical-surgical inpatients to psychiatric status constituted the next most frequent patient admission group to the scatter-bed program (21–31 percent).

The significant difference in the number of female and male patients admitted to the program is striking, even in comparison with the normally higher percentage of women admitted to traditional psychiatric units. The overwhelming proportion of white patients admitted (81–86 percent) over black patients (11–16 percent) and other groups (2–4 percent) reflects the distribution of the local upper eastside Manhattan ethnic population, the distribution of private practice ethnic patients, and the absence of Medicaid patients and involuntary admissions. Age breakdowns of the admissions are not shown in the table.

The statistics on admitting diagnoses in the scatter-bed program reveal a preponderance of depression (55–71 percent). Other diagnoses of psychosis (mania, schizophrenia, schizoaffective disorder, and other psychoses) constitute the next most frequent category of admissions (16–29 percent). Alcoholism (3–8 percent) and substance abuse (3–6 percent) form the third most frequent diagnostic grouping of patients admitted to the program.

The average length of stay of the scatter-bed patients was remarkably short, (14.7–17.6) days, compared with those of acute care psychiatric units in the New York metropolitan area (17–31 days). The fact that the program's lengths of stay have been decreasing in recent years is in no small part a consequence of the active efforts of the PSRO at the Lenox Hill Hospital and the increasing awareness of the role of the PSRO by attending physicians and other hospital personnel.

The insurance coverage of the program's psychiatric patients reflects a preponderance of Medicare and Blue Cross/Blue Shield third party payers. The absence of Medicaid is again striking.

The discharge dispositions of the great majority of the psychiatric patients to their homes and to a resumption of private outpatient management reflects the type of social and economic support structures enjoyed by these individuals. Significantly, transfers to local segregated psychiatric units occurred much more frequently in the first two years of the program (7 percent and 5 percent) than in subsequent years (1–2 percent). This is a consequence of the attending physicians' increasing familiarity with the scatter-bed system and the disappearance of many of the initially perceived clinical limitations.

Over the seven years that the Lenox Hill scatter-bed program has provided services, its capability to admit patients with affective disorders, even with high suicidal risk, has been impressive. Such admissions require that the admitting physician order a private duty nursing aide and that there be close monitoring of the patient by the floor nursing staff. In these situations, aggressive management by the admitting physician is especially important. In fact, among the more than 1,600 patients admitted over the seven years, there have been no suicidal deaths.

The Lenox Hill scatter-bed program is especially clinically suitable to the needs of patients with mixed psychiatric-medical diagnoses, paranoid disorders, depression, anorexia nervosa, and alcoholism. On the other hand, patients with more bizarre, agitated, or disorganized symptoms of schizophrenia are problematic for management on the open general care floors of the system. Their presence in semiprivate beds next to medical patients has proven difficult for such patients, their families, and their physicians. Interestingly, in contrast, the medical-surgical nursing staff have adapted well to all clinical categories of patients admitted to the program.

Patients with substance abuse problems have proven difficult to manage on open units. In some cases, the admission of such patients has led to the appearance of illicit drugs on the medical floors—a most disturbing development. In keeping with the initial design of the program, no involuntary patients or violent patients have been admitted.

The program has been fortunate in being able to maintain a stable, dedicated mental health team; its members are in large part responsible for the smooth and effective operation of the program. Good working, coordinative relationships have developed between the team and the private psychiatric attendings. Its members have been especially useful in fostering the accepting manner in which the program has been greeted by the medical-surgical nursing staff and other support personnel of the hospital.

Discussion: Advantages and Disadvantages of the Psychiatric Inpatient Scatter-Bed Program

Based on the experiences described in the above case study, there are clearly many advantages in the use of scatter-bed services over more traditional psychiatric inpatient units. However, it is also clear that there are significant weaknesses and limitations to such nonsegregated psychiatric services, which need careful attention.

Advantages and Strengths

First, the nonsegregated admission of patients with primary psychiatric disorders to general care units decreases the stigmatization that many individuals attach to psychiatric hospitalization. It eases the process of admitting many patients who hesitate or openly refuse to be hospitalized on discrete psychiatric units (paranoid patients). Also, the patients' family members and friends often feel more comfortable about visiting them on open medical units.

Second, a scatter-bed system avoids many of the problems created or reinforced by the behaviorally aberrant subcultures on psychiatric units. There is in fact significantly less behavioral deviancy tolerated on open general care units compared with psychiatric units, where such behavior is "understood." The healthy reality orientation fostered by the presence of acutely medically ill patients on the same units provides the psychiatric patients with a more realistic perspective on their own difficulties.

Third, the familiarity of specialty nurses and physicians with general care unit milieus removes many of the psychological barriers to the involvement of these professionals in the care of psychiatric patients on scatter-bed services. Many nonpsychiatric professionals do not like, and sometimes openly avoid, providing consultations to patients on psychiatric units.

Fourth, the design of a scatter-bed program minimizes differences in the admission and in-hospital management of psychiatric patients and other medical patients and thus serves to integrate psychiatry more closely in the medical world of the general hospital.

Fifth, scatter-bed services facilitate the training of nonpsychiatric house staff, attending physicians, nursing staff, and other support personnel in the recognition of and management of patients with emotional disorders. This occurs as a result of their primary clinical involvement with such patients, under the supervision and support of psychiatric staff. Undoubtedly, this increased amenability to psychiatric training has a positive impact on the approaches of these professionals to the emotional experiences of medical-surgical patients to whom they also provide care.

Sixth, a scatter-bed program serves as an ideal clinical care system for the diagnostic and treatment needs of patients with combined medical-psychiatric problems. The elderly patient and patients with anorexia nervosa, alcoholism, organic states, and other disorders are particularly benefited in such a program. Conversions between medical and psychiatric statuses are accomplished with minimal changes, since the patient is not physically transferred to a different bed or unit.

Seventh, the mobility of the inpatient mental health team and its involvement with care providers throughout the hospital promote the integration of this psychiatric team with, and its acceptance by, medical-surgical personnel.

Eighth, the training of undergraduate, third-year medical student clerks on a scatter-bed service has major benefits. These students come to see their psychiatric inpatient rotation as similar to that in other clinical clerkships. Compared with their colleagues with clerkships on segregated units, they have less of a tendency to segment psychiatry off into a category that is essentially different from that of other specialties.

Disadvantages and Limitations

First, during periods of high occupancy of medical-surgical beds, there are significant difficulties in admitting emergency and acute psychiatric patients within a period of time consistent with the needs of their clinical presentations. This is due to the fact that the medical-surgical beds are not reserved specifically for psychiatric patients but rather are part of the pool of general medical case beds.

Second, a scatter-bed program clearly cannot provide in-hospital psychiatric management for all types of acute problems and diagnoses. Disorganized or bizarre schizophrenics, many acute manics, substance abusers, involuntary and violent patients, and some patients with impulse disorders and acting-out behaviors cannot be effectively managed on an open, scatter-bed program.

Third, scatter-bed programs tend to operate more on a medical-model basis than on the basis of a therapeutic community or token economy, both of which require more controlled psychiatric units.

Fourth, as the patient census increases, the logistical problems of transporting patients to and from the medical-surgical floors to the psychiatric treatment area become more time-consuming and difficult. The important factors here are (1) the location of the psychiatric inpatient treatment area relative to the floors to which the patients are admitted and (2) the accessibility of this area to those floors.

Fifth, in the great majority of states, scatter-bed programs may not be certified by the state mental health authority, thereby making Medicaid patients ineligible.

Sixth, the current guidelines that govern psychiatric residency training accreditation do not seem to approve of scatter-bed programs to satisfy requirements for inpatient experience. Consequently, scatter-bed programs may have to remain based on a system of private practice or salaried attendings until the guidelines are clarified on this point.

Seventh, the absence of psychiatric resident staffing for scatter-bed programs makes a true 24-hour/day, 7-day/week admission system to such a service impossible for many physicians. Consequently, evenings, nights, and weekend and holiday periods are weak in regard to the smooth admission of emergency patients to such programs.

Formally Developed Psychiatric Scatter-Bed Programs Versus Nonprotocol Systems

Many of the patients with primary psychiatric disorders who are admitted on a nonsegregated basis to general hospitals are apparently admitted to what we call nonprotocol programs, that is, programs without clinical admission guidelines, treatment criteria (utilization review), quality assurance procedures, or perhaps even designated hospital-based psychiatric professional staff. The advantages of the kind of scatter-bed program developed at Lenox Hill Hospital over these types of nonprotocol programs are several. First, a scatter-bed program has stipulated guidelines that address the admission screening process of "clinically appropriate" patients in a manner that is consistent with the inherent limitations of the milieu of an open medical unit.

Second, the hospital-based multidisciplinary mental health team in a scatter-bed service provides many of the requisite administrative and clinical management services necessary for an effective in-hospital diagnostic and treatment program. These include group and activity therapies, psychiatric nursing care, ECT, quality assurance, utilization review, and discharge planning. In short, a scatter-bed arrangement makes it possible to provide a substantial, structured inpatient care program.

Third, a scatter-bed program provides the necessary liaison support and education of nonpsychiatric medical and nursing staff of the general care units. This includes mental health staff availability for emergencies and crises of psychiatric inpatients.

Fourth, in such a program, there is close coordination with and support of the psychiatric consultation-liaison service by the inpatient mental health team, which translates into significant advantages over a nonprotocol system.

Finally, with the increasing emphasis of government and other third party payers on the quality and appropriateness of various in-hospital clinical services, the lack of organized therapeutic programs in nonprotocol scatter-bed operations is likely to be the focus of growing attention and concern. Such programs will have to demonstrate that they render services that compare favorably with those provided in more traditional psychiatric units.

SUMMARY

It is well-documented that, today, patients with primary psychiatric disorders are admitted more frequently to nonsegregated, open medical-surgical wards of general hospitals than to segregated psychiatric units. This is a remarkable situation, in that the accepted standard of psychiatric inpatient care is that provided in segregated units. In fact, little is known about the clinical services that patients receive in nonsegregated programs. In the absence of descriptions in the literature of specific programmatic support for group and activity therapy, specialized nursing and social work care, given the generally inadequate physical facilities for psychotherapy and the relatively rigid schedules of most psychiatrists, it is reasonable to assume that the primary treatment modality in scatter-bed programs is pharmacotherapy. However, much research is still needed to determine whether such scatter-bed psychiatric inpatient care constitutes an effective level of management for the large numbers of psychiatric patients who are admitted to general hospitals.

REFERENCES

1. J.R. Ewalt and P.L. Ewalt, "History of the Community Psychiatry Movement," *American Journal of Psychiatry* 126 (July 1969).

2. G.H. Flamm, "The Expanding Roles of General-Hospital Psychiatry," *Hospital and Community Psychiatry* 30 (March 1979).

3. M.H. Greenhill, "Psychiatric Units in General Hospitals: 1979," *Hospital and Community Psychiatry* 30 (March 1979).

4. R.F. Mollica, "From Asylum to Community: The Threatened Disintegration of Public Psychiatry," *New England Journal of Medicine* 308 (7): 367–373.

5. L.D. Ozarin and C.A. Tube, "Psychiatric Inpatients: Who, Where and Future," *American Journal of Psychiatry* 131 (January 1974).

6. P.H. Person, Jr., P.L. Hurley, and R.H. Giesler, "Psychiatric Patients in General Hospitals," *Hospitals* 40 (16 January 1966).

7. Joint Commission on Mental Illness and Health, *Action for Mental Health: Final Report* (New York: Basic Books, 1961).

8. Greenhill, "Psychiatric Units."

9. G.L. Klerman, "National Trends in Hospitalization," *Hospital and Community Psychiatry* 30 (1979): 112.

10. C.A. Kiesler and A.E. Sibulkin, "Episodic Rate of Mental Hospitalization: Stable or Increasing?" *American Journal of Psychiatry* 141 (January 1984).

11. C.A. Kiesler and A.E. Sibulkin, *People, Clinical Episodes, and Mental Hospitalization: A Multiple-Source Method of Estimations in Advances in Applied Social Psychology,* ed. R.F. Kidd and M.J. Saks (Hillsdale, N.J.: Lawrence Erlbaum Associates, 1983).

12. Ibid.

13. P. Castelnuovo-Tedesco, "Care of Female Psychiatric Patients, Including the Acutely Disturbed, on an Open Medical and Surgical Ward," *New England Journal of Medicine* 257 (17 October 1957).

14. Ibid., 752.

15. F.J. Ayd, "Psychiatric Patients on General Medical Wards," in *Frontiers in General Hospital Psychiatry,* ed. L. Linn (New York: International Universities Press, 1961).

16. P.W. Dale and H.S. Wright, "The Care of Psychiatric Patients in a General Hospital without Special Facilities," *American Journal of Psychiatry* 118 (1962).

17. N.S. Wright and P.W. Dale, "A Psychiatric Service as an Integral Part of a Community General Hospital," *Psychiatry in Medicine* (1 April 1970).

18. G.R. Reding and B. Maguire, "Nonsegregated Acute Psychiatric Admissions to General Hospitals—Continuity of Care within the Community Hospital," *New England Journal of Medicine* 289 (26 July 1973).

19. L. Mutty, Correspondence, *New England Journal of Medicine* 289 (8 November 1973).

20. W. Anderson, Correspondence, *New England Journal of Medicine* 289 (8 November 1973): 1042.

21. A. Werner, F.A. Knorr, and J.M. Stack, "Psychiatric Services in a Rural General Hospital," *International Journal of Psychiatry in Medicine* 8 (1977–1978).

22. R. Radman and S. Davidson, "Short-Term Treatment in a General Hospital Following a Suicide Attempt," *Hospital and Community Psychiatry* 28 (July 1977).

23. P.R. Smith, "Nonsegregation of Psychiatric Patients in a General Hospital," *Journal of Psychiatric Nursing* 17 (February 1979).

24. Personal communication from the Manhattan Borough Coordinator, New York City Department of Mental Health, Mental Retardation, and Alcoholism Services, 1978.

25. Lenox Hill Hospital, Department of Medicine, "Protocol for the Admission and

Treatment of Patients with Primary Psychiatric Disorders to Lenox Hill Hospital on an As-Available General Care Bid Basis " (New York: Author, May 1978).

26. Lenox Hill Hospital, "Lenox Hill Hospital Psychiatric Physician Care Criteria for Utilization Review " (New York: Author, March 1978).

27. Lenox Hill Hospital, Department of Medicine, "Lenox Hill Hospital Psychiatry Service Electroconvulsive Therapy (ECT) Policies and Procedures " (New York: Author, May 1978).

Chapter 3

Psychiatric Consultation-Liaison Services

Larry S. Goldblatt, M.D.

INTRODUCTION

Much has been written about consultation-liaison psychiatry, its origins, development, objectives, modes of functioning, accomplishments, and problems. Lipowski[1-4] and others[5-11] have provided excellent reviews. Most of these writings reflect the situation of the institutions from which they emanate. By and large, the authors are based in university hospitals. The principal activities of these institutions are education and research, with service an important but secondary source of esteem and morale for the medical faculty. Out of a total American general hospital population of 5,500, these institutions number approximately 200. Little has been written about consultation-liaison psychiatry in the other 5,300 general hospitals across the country. In these hospitals, medical education is part of the programmatic agenda, but clinical services to the community are, without doubt, their principal *raison d'être*. Moreover, the quality of clinical services provides their major sources of funding and professional recognition.

Lenox Hill Hospital developed as an acute care community hospital that emphasizes primarily clinical services. However, in recent decades graduate medical education has come to play an increasingly important role in the hospital. In 1982, this culminated in a formal affiliation agreement with New York Medical College, transforming Lenox Hill into a "university teaching hospital." Yet, in spite of this affiliation, the hospital has very much retained its primary character as a community-based, voluntary facility, with a very strong private practice medical tradition among its more than 750 voluntary attending physicians and allied health professionals.

To review briefly, Lenox Hill Hospital is of moderate (698 beds) size, located on the upper east side of New York City, serving the entire metropolitan area but dedicated to enhancing health and providing health care in its own community. It is considered a university teaching hospital but in the affiliate, more than the primary, sense. It is involved with undergraduate medical and postgraduate residency education, but these training programs are largely supported by the activities of private practitioners, as opposed to full-time salaried medical faculty. The hospital has 27,000 admissions per year, of which 92 percent are private patients whose care is provided by voluntary attending physicians. These patients are cared for on "private" floors, where their attending physicians are solely responsible for management decisions, and on "regional" floors, where private patient care is provided by house staff physicians in collaboration with private attendings. Usually, the regional floors have the sickest of the private patients (exclusive of those admitted to critical care areas) because of the full and active participation of the medical house staff in their care.

The remaining eight percent of the patients constitute nonreferred or "service" cases. These are patients who are admitted through the emergency room or the outpatient clinics and do not have or request a private physician. They are assigned to the "service" wards and are cared for by the medical house staff under the supervision of an attending. The hospital has ten free standing residencies in the clinical specialties of internal medicine, general surgery, pediatrics, plastic surgery, obstetrics and gynecology, orthopedics, urology, ophthalmology, radiology, and pathology. In addition, there are three affiliated residency programs in psychiatry, anesthesiology, and otolaryngology. The residents in these programs are under the direction of salaried departmental directors and their clinical teaching staffs, most of whom teach on a voluntary basis in exchange for hospital admitting privileges. Approximately 25 percent of these 1,960 service admissions receive psychiatric consultation services, which totaled 1,200 in 1984. These services are formally provided by the Psychiatric Consultation-Liaison Service.

Like most general hospitals throughout the United States, Lenox Hill does not have a free-standing psychiatric residency training program or a multitude of salaried attending psychiatrists to supervise, teach, and provide specialized clinical services. There are a total of six salaried psychiatrists in administrative and clinical capacities on the hospital staff:

- Administrative
  1. attending-in-charge—20 hours/week
  2. chief of Psychiatric Consultation-Liaison Services—15 hours/week
  3. chief of Psychiatric Inpatient Services—30 hours/week
  4. coordinator of psychiatric education—25 hours/week

- Clinical
  1. psychiatric clinic adult staff psychiatrist—12 hours/week
  2. psychiatric clinic child staff psychiatrist—18 hours/week

The Psychiatry Service has two full-time and two part-time residents on rotational assignment from the New York Medical College. The hospital has historically relied upon members of the voluntary psychiatric attending staff to provide consultation-liaison services throughout the institution. However, as service consultations increased over the years and other psychiatric clinical and training programs were established, it became clear that the small core of salaried psychiatrists and one full-time psychiatric resident assigned to the service could not meet the requests for consultations.

Our challenge was to develop a model that emphasized and encouraged continuing participation by the psychiatrists and psychologists on the voluntary staff in a manner that yielded quality comprehensive clinical services while maintaining continuity of interest, performance, and high morale. The programmatic structure, procedures, and processes that were developed to meet this challenge may well serve as a model for the many general hospitals that are faced with similar limitations.

A CASE STUDY: THE LENOX HILL HOSPITAL CONSULTATION-LIAISON SERVICE

Developmental History

A review of Lenox Hill Hospital annual reports from 1903 to 1935 reveals that there were only three physicians performing psychiatric consultation work during that period. From 1935 to 1973, psychiatry at the hospital was largely limited to the services provided in the outpatient clinic (see Chapter 4). Certified social worker psychotherapists counselled clinic outpatients, with limited back-up services provided by psychiatrists. Psychiatric involvement in other care areas of the hospital was very sparse, occurring mainly on an as-needed basis for crises or emergency situations. These situations characteristically focused on acutely psychotic patients on the medical wards, patients wanting to sign out against medical advice, evaluation of patients admitted to the intensive care unit (ICU) after having overdosed in suicide attempts, patients who were thought to be actively suicidal, and so on. But there was no organized and adequate consultation system for referral or follow-up of these patients.

In the late 1960s, two voluntary psychiatrists at Lenox Hill began to work on their own initiative on specific inpatient units. These physicians attended medical conferences and consulted with patients of the Obstetrics and Gynecology Department and the Plastic Surgery Service. In 1973, a third consultant joined the attending staff; this professional became involved with liaison work to the nursing staff of the ICU and provided consultations throughout the hospital. Between May 1973 and July 1974, the volume of consultations increased so much that these attendings became convinced of the need for a more organized consultation system. A formal program proposal for a Psychiatric Consultation-Liaison Service was developed by the group with support from the Department of Medicine (see Chapter 1). The proposal, as approved by the medical board, included the funding of a part-time (15-hours-per-week) position of chief of the new service.

The Psychiatric Consultation-Liaison Service was formally initiated in July 1974, when Allen H. Collins became its first chief. Over the next five years, many additional voluntary psychiatrists were recruited to join in the work of the service. These staff members enabled the program to expand its services to new inpatient wards in response to expressed needs. While all of these general psychiatrists were well-trained, few of them had specific or extensive consultation-liaison training or experience. Nevertheless, they were assigned as consultants to a variety of general care units and specialized care areas throughout the hospital.

During this time, it was clear that the consultation-liaison service was providing the lead for the development of psychiatry at the hospital, and many outside psychiatrists sought to join the attending staff in the hope that they could participate in this process. Their motivations were varied, but most desired one or more of the following:

- the stimulation of working with colleagues in an area that promotes collaboration with other physicians
- the opportunity to be involved in traditional medicine after having been disappointed by the community mental health movement
- a resource network for patient referrals
- a return to a general hospital setting with its multispecialty collaboration in the treatment of patients

The smooth growth and development of the consultation-liaison service were strained by inadequacies in other areas of the Psychiatry Service. The absence of training programs and inpatient services, the minimal availability of emergency coverage, and the limited outpatient services all contributed to the problems. Many of the voluntary attendings, unable to maintain adequate levels of interest and involvement, resigned after brief tenures.

The development of the Inpatient Scatter-Bed Service (1978), the initiation of training programs with New York Medical College (1978), and the revitalization of the Outpatient Clinic (1979–1980) all served to enhance the workability of the consultation-liaison service. In June 1978, Dr. Collins was promoted from chief of consultation to attending-in-charge of the entire

Psychiatry Service. A search committee for a new consultation service chief was subsequently established; and, in September 1979, the author was selected. In the context of the major administrative reorganizations that were occurring in the Psychiatry Service, the author was given full administrative responsibility and authority to provide executive leadership in the following four program areas:

1. evaluating the existing staff and programs
2. reorganizing them to perform assigned functions more effectively
3. expanding programs to meet requests for more consultation-liaison services
4. moving into areas that were presently not serviced

The evaluation process involved numerous meetings with the voluntary attending psychiatrists participating in the service, the chiefs of the nonpsychiatric clinical departments and services, members of the Department of Nursing, members of the Department of Social Work, and the chiefs of consultation-liaison services of other hospitals.

Continued efforts were made to provide liaison services to existing inpatient units, and plans were formulated to expand these to include every inpatient and outpatient service of the hospital. Administrative and interpersonal support was extended to the liaison-consultants to enable them to service the rest of the hospital staff and patients. From the outset, a great deal of time and energy was allocated to the support, education, nurturance, and administrative back-up of the attending staff.

In 1979, 16 voluntary attending psychiatrists participated in the clinical activities of the consultation-liaison service. They were assigned to the ten principal medical-surgical inpatient services. However, it was discovered that eight of the consultants had become uninterested and were performing little service. Meetings were held with these individuals, and agreement was reached to transfer their service assignments to the outpatient clinic or the newly organized Teaching Service. Those remaining on the consultation-liaison service were strongly encouraged and reassured. Selected consultants who had joined the Psychiatry Service in the pre-1979 period and had been assigned to the outpatient clinic were invited to transfer their hospital involvement to the consultation-liaison service, and three attendings were thus recruited. In order to expand clinical operations properly, a major effort was made to recruit from the outside additional psychiatrists with consultation-liaison training and/or experience. The teaching conferences that had been established in 1978 for medical students were expanded to include psychiatric residents and attendings. To make these conferences more professionally attractive and stimulating, it was necessary to formalize the protocols, invite outside guest case discussants and presenters, and select clinical topics of interest and relevance.

At the same time, a major change began in the way the service operated. The model that operated prior to 1979 (Model I) involved voluntary attendings exclusively. In Model I, the attendings provided (1) direct consultation to patients, (2) liaison education to hospital professional and support staff, and (3) support of the primary health care team on the hospital units. Model II, which began in 1979, was a mixed model. Many voluntary attendings continued in the same mode as previously. But they also began to supervise a PGY-2 psychiatric resident, who served in a four-month consultation-liaison rotation from the New York Medical College Valhalla campus, and two third-year medical students on a two-month psychiatric clerkship. The new resident and medical students, under the supervision of attending psychiatrists, began to see patients on some of the inpatient medical-surgical units. At the same time, several of the voluntary attending psychiatrists continued their consultation-liaison work in other clinical areas; hence, the "mixed" Model II.

Current Operations

Organizational Structures and Administrative Relationships

Today, the Psychiatric Consultation-Liaison Service functions as an integral part of the Psychiatry Service. It is a clinical service division, along with the Outpatient Clinic and the Inpatient Scatter-Bed Service. The chief of the service reports to the attending-in-charge of the Psychiatry Service and oversees all consultation-liaison activities. These include:

- routine consultation and follow-up
- emergency consultation
- liaison services
- consultation-liaison training of psychiatric trainees
- supervision of the fee collection system of third party reimbursements for "service" consultations

These activities take place on the service wards, private floors, outpatient clinics, and the emergency room and are performed by staff consisting of psychiatrists, psychologists, nurses, and social workers. The chief of the service works closely with the coordinator of psychiatric education in the training of the medical students and psychiatric residents assigned to the service. All salaried and voluntary professional staff who perform private patient consultations are administratively responsible and accountable to the chief. The Psychiatric Emergency Service (see Chapter 5) and a newly initiated Pain Evaluation and Treatment Service (PETS), with its own clinical coordinator, also operate under the administrative and supervisory control of the chief of the consultation-liaison service. The chief functions in the role of liaison professional to the other clinical and administrative departments of the hospital on consultation-liaison matters and often meets with administrative counterparts in these departments to discuss problems or plan new programs. Whenever these discussions involve the activities of other divisions of the Psychiatry Service, close coordination is effected with the other Psychiatry Service administrative staff. The chief's other responsibilities include (1) linkage to other hospitals, through their directors of psychiatric emergency services, to facilitate emergency room patient transfers; (2) linkage to the directors of consultation-liaison services and psychiatric inpatient services of other hospitals to facilitate the transfer of "medical" patients who are seen in consultation and require more intensive psychiatric hospital care than can be provided at Lenox Hill; and (3) representation of the service at meetings nationally and throughout the metropolitan area.

Staffing

The consultation-liaison service is staffed by mental health professionals and trainees, most of whom devote part of their time to consultation-liaison work and the remainder to other psychiatry service program areas. Some are salaried, but the majority are voluntary staff (see Tables 3–1 and 3–2). Of the entire staff, 23 are voluntary attending psychiatrists who provide a total of 47 hours per week of professional activity in direct patient consultations on "service" cases, liaison (indirect) education-support to medical-nursing staff, and supervision of trainees at the resident and medical student levels. The participation of these 23 voluntary attendings has enabled the consultation-liaison service to provide a wide range of programs and services. The value of this staff cannot be overemphasized.

The coordinator of psychiatric education works closely with the chief of the consultation-liaison service in planning the consultation-liaison experience for the psychiatric residents and medical students, co-leading a consultation-liaison conference on the neurology unit, and presenting lectures and reading seminars on consultation-liaison psychiatry to the trainees. The clinical psychologist co-leads the neurology unit conference and provides psychological testing upon request. The mental health nurse specialists provide liaison education to nursing staff and patient consultations when requested by nursing. They often serve as liaison between nursing staff and

Table 3–1 Psychiatric Consultation-Liaison Service Professional Staff: Hours per Week by Activity

Position/Activities Title	Admini- stration Hrs./Wk.	Teaching Hrs./Wk.	Liaison Hrs./Wk.	Consultation to Service Patients Hrs./Wk.	Psychological Testing Hrs./Wk.
Chief of service	10	5	2		
Coordinator of psychiatric edu- cation	4	3	1		
Voluntary attend- ing psychia- trists (23)		10	29	8	
Clinical psycholo- gist			1		1
Mental health nurse special- ists (2)			10	4	
Activities thera- pist			1		
Psychiatric (PGY- 2) resident			2	25	
3rd-year medical students (2)				10	
Total hours per week	14	18	44	47	1

the psychiatric consultants. The coordinator of therapeutic activities leads a weekly activity therapy group on the general surgery and urology unit. The psychiatric resident and medical students perform consultations, make follow-up visits, and participate in multidisciplinary treatment planning meetings on several service units.

Service Setting

Consultation-liaison service activities are conducted in a variety of areas within the general hospital setting. The hospital is composed of six connecting wings around a central core, occupying an entire city block. General acute care and specialized beds are located on 19 nursing units on nine floors. Each unit is composed of 20 to 36 beds. The beds are almost all in semiprivate rooms, with a sprinkling of private rooms. Each unit has its own nursing station, examining room, conference room, and patient/visitors lounge area. The medical-surgical units are divided into three categories,

Table 3–2 Psychiatric Consultation-Liaison Service, On-Call Emergency Service Professional Staff: Activities and Hours per Week

Title	Activities	Hrs./Wk.
Weekdays:		
Clinic staff psychiatrists (2)	on call throughout hospital, including ER	9–1, 2 days 1–5, 2 days
Psychiatric residents (2)	on call throughout hospital, including ER	9–1, 3 days 1–5, 3 days
Clinical psychiatric social worker	psychosocial consultations, dispositional arrangements in ER	9–5 daily
	rape intervention program in ER	9–5 daily
Outpatient mental health nurse specialist	scheduling of emergency on-call coverage	9–5 daily
	psychiatric and psychosocial ER interventions, triage consultations, dispositions	9–5 daily
Chief of service	psychiatric back-up for all areas	9–5 daily
Evenings and weekends/ holidays:		
Voluntary attending psychiatrists (35)	on call throughout hospital, including ER	Rotate coverage for 1-wk periods 5 P.M.–11 P.M. weekdays 9 P.M.–11 P.M. weekends/ holidays
Chief of service	back-up for voluntary attendings	24 hrs/day 48 weeks/year

based on the physician(s) responsible for providing patient care services ("private," "regionalized," "service"), but all units are physically similar.

The outpatient department clinics are located on the first five floors of the Lachman Pavilion, the first floor of which is allocated to administrative functions and the Emergency Department. Liaison meetings are conducted in the conference room of the unit to which a consultant is assigned. In the absence of such a conference area, the liaison meetings are held on 11 Lachman where the consultation-liaison service is based.

Inpatient consultation generally occurs at the bedside or in the unit examining room, conference room, or head nurse's office. In view of the fact that most patients are located in semiprivate rooms and other areas of the units are highly utilized, the need for complete privacy for psychiatric consultations can present problems. The more ambulatory the patient, the greater the number of options there are for consultation to occur in a completely private space. Psychiatric consultation services provided to out-patient department clinic patients do not pose as great a problem; these patients are seen without difficulty in clinic area examining rooms, staff offices, or conference rooms.

A large part of the administrative activities of the service are conducted on 11 Lachman where the service is based, along with other psychiatric programs, exclusive of the Outpatient Clinic. This floor houses the adminis-trative offices of four program directors, including the chief of consultation-liaison, three offices for the inpatient scatter-bed staff (nursing staff, coordinator of therapeutic activities, social worker), and one office shared by the psychiatric resident and medical students. The office manager/secretarial services are located in two other offices. A large conference room serves as an all-purpose space for various psychiatry service activities, meetings, and conferences. The physical proximity of the program directors and professionals involved in various psychiatry service activities substan-tially improves channels of communication and collaboration.

Clinical Service Consultations

The consultation-liaison service currently provides direct consultation evaluations and follow-up visits and extends liaison-education support to most clinical services of the Lenox Hill Hospital. This is accomplished by assigning professionals to specific areas and time periods, as shown in Table 3-3.

Initial consultations and follow-up visits to service patients are done upon request on an as-needed basis. Service is provided on these cases by staff described above. Services to private patients are provided by private psychi-atric consultants requested by the patients' primary physicians on a fee-for-service basis.

Routine Consultations on Service Cases: In 1984, psychiatric consulta-tions to service cases included 376 initial evaluations and 851 follow-up visits. In Table 3-4, these figures are compared with those of the ten previous years.

Table 3-3 Clinical Service Assignments in the Consultation-Liaison Service

   A. Consultation & liaison units/services:
      1. Neurology unit
      2. GI—Inflammatory Bowel Disease Service
      3. ENT cancer team
      4. Renal hemodialysis
      5. Cardio-Thoracic Surgery Service
      6. Radiotherapy
      7. Service medicine units
      8. Pain Evaluation & Treatment Service
      9. Pediatrics unit
      10. Progressive coronary care unit
      11. General surgery unit
      12. Urology
   B. Consultation only:
      1. Neurology Clinic
      2. Methadone Clinic
      3. Ob-Gyn Psychosomatic Clinic
      4. Urology Impotence Clinic
      5. Employee Health Clinic
      6. Pediatric Allergy and Neurology Clinic
      7. Emergency Department
   C. Liaison only:
      1. Ob-Gyn Service
      2. Progressive coronary care team
   D. As-needed consultation:
      1. Intensive care unit
      2. Acute coronary intensive care unit
      3. Plastic surgery
   E. As-needed liaison:
      1. Regional medical floors
      2. Labor and delivery unit
      3. Neonatal intensive care unit

These services were provided by the 23 voluntary attending consultants and the residents and medical students under their supervision. In direct patient care services, the attending consultants collectively provided 8 hours per week, the psychiatric resident 25 hours per week, and the two medical students 10 hours per week. The trainees are supported by 10 hours of supervision per week from the attending psychiatrists. Thus, on an annual basis, there are 1,200 consultation visits provided by 3,000 hours of paid and voluntary time. This is exclusive of the 14 hours/week of salaried administrative time provided by the consultation-liaison service chief.

The impressive growth of consultation services in the decade 1974–1984 reflects:

- the formalization of the program in 1974 with specific policies and procedures
- the reorganization in 1979–1980 in which existing services and staff were reevaluated, thereby permitting new programmatic recruitment and expansion
- able and dedicated leadership, with strong administrative support from the Psychiatry Service, Department of Medicine, other clinical departments, and the hospital administration
- the addition of several levels of educational activities, including undergraduate medical student, psychiatric resident, and continuing in-service education for attending psychiatrists, psychologists, and nurse clinicians
- recognition by medical-nursing personnel of the need for such services on the medical-surgical inpatient units, outpatient clinics, and emergency room
- the provision of quality and relevant consultation clinical care, which reinforced the credibility of the service throughout the hospital

A striking statistical trend is seen in the period 1979–1984, when initial evaluation visits declined from 537 to 376, a decrease of 30 percent. This occurred in the context of a 195 percent increase in follow-up visits. This interesting mix of figures may have resulted from the shift in program from Model I (all voluntary attendings) to Model II (mixed voluntary attendings

Table 3–4 Psychiatric Consultation-Liaison Service, Direct Consultation Visits to Patients: 1974–1984

Year	Initial Evaluation	(% change from previous year)	Follow-up Visits	(% change)	Total Visits	(% change)
1974	197		69		266	
1975	277	(+35)	57	(− 18)	324	(+22)
1976	339	(+27)	61	(+ 7)	400	(+23)
1977	376	(+11)	171	(+280)	547	(+37)
1978	444	(+18)	297	(+174)	741	(+35)
1979	537	(+21)	288	(− 4)	825	(+11)
1980	518	(− 4)	545	(+ 89)	1,063	(+29)
1981	437	(−16)	688	(+ 26)	1,125	(+ 6)
1982	399	(− 9)	653	(− 6)	1,052	(− 7)
1983	276	(−31)	932	(+ 42)	1,208	(+15)
1984	376	(+36)	851	(− 9)	1,227	(+ 2)

and supervised trainee-residents and students). The trainees are in attendance at the hospital eight or more hours a day, five days a week. This enables them to provide closer contact and follow-up care to patients than the voluntary attendings, who are in attendance for only one to two hours a day, two days a week. However, as a rule, trainees feel less comfortable than experienced attendings in engaging new clinical situations. This attitude, which varies from mild discomfort to gross avoidance, is communicated in a variety of ways to requesting medical physicians and nursing personnel. It might be manifested in a delay in responding to consultation requests, in a failure to speak with requesting physicians and nurses before and/or after the patient is seen, in the absence of active case-finding activities on the units, in subtle interpersonal cues manifested during the consultation process toward unit personnel, or, finally, in inadequate evaluation or consultation notes. In any event, once the initial evaluation visits have been made by the trainees, their anxiety subsides and they are able to continue seeing many of the patients in follow-up. This change is reinforced by the supervisory process.

The discrepancy between decreased initial evaluation visits and increased follow-up visits may also be due to medical-nursing professionals on the units not being as quick to request psychiatric consultations from trainees as they did from attending physicians. This underscores the importance of making it known to these professionals that all trainees are closely supervised by attending psychiatrists, which can result in effective, helpful consultations. The 36 percent increase in initial consultations in 1984 relative to 1983 reflects the results of our efforts in addressing these difficulties with supervisors, the inpatient mental health nurse specialist, trainees, and ward medical-nursing personnel.

As noted earlier, these figures represent service to approximately eight percent of the total inpatient population at Lenox Hill. Precise figures are not available on the number of psychiatric consultations provided to "private" inpatients. But it is our distinct impression that the number of private consultations has probably tripled or quadrupled over the same decade. At the same time, the quality of consultation care appears to have improved dramatically to both the "service" and "private" patient sectors, because of the increase in the number of requests, the decrease in the number of complaints, and the addition of well-trained, experienced psychiatric consultants.

It is also useful to study the distribution of "service" contacts by specific clinical services over the seven-year period, 1978–1984. The relevant figures are shown in Table 3–5. As can be seen, contacts with general medical service patients have grown steadily, increasing over the seven-year period by 129 percent. This growth reflects the fact that the medical floors serve as the principal area for the teaching of consultation-liaison psychiatry to psychiatric residents and medical students. Similarly, the significantly increased activity to the Neurology Service reflects the fact that this service has become the second most important area for training. Joint "walk rounds" with a neurology attending and a psychiatric attending are held once per week. These professionals also co-lead a weekly biopsychosocial conference for the house staff.

The Renal Hemodialysis Service has shown no consistent growth over the period; it has had a rather stable patient population for several years. Most of the consultation-liaison work done on the renal unit is with the staff, to help deal with burn-out and staff reactions to the occasional death of a long-term patient. New patients are accepted only when an old patient has had a successful transplant, has relocated, or has died (see Chapter 9).

The diagnoses of the patients seen by the psychiatric consultants include adjustment disorders with anxiety and depression, organic brain syndromes, personality disorders, substance abuse disorders, psychophysiologic disorders, schizophrenia, and affective disorders. The percentage breakdowns of these diagnoses are shown in Table 3–6.

Requests for routine consultation are made by the medical and surgical physicians primarily responsible for the care of patients. Frequently, case finding is done by nurses and social workers. For routine consultation requests on "service" cases, the consultees telephone the Psychiatry Service office or send in written consultation request forms. The consultation-

Table 3–5 "Service Case" Consultations of the Psychiatric Consultation-Liaison Service, by Clinical Service

Name of Service	1978	1979	1980	1981	1982	1983	1984
General medicine	275	313	425	451	566	622	630
Neurology	29	43	52	55	49	104	156
Renal hemodialysis	25	31	21	21	35	15	20
General surgery	109	117	125	118	86	140	80
Orthopedics	33	44	34	32	25	13	35
Obstetrics and gynecology	9	23	29	82	16	48	19
Critical care (ICU)	43	15	56	29	26	27	50
Pediatrics	14	23	26	18	0	12	15
Methadone clinic	—	—	62	74	40	68	98
Emergency room	87	197	186	119	134	124	77
Employee health clinic	—	—	—	—	—	15	10
ENT							23
Ophthalmology							10
Other	117	4	26	69	75	20	4
Totals	741	810	1,042	1,068	1,052	1,208	1,227

liaison service then forwards the request to the appropriate consultant. Occasionally, the consultee is given or knows the name and telephone number of the assigned consultant so that direct contact can be accomplished more quickly.

Until 1980, the Psychiatric Consultation-Liaison Service was primarily inpatient-unit oriented. Over the past four years, however, an increasing number of medical and surgical outpatient clinics have been included in the service. Psychiatric consultants are assigned for on-site attendance on the specialty clinics, as listed in Table 3–3.

Patients may be referred to the Psychiatric Outpatient Clinic from any part of the hospital. Referrals from other clinics of the Outpatient Department have always been a major source of new patients. Having consultants on-site in these clinics has in fact increased the number of evaluations being requested. It has also circumvented many of the problems of patient non-compliance with referral to the Psychiatric Clinic for evaluation. For those clinics that do not as yet have a specifically assigned psychiatric consultant, the outpatient mental health nurse specialist provides the clinical linkage. Patients are initially seen by this professional, and further involvements with psychiatric consultants are arranged, as indicated.

Routine Consultations on Private Cases: Routine consultations to private cases are generally negotiated directly between the physician-consultee and the psychiatrist-consultant. There are, however, occasions when the chief of the service is contacted for purposes of recommending a specific individual for a case. At these times, referral is made on both a rotational and subspecialty basis. For example, a physician seeking consultation for a patient with terminal renal disease may be referred to the consultant assigned to the Renal Hemodialysis Unit.

Table 3–6 Diagnoses of Patients Seen in Psychiatric Consultation: 1984

Diagnosis	Percentage
Adjustment disorders	30.0
OBS	13.0
Personality disorders	17.0
Substance abuse disorders	11.0
Psychophysiologic	0.1
Schizophrenia	5.0
Affective disorders	5.0
(mainly major depressive disorders)	
No psychiatric diagnosis	3.0
Other	4.0
Reactive depression	12.0
	100.0

On the Cardio-Thoracic Surgery Service (see Chapter 9), a new and very skilled consultant was assigned in 1981. This professional developed a unique system with the chief of cardiovascular surgery: Almost every patient admitted to the service is seen in preoperative evaluation, and close postoperative recuperation is observed for signs of emotional difficulties, which signal the intervention of the consultant. There has been a remarkable growth in the number of consultations provided on this service over the past three years. By convention, these consultations are not included in the service statistics because they are primarily private.

All psychiatric consultation services within the hospital, service and private, are technically under the supervision of the chief of the consultation-liaison service. However, for the great majority of private consultations, which are provided by board-certified attending psychiatrists, supervision is neither necessary nor desirable. The chief of service is available for any help to these attendings, and such help is provided on a peer supervisory basis.

Emergency Consultations to "Service" and "Private" Cases: Emergency consultation to the Emergency Department is more fully described elsewhere (see Chapter 5). Here, it should be noted that the system of providing emergency psychiatric consultation to medical-surgical inpatients is identical to that in the ER consultation system, with one exception: During 9 A.M. and 5 P.M., emergency consultations to service medical-surgical unit patients are covered by the psychiatric resident assigned to the consultation-liaison service. If a member of the voluntary psychiatric attending staff has not been called directly by the nonpsychiatric physician or the psychiatrist is unable to respond quickly enough to address the situation, emergency consultation to the private patient is arranged by the chief of the service.

Psychiatric Liaison Activities

In the philosophy of the service, liaison and consultation are inextricably bound together. Over half the members of the voluntary psychiatric attending staff request to be assigned to the consultation-liaison service. All attendings who receive assignments perform liaison activities with the staff of a particular unit on a regular basis. The mix between liaison ("indirect") and consultation ("direct") work varies according to the inpatient ward or clinic unit of assignment and the training and personality of the professional involved. In addition to this clinical work, some consultants serve in liaison capacities with hospital-wide administrative and planning groups, including committees of the medical board.

As a rule, trainees (including the PGY-2 psychiatric residents and third-year medical student clerks) are not encouraged to become involved in more extended liaison activities. They are encouraged to provide liaison work that is a necessary part of a good psychiatric consultation service; direct preconsultation and postconsultation, person-to-person discussions with the physicians and nursing staff who care for the patients are in fact strongly encouraged. However, we have found that the trainees lack the requisite professional knowledge and experience necessary to provide noncase-oriented liaison education and support to floor professional staff. A limited number of trainees have been exceptions to the rule, and we have supported these individuals in specific liaison interests.

Attending consultants are encouraged to be actively involved in their assignments. We have found that the degree of a consultant's clinical involvement depends a great deal on the personalities of the key persons involved and how they relate to each other. Indeed, these factors are much more important than the specialty of the assigned service or the training and experience of the consultant. Some nonpsychiatrists are very open to involvement with psychiatric staff. Some consultants with very good social skills adapt well to liaison work, even without formal training. The relevant social skills include a fluid and relaxed interpersonal manner, the use of nonjargon language, a directness of approach, and an action-intervention orientation.

The most effective liaison relationships seem to occur within disciplines. Generally, the psychiatrists on the service prefer to engage in liaison activities with other physicians, and they manage these relationships better than do nonphysician consultants. The inpatient mental health nurse specialist does a significant amount of liaison with medical-surgical nursing staff colleagues and is highly regarded as a valuable resource by them (see below).

Liaison Nursing

Liaison nurses are an active and important asset of the consultation-liaison service. The Psychiatry Service has two mental health nurse specialists, one for inpatient programs and the other for outpatient/emergency programs. Both perform consultation and liaison activities where appropriate and as indicated in their respective areas. They work closely with the chief of the consultation-liaison service. Both serve frequently in liaison between the psychiatrists of the service and the staff of the Nursing Department.

The inpatient mental health nurse specialist spends one hour a week in supervision with a voluntary psychiatric attending who has subspecialty expertise in group process and training. Group work with nursing staff constitutes a large part of this specialist's consultation-liaison work. The specialist performs 75 patient evaluation and follow-up visits annually, at the request of medical-surgical nurses. These services are requested in situations in which the medical-surgical nurses have difficulty managing or understanding a patient, when they need assistance in convincing the patient's physician that psychiatric evaluation is needed, or when other professional and personal problems arise. Over the years, the inpatient mental health nurse specialist has performed these services with ever-increasing frequency.

Conferences and Presentations

Consultation-liaison topics are presented in various conference and presentation settings at Lenox Hill Hospital. Consultation-liaison case conferences are held monthly. At these conferences, a patient is presented by a trainee or attending; this is followed by an interview and discussion conducted by an invited psychiatrist. Consultation-liaison attendings or psychosomatic clinicians and researchers from other hospitals are invited to lead these conferences.

The monthly service attending luncheon provides a forum for informal case presentations, administrative and planning discussions, outside speakers on topics related to private practice, journal article reviews, and reports on outside meetings. The tone is informal, and the atmosphere is supportive. A major goal is to develop and maintain group cohesion for mutual support. Another goal is to develop a less-formal setting for in-service education at the attending level.

Psychiatric service meetings are held on a monthly basis. Several of the ten presentations made each year at these meetings are on consultation-liaison topics. These presentations have involved nonpsychiatric physicians of the hospital (or outside institutions) who discussed their clinical or research work or their involvement with psychiatric issues. The discussions of their perceptions of the use of psychiatry in their work have led to the development of new liaison opportunities. In fact, the liaison program with the inflammatory bowel disease section of the Gastroenterology Service grew out of one such presentation. One of the main goals of these meetings is to give some continuing education in the psychiatric area to psychiatric attendings who are not actively involved in the consultation-liaison service and who perform only occasional consultations on medically ill patients. Psychiatric presentations are also cosponsored by the consultation-liaison service at least annually at the combined medical-surgical grand rounds of each department.

Finally, trainees make weekly rounds with the chief of the service and the inpatient mental health nurse specialist on all patients being followed. These rounds allow trainees to see case material of their fellow trainees, which broadens their exposure and enables them to see liaison and case finding in action.

Supervision of Psychiatric Trainees

The attending consultants who are primarily involved in liaison and consultation with the clinical services are generally not involved in the teaching and supervision of psychiatric trainees. Other members of the consultation-liaison service are assigned for this purpose, meeting with the psychiatric resident and medical students to discuss cases. Each trainee is individually supervised two to three hours a week, and all trainees meet as a group for one hour of supervision each week. This supervision emphasizes psychiatric history taking, mental status evaluation, DSM–III diagnosis, dynamic case formulation, treatment recommendations, communications skills and procedures with medical-surgical physicians and nursing and social work staff members, countertransference issues, and psychophysiologic research and psychosomatic theory. The trainees are required to have supervision on each case they see. The name of the supervisor is included in the first note written on the case. All consultation and follow-up notes are reviewed and countersigned by the case supervisor at each supervisory hour. Additional supervision is given on rounds with the chief of service and the inpatient mental health nurse specialist. Supervision and other elements of the educational program of the service are jointly administered by the chief of the service and the coordinator of psychiatric education.

Funding Issues

Adequate funding is required even for a consultation-liaison service in which 40 percent of the staffing time is provided by voluntary attendings and trainees. The funding for the service is in three categories:

1. funds from the hospital operating budget, for salaries, stipends, and supplies
2. funds obtained through donations and bequests to the Psychiatry Service from benefactors
3. funds generated from consultations provided to service cases.

The funding provided by the hospital operating budget for psychiatry supports the professional positions relating to the service. These are shown in Table 3–7.

Table 3-7 Lenox Hill Hospital Operating Budget for
Consultation-Liaison Staffing

Position	Hrs./Wk.	Annual Salary
Chief	15	$18,000.00
Coordinator of psychiatric education	8	9,600.00
Coordinator of therapeutic activities	2	1,000.00
Office manager	6	4,000.00
Senior secretary	6	3,000.00
PGY-2 psychiatric resident	30	18,000.00
Chief psychologist	2	2,000.00
Inpatient mental health nurse-specialist	7	5,000.00[a]
Outpatient mental health nurse-specialist	5	4,000.00[a]
Total		$64,600.00

[a]These funds are provided through the Department of Nursing.

Funds collected from third party insurers for services rendered to service cases amount to $8,000–$10,000 per year. The services to service patients are provided by fully trained attendings or by trainees under their supervision. By hospital regulation, service patients who have insurance coverage can have their third party insurers billed by a fiduciary agent on behalf of the attending psychiatrist involved. The rate of reimbursement depends on the kind of service rendered and the rated experience of the consultant. Consequently, the services rendered by attendings and trainees are billed at different levels. Because many of the service cases do not have insurance, the average reimbursement collected for a consultation service is $10 per visit. The service monitors billing and collections and makes a continuous effort to improve the efficiency of the system in order to maximize collections.

Evaluation of Services

Evaluation activities provide necessary feedback to the service chief, showing (1) the extent to which direct clinical consultation services and indirect liaison educative support services are being provided; (2) the areas of the hospital to which these services are provided; (3) the quality of the services, as perceived by requesting medical-nursing staff and patients; (4) the strengths of each program; and (5) any problem areas. It is also important to assess these aspects of service delivery from the perspective of the voluntary psychiatric attending staff and psychiatric resident trainees who provide the program. Comparisons between the various groups produces valuable data that are used to explore discrepancies in views and to modify programs, as necessary.

One of the principal tasks of the service chief is to monitor the consultation-liaison programs of the service. This assessment and evaluation activity requires specific procedures and mechanisms. For example, ongoing statistical charting of all initial and follow-up consultation visits is maintained. The chart information includes the name of the patient, the ward/clinic where the service is performed, the identity of the requesting professional(s), the reason(s) for the request, the DSM III diagnostic impression, treatment recommendation(s), and dispositional recommendation(s). These data are currently being computerized from a manual system.

In addition, weekly meetings are held with the psychiatric resident. These meetings deal with inquiries concerning the extent of the services provided, the quality of the experiences, and the particular gratifications and problems encountered. Supplementing these meetings, the weekly Executive Committee meetings frequently focus on programmatic services in consultation-liaison psychiatry, particularly on problems that have arisen, hospital areas that need new or additional services, and coordination difficulties with psychiatric or other programs. At the end of each calendar year, the service chief presents a formal report of program operations to the committee for the previous 12-month period. This report includes directions for the following year.

Bimonthly meetings are held with the attending-in-charge of psychiatry. These meetings focus on specific issues of program development and any problem areas that have been encountered. The participation of members of the voluntary attending staff in consultation-liaison service activities is also routinely discussed. In addition, monthly luncheon meetings with members of the voluntary psychiatric attending staff who participate in service activities provide the chief with an overall assessment of these professionals' enthusiasm and motivation, any problems they are encountering, and possible modifications needed in existing services. These periodic meetings are supplemented by weekly meetings with the coordinator of psychiatric education, during which the activities of the resident trainee on the service are discussed.

Periodic meetings with medical-surgical departmental directors and section chiefs focus on specific problem areas in existing programs and the need to expand or otherwise modify consultation-liaison services to that clinical administrator's area. There are also informal, periodic meetings with inpatient unit/clinic medical house staff, nursing staff, and social work staff to discuss their perceptions of service activities and personnel. Finally, the service has occasional meetings with outside professionals of other institutions to aid in evaluating a facet of the service that needs modification.

These various program assessment and evaluation activities have resulted in:

- changes in specific voluntary attendings assigned to the service
- expansions of activities to the outpatient department clinics
- changes in the administrative overview of the on-call consultation system to the ER and inpatient wards
- establishment of a new (inpatient) Pain Evaluation and Treatment Service (PETS)

SUMMARY

The emergence of psychiatric consultation-liaison programs in general hospitals over the past two decades is a manifestation of the remedicalization of the specialty of psychiatry. In many institutions, these programs have provided the clinical leadership for departments of psychiatry. They have strengthened the discipline in its transactions with other medical-surgical specialties.

These successes of consultation-liaison psychiatry are due principally to the relevance of the clinical and support/liaison services the field has provided to patients and their families and to physicians and nursing personnel. Liaison psychiatrists have become progressively involved in the training of undergraduate medical students, physicians-in-training, and post-graduate doctors in psychosomatic interfaces between the various medical disciplines. Technological advances in psychiatry, including psychopharmacologic agents and diagnostic tests, and the emergence of biopsychosocial concepts throughout the field of medicine have brought psychiatry and medicine's other specialties closer together.

The Voluntary Staffing Model

The initiation of the Psychiatric Consultation-Liaison Service at Lenox Hill Hospital did not result from generous federal grants or other outside funding. Rather, it was the creation of members of the voluntary psychiatric attending staff who strongly felt the need to provide such a program. The same psychiatrists have continued to provide the principal staffing support for the comprehensive clinical services and training activities that have evolved over the past decade. The single salaried professional who has provided administrative direction for the service since its inception is the part-time chief. Other salaried staff involved with the service have been recruited from other psychiatric clinical and teaching programs, insofar as these have intersected with consultation-liaison activities.

Thus, the service's organizational model is primarily one of voluntary psychiatric professional staffing, relying on a minimum of expensive salaried support. The author believes that a great many acute care general hospitals across the country can utilize this structural model in developing similar psychiatric consultation-liaison programs. Not incidentally, the current institutional health care emphases on quality assurance, cost containment (problems with lengths of stay), legal liabilities, and medical-nursing staff support are all positively impacted by the services of the voluntary model.

Advantages

The voluntary staffing model has in fact several distinct advantages. Within its inexpensive context, the part-time salaried chief functions as an active member of the voluntary attending staff. This dual professional identity provides him with a first-hand knowledge of the difficult and complex clinical issues of practice in the hospital and office settings. It allows for greater collegiality with staff members, who are also primarily private practitioners. It affords opportunities for the chief to refer private consultations to these colleagues and to provide them with peer supervisory assistance on difficult cases. It has been frequently observed that physicians who give up clinical medicine entirely to become full-time administrators tend to forget the demands of the day-to-day clinical world. This can in fact become administratively disastrous for a clinical service chief who must rely on the consistent enthusiasm and dedication of voluntary professional staff.

The chief's clinical skills permit a realistic assessment of the quality of care, the discovery of unmet needs that require additional services, and the personal provision of clinical services in areas of particular interest and in emergency situations when no other staff are available. This hands-on approach has come to be respected by psychiatric and nonpsychiatric colleagues throughout the institution.

Another advantage of the voluntary staffing model is that the members of the voluntary psychiatric attending staff are provided the means to establish and maintain relationships with physicians, nurses, social workers, and others who can serve as potential referral sources. The liaison psychiatrist also comes to know many other medical specialists to whom patients can be referred and thus can establish a more comprehensive medical network within which to practice. These relationships serve to break down the isolation of private office practice. The opportunity for professional contacts is further stimulated through teaching conferences, consultations with colleagues, and student supervision.

For trainees, the model provides learning experiences in a setting in which many are likely to find themselves upon completion of training. Their supervisors are practitioners in the "real world" and thus can serve as role models for future professional identification.

Finally, for all professional staff members—physicians, social workers, psychologists, nurses, activity therapists—the model provides the opportunity to work in a multidisciplinary environment. The heterogeneity of viewpoints inherent in such an environment can be of great learning value, especially in a milieu that stresses collegiality. The stimulation afforded by such an atmosphere can substantially raise morale and reduce clinical burnout.

Limitations

There are, however, certain difficulties with the voluntary staffing model for a psychiatric consultation-liaison service. First, the part-time salaried nature of the position of chief and the absence of any additional administrative supporting staff who are clearly assigned to the service place great demands on the program clinician-executive. This is especially true during periods of demanding administrative undertakings, such as the initiation of a new program, the assessment and modification of problematic services, or the performance evaluation of "difficult" attendings. In an institution in which consultation-liaison services have become comprehensively developed, the chief's areas of responsibilities can expand considerably and present major challenges in the context of a time-limited administrative position.

Second, the voluntary psychiatric attendings who provide the staffing for much of the program are independent practitioners, with limited accountability to the chief. The chief's ability to negotiate tactfully is an essential interpersonal skill in such a situation. The chief must utilize a variety of administrative, clinical, and teaching skills to provide professional and economic gratifications for the attendings. Group leadership skills for developing attending and trainee staff camaraderie and cohesion are also essential.

Third, it is not easy to recruit attendings who can adapt to the demands of consultation-liaison work in the general hospital setting. Many psychiatrists who are not specifically trained in consultation-liaison psychiatry—especially those who graduated from residencies more than 15–20 years ago—find the work difficult and discouraging. The few who have received subspecialty training rarely seek voluntary positions in the field. Thus, the recruitment of a capable professional staff and the maintenance of morale are major activities of the service chief. Special screening and interviewing techniques have been developed (see Case Study 2 in Chapter 1) to improve our ability to select qualified voluntary staff who can meet the challenges of the clinical tasks and consequently continue to be active at the hospital. Maintaining a cadre of enthusiastic and dedicated voluntary staff is in fact probably the most important job of the service leadership. It entails monitoring attendings' satisfactions with their experiences, keeping track of how enjoyable their student/resident supervisions are, assessing their needs for continuing education, and tactfully inquiring what their referrals of private patients have been. All of these are important in supporting them and keeping them active. In all these ways, the chief functions as facilitator and advocate of the voluntary attending staff.

Fourth, the voluntary attending model poses problems in maintaining adequate consultation coverage for emergency psychiatric situations. This issue is addressed in detail in Chapter 5.

Maintaining Credibility and Viability

The credibility of the consultation-liaison service throughout the hospital ultimately depends upon the quality and availability of the services that are provided. The manner in which these services are presented is also important. In both these areas, the maintenance of an active and collaborative set of relationships with the rest of the Psychiatry Service and with other clinical departments and support services is essential. The ability of the program to provide leadership for the development and expansion of other psychiatric programs in the institution is facilitated by such relationships.

The support of the attending-in-charge of the Psychiatry Service has been critical to the leadership of the Psychiatric Consultation-Liaison Service. Regular exchanges of views, problem-solving sessions, mutual advocacy in improving and expanding programs are concrete manifestations of this support. The fact that the position of attending-in-charge is half-time, with its own severe administrative demands, magnifies greatly the administrative stresses amid severe time constraints that are involved.

In this context, helpful support has come from consultation-liaison colleagues in local and national liaison societies. The periodic meetings and conferences conducted with chiefs of nonpsychiatric clinical departments have also been exceedingly useful in obtaining feedback about needs and desirable services from the consultees' perspectives. The potential for similar sources of support exists in every general hospital.

There are also financial incentives for becoming involved in consultation-liaison activities in the general hospital. The potential for developing strong referral sources from multispecialty physicians with large private practices is very great. These referral networks can have a profound impact, not only on the financial viability of one's private practice, but also on the context in which one practices the psychiatric specialty. A steady stream of new patients facilitates a practitioner's orientation to shorter periods of treatment. This is particularly important in the context of the continuing evolution of the health care bureaucracy's concerns with cost containment. The fact that this evolution is currently limited to in-hospital practice does not preclude its eventual extension to the office setting. The days of long-term, open-ended psychotherapy with most patients may be fast approaching their end. The active involvement of psychiatric practitioners in consultation-liaison services in general hospitals will become increasingly important as these developments evolve.

Finally, as the national debate continues between psychiatrists and their nonmedical mental health professional colleagues about who is best trained to render services, the natural roles of psychiatrists as medical specialists along with internists and surgeons in the general hospital setting becomes clearer. The invocation of the importance of medical training by generations of psychoanalysts, to distinguish themselves from their "lay" colleagues, has particular relevance for the psychiatric generalists of today. This is becoming especially true as psychiatry becomes remedicalized and medicine becomes psychosocialized. Modern consultation-liaison psychiatry has accomplished what the psychosomatic researchers and clinicians of the 1930s and 1940s could not: the development and operational testing of multifactorial conceptual models of disease etiologies, research designs, and techniques and the establishment of practical intervention strategies that are clinically relevant to medicine.

REFERENCES

1. Z.J. Lipowski, "Review of Consultation Psychiatry and Psychosomatic Medicine," *Psychosomatic Medicine* 29 (1967): 153–171.

2. Z.J. Lipowski, "Review of Consultation Psychiatry and Psychosomatic Medicine II," *Psychosomatic Medicine* 29 (1967): 201–224.

3. Z.J. Lipowski, "Review of Consultation Psychiatry and Psychosomatic Medicine II: Theoretical Issues," *Psychosomatic Medicine* 30 (1968): 395–422.

4. Z.J. Lipowski, "Consultation-Liaison Psychiatry: An Overview," *American Journal of Psychiatry* 131 (1974): 623–629.

5. J.S. Eaton, Jr., et al. "The Educational Challenge of Consultation-Liaison Psychiatry," *American Journal of Psychiatry* 134 (1977): 20–23.

6. W.M. Glazer and B.M. Istrachan, "A Social Systems Approach to Consultation-Liaison Psychiatry," *Journal of Psychiatry in Medicine* 9 (1978–1979): 33–47.

7. M.Y. Greenhill, "The Development of Liaison Programs," in *Psychiatric Medicine,* ed. G. Usdin (New York: Brunner-Mazel, 1977), 115–191.

8. C.P. Kimball, "Conceptual Developments in Psychosomatic Medicine: 1939–1969," *Annals of International Medicine* 73 (1970): 307–310.

9. R.O. Pasman, ed., *Consultation-Liaison Psychiatry* (New York: Grove & Stratton, 1972).

10. J.J. Strain and S. Grossman *Psychological Care of the Medically Ill: A Primer in Liaison Psychiatry* (New York: Appleton-Century Crofts, 1975).

11. M.H. Greenhill, "Liaison Psychiatry," in *American Handbook of Psychiatry,* 2nd ed., vol. 7, ed. Silvano Arieti and H. Keith Brodie (New York: Basic Books, 1981), 672–702.

Chapter 4

The Management of Psychiatric Outpatient Services

Martin H. Greenstein, A.C.S.W.

INTRODUCTION

The administration of psychiatric outpatient services in the general hospital poses a special challenge when the organization does not have, as a major investment, the provision of mental health services. The Psychiatric Outpatient Clinic at Lenox Hill Hospital is not supported by federal grants or local governmental funding, except indirectly through Medicaid and Medicare reimbursement. The clinic's funds are provided through the general hospital operating budget and from a small number of private special funds designated for particular teaching or patient care activities. The self-pay, Medicare, Medicaid, and other third party insurance fees generated by clinic visits have not historically offset the operating expenses. This reality is a major aspect of the administrative challenge.

Bachrach notes that, though it is often overlooked, the general-hospital-based psychiatric outpatient clinic nevertheless provides a considerable amount of care.[1] This author goes on to note that the lack of literature on general hospital outpatient psychiatric clinics is especially interesting in view of the current emphasis on continuity of care by service planners and providers. Bachrach suggests that "either the importance of outpatient care in the spectrum of psychiatric services is seriously overlooked or else the service providers are too deeply involved in clinical and/or administrative responsibilities to take the time to write about them."[2] Indeed, both possibilities may be true. This author must include himself (up to this time) among those who have been too deeply involved in day-to-day issues of service delivery to take the time to write about them.

Another aspect of this problem can be seen from the perspective of governmental and quasi-governmental planning organizations. Continuity of care is a problem in the context of deinstitutionalization. Patients discharged from state hospitals, especially in large urban areas, often do not receive the care they need in the communities to which they are discharged. However, continuity of care has generally not posed problems for medical inpatients in general hospitals who require psychiatric consultations and need follow-up care or for the large numbers of patients who attend medical-surgical clinics and require outpatient psychiatric services.

The Psychiatric Outpatient Clinic at Lenox Hill Hospital serves many patients who are treated medically as inpatients or as outpatients in other clinical departments of the hospital. These patients constitute a diverse group with a wide range of medical and psychiatric diagnoses. Many do not live within the mental health catchment area of the hospital designated by the local planning bodies (New York City Department of Mental Health and Mental Retardation Administration). In any case, though constituting a very high proportion of the clinic's caseload, they are not emphasized as a priority group meriting special attention for government funding or special services. The diversity of the patients' diagnoses, ages, ethnic backgrounds, and location of residence makes it difficult to draw the interest of those agencies that offer funding targeted at specific patient groups, such as the deinstitutionalized, the elderly mentally ill, children, adolescents, and so on. Attention to continuity of care from medical to psychiatric, from inpatient to outpatient, should be, however, a priority for providers in the general hospital.

The Psychiatric Outpatient Clinic at Lenox Hill is a modest-sized service with an annual volume of over 6,000 patient visits. There are approximately 300 active patients at any given time, and approximately 1,000 patients who are provided psychiatric evaluation and/or treatment services each year. Additional patients receive brief telephone or in-person screening interviews but are not included in the active caseload because they are referred to other facilities more appropriate to their needs.

The patients span the spectrum of ethnic and socioeconomic backgrounds, although a majority are in the poverty group. Approximately 60 percent of the patients receive Medicaid and other forms of public assistance; 35 percent pay fees on the lowest end of the clinic sliding scale. Only a few calls and applications are received from people who can afford usual and customary private fees.

The staff members vary by professional discipline, hours worked per week, salaried or voluntary status, and clinical department of accountability (nursing, social work, psychiatry).

HISTORICAL PERSPECTIVE

The Psychiatric Outpatient Clinic was established in the early 1930s, in part as a response to a request from a settlement house that was taking in homeless boys and men during the Depression. Patients were referred by the settlement house, local churches, other social welfare organizations, and by other clinical departments of the hospital. In its early stage, the clinic was open only three days a week. It was staffed by a psychiatrist, two psychologists, a social worker, and voluntary social workers and clerical staff. In 1934, additional psychiatrists were added to the staff. Community service was emphasized, and referring organizations were invited to partici- pate in case conferences. As the caseload grew, the representatives of the referring organizations were asked to carry their own patients under the supervision of the clinic staff. No outside funding was available, and through the mid-1950s, the clinic continued to be supported, by and large, from hospital funds. In 1956, the clinic applied for and obtained a contract with the New York City Community Mental Health Board. This contract provided funding for substantial additional staff, including social workers, psychologists, and clerical support. One of the social workers became the administrative head of the clinic. In 1976, during the height of the New York City fiscal crisis, the city failed to renew the contract. Four of the five social workers in the clinic at that time were reassigned to other areas of the hospital. One full-time social worker remained in the clinic, along with the chief psychologist, part-time psychiatrists, and voluntary attendings.

In 1978, an attempt was again made to revitalize the clinic with the hiring of a part-time attending psychiatrist in charge and, soon thereafter, the hiring of a full-time coordinator (the author). At this time, the clinic was reorganized into a system of "tracks" for subspecialty treatment in the areas of sex therapy, biofeedback, behavior therapy, learning disabilities evalua- tion, psychopharmacology, short-term therapy, and psychoanalytically ori- ented psychotherapy. This system was not successful, at least in part because it left little room for the many patients whose diagnoses and treatment needs did not fit into the highly compartmentalized categories.

The system was also problematic because the initial evaluators of the patients did not feel that the specialty treatment options were primarily what the patient needed. The evaluators tended to recommend treatment modali- ties with which they were most familiar or comfortable. An evaluator whose primary treatment orientation was psychoanalytically oriented psychother- apy was not likely to assign a patient to biofeedback for the treatment of an anxiety disorder.

Additionally, the subspecialty staff members were primarily new volun- tary attending psychiatrists and psychologists who were not well-known to the evaluators who had been with the clinic for many years. There were occasions when a patient was referred for the subspecialty treatment but was found by the subspecialty practitioner to be unsuitable.

All too often, the patients seemed to have complicating medical illnesses, unclear or multiple psychiatric diagnoses, and psychosocial problems. The majority of the patients were poor, on public assistance, with high levels of psychosocial stress. Many of the patients required ego-supportive, open-ended psychotherapy; but this therapeutic option was severely limited in the subspecialty system, where most of the available staff time was consumed by the specific treatment tracks. The result was a long waiting list for psychotherapy and unfilled openings for the subspecialists. In light of this experience, it was decided to abandon the subspecialty model and return to the general treatment model, with the subspecialties available adjunctively on a more limited basis.

Rich et al. found that certain requirements of scale and expertise must exist for subspecialty units to succeed. Even when such a system can be established, because of inevitable diagnostic uncertainties, a general clinic must still be available for the patients.[3] The experience at Lenox Hill confirms their observation that, for subspecialty divisions in mental health services to succeed, there must be a sufficient number of patients who might profit from such services, sufficient staff interest and expertise, and the will to develop them.[4]

In 1980, after reverting to the general psychiatry model, the clinic was again expanded. The staff was increased by two part-time psychiatrists and two part-time psychologists. This expansion was necessary in order to comply with increasingly stringent staffing standards of the New York State Office of Mental Health. Compliance with the new standards was essential in order for the clinic's operating certificate to be renewed. The new positions, including that of a psychiatric nurse clinician, were totally funded by the hospital. Since 1980, the staff levels have remained stable.

ADMINISTRATIVE STRUCTURE

The Psychiatric Outpatient Clinic is a component of the Psychiatry Service, which is a section of the Department of Medicine. The clinic's strategic planning and major operational issues are addressed in the context of a collegial executive committee in which the coordinator of the clinic participates with the attending-in-charge and the coordinators and chiefs of the other service components. This managerial group ensures effective coordination among the various components.

The organizational chart in Figure 4–1 shows the clinic's administrative structure. The coordinator is the administrative head of the clinic, with responsibility for day-to-day operations, program planning, budget preparation and negotiation, compliance with governmental regulations, trouble shooting, customer service, and some clinical duties. The coordinator chairs

Figure 4–1 Organizational Chart of the Psychiatric Outpatient Clinic

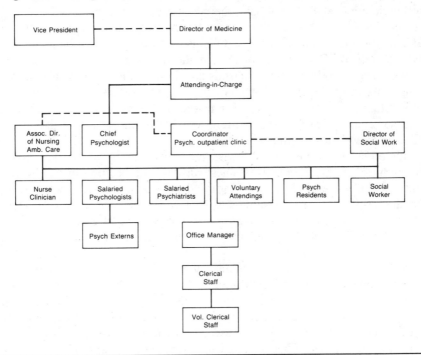

the monthly clinic staff meetings which are attended by all salaried staff. The coordinator also meets with the clerical staff on supervisory matters, including annual performance appraisals and salary reviews. The coordinator reports to the attending-in-charge of the Psychiatry Service but also is authorized to work directly with the vice-president for psychiatry and other administrative staff of the hospital. The coordinator also represents the Psychiatry Service at monthly hospital department head meetings, chaired by the hospital president.

The clinic has a complex relationship with the hospital administration. Traditionally, it has not operated under the administrative supervision of the director of medical/surgical services and other ambulatory care areas. While it functions in part with the same administrative structure that exists in those areas—for example, for registering, setting fees, and billing patients—it functions very differently in other ways—for example, in hours of service, patient scheduling patterns, staffing, and record keeping. It has thus remained under the jurisdiction of the vice-president for psychiatry (and medicine).

There are some problems with this arrangement, especially insofar as the psychiatric clinic staff do not have the necessary direct input and flexibility in determining patient fee scales. Generally, however, relationships with the staffs of the other clinics are good. This is evident in the fact that the medical/surgical clinic staffs are among the major sources of our patient referrals. The medical/surgical referrals are, in fact, the predominant source of our walk-in applications. Patients are sent directly from these clinics to the Psychiatric Outpatient Clinic for intake and evaluation. A phone call from the referring staff person is preferred, but often the patient is simply told to go directly to the clinic.

With other department heads who have staff assigned to the clinic, relationships are more sensitive. These include the relationships with the mental health nurse clinician (nursing) and the social worker (social work) who are responsible and accountable to the directors of their respective departments. Day-to-day performance, overall performance appraisals, hiring, and termination decisions must be carefully negotiated with these directors.

Excellent relationships are maintained with the associate director of nursing for ambulatory care and the director of social work. Recently, as clinic coordinator, the author worked with the associate director of nursing to develop a system of "capturing" psychiatric consultations provided on-site in the medical/surgical clinics. These consultations to patients had previously been lost for the clinic's statistical and fiscal purposes. They are now tallied, billed, and identified as psychiatric outpatient visits. Copies of all ambulatory psychiatric consultations are sent to the clinic for tabulation.

The director of social work participates in the activities of the clinic as the supervisor of the assigned social worker. That director also participates as a member of the Special Review Committee which, as part of the quality assurance system mandated by New York State, reviews all untoward incidents and recommends policy and procedural changes as necessary.

STAFFING

The salaried staff of the clinic consists of psychiatrists, psychologists, social workers, a psychiatric nurse clinician (or specialist), and three clerical staff (see Table 4–1). There are two salaried part-time psychiatrists (12 hours/week and 18 hours/week) who are equal to .9 full-time equivalents (FTE). The clinic has four salaried psychologists (one of whom is the chief psychologist of the Psychiatry Service), constituting 1.8 FTE.

In addition to the professional salaried staff, the professional staff in training includes a psychiatric resident (full-time) and two psychology

Table 4-1 Staffing Chart of the Lenox Hill Hospital Psychiatric Outpatient Service

Title/Discipline	Hrs./Wk.	Reports to
Salaried Staff:		
Coordinator/Social Work	30	attending-in-charge, Psychiatry Service
Chief Psychologist	20	attending-in-charge
Psychiatrist (part-time)	12	coordinator/attending-in-charge
Psychiatrist (part-time)	18	coordinator/attending-in-charge
Social Worker	35	coordinator/director of social work
Nurse Clinician	35	coordinator/associate director of nursing
Associate Psychologist	11	coordinator/chief psychologist
Clinical Psychologist	15	coordinator/chief psychologist
Clinical Psychologist	18	coordinator/chief psychologist
Trainee Staff:		
Psychiatric Resident	35	coordinator/director of psychiatric education
Psychology Extern	16	coordinator/chief psychologist
Psychology Extern	16	coordinator/chief psychologist
Voluntary Attending Staff		
Psychiatrists (12)	36	coordinator/attending-in-charge
Psychologists (7)	21	coordinator/chief psychologist
Clerical Staff		
Office Manager	35	coordinator
Receptionist	35	office mgr./coordinator
Clerk Typist	35	office mgr./coordinator

externs (part-time). In addition to the 19 voluntary attending psychiatrists and psychologists, who are not salaried, there are a number of licensed (multidisciplinary) mental health professionals who, as part of their post-graduate psychotherapy training, provide psychotherapy to clinic patients.

The clinic has a total of 36 staff members in professional, trainee, and clerical categories. Among these staff members, 205 professional hours per week are devoted to patient care. The clinic's limited staff resources are maximized through the use of:

- nonsalaried voluntary attending staff to provide direct service and supervision of trainees
- nonsalaried trainees, that is, psychology externs, who are enrolled in graduate psychology programs and eager to obtain supervised direct service experience in advance of their internships
- psychiatric residents (PGY 2 and 3) who require outpatient training on rotation from the affiliated medical school residency program (New York Medical College Psychiatric Residency Training Consortium)

- an experienced mental health nonphysician professional to direct the program
- experienced staff—salaried and voluntary—to supervise trainees, lead teaching conferences, direct disposition conferences, and provide group supervisions

The nonsalaried voluntary attending staff are psychiatrists (largely board-certified) and licensed clinical psychologists who are afforded privileges at the hospital in exchange for clinic (or other service) patient care or supervisory responsibilities. The psychiatrists may admit patients to the inpatient scatter-bed program described in Chapter 2. The clinical psychologists may provide testing and psychotherapy services to inpatients, although they do not have admitting privileges. The voluntary staff members are generally willing to provide direct service to patients in the Psychiatric Outpatient Clinic, unless their clinical interests and expertise are in other areas, such as consultation-liaison or education.

The willingness of experienced psychiatrists and psychologists to provide three hours a week of voluntary clinical service or supervision derives from the high regard in which Lenox Hill Hospital is held in the community and region, its high quality of patient care, and the opportunity for private practitioners to meet and interact with colleagues in a way that is not possible in solo or group private practices. The patient services provided by the voluntary attending psychiatrists include initial psychiatric evaluations, psychopharmacological evaluations, and follow-up visits. The attending psychiatrists usually prefer not to treat ongoing psychotherapy patients. The voluntary psychologists, in contrast, do provide some direct psychotherapy to patients, especially children. The voluntary psychologists generally prefer not to provide psychological testing on a nonprivate (service) basis.

In the development of the various training programs at Lenox Hill Hospital, didactic teaching or supervision has been the preferable assignment for most voluntary staff members. This type of supervision of trainees is generally a more fulfilling assignment than clinical service; it thus alleviated a significant morale problem that existed among the voluntary staff prior to 1980 (pretraining era). Such supervision provides an activity that is often different from what the clinic's experienced professionals do in their private practices. It offers the opportunity to contribute to the training of coprofessionals through a collaboration and sharing of responsibility for patient care. Various members of the voluntary staff have subspecialty expertise within their fields and are able to provide teaching in a more specialized clinical area, for example, psychopharmacology, group therapy, family and child therapy, sex therapy, forensic psychiatry, learning disabilities, and short-term dynamically oriented psychotherapy.

The importance of utilizing the resources of the voluntary staff cannot be overstated. This utilization is optimal when the facility and the individual staff member believe that they are mutually benefiting from the arrangement.

Problems do arise, however, when voluntary staff do not feel they are getting what they want and need. Voluntary professionals who joined the clinic staff expecting to get referrals of private patients have at times been disappointed. The disappointment was often manifested in poor attendance, tardiness, poor work quality, and lack of interest in their clinic responsibilities. In this context, an attempt is made to provide all new or prospective voluntary attendings with an orientation that notes the limited opportunities for private referrals but stresses the potential areas for satisfaction.

FORMS OF THERAPY OFFERED

Patients are offered various forms of therapy, including individual long-term or short-term psychotherapy, group therapy with six different group compositions, family therapy, couples therapy, behavioral therapy, biofeedback, stress reduction and relaxation training, and psychopharmacology.

Individual long-term psychotherapy is provided by all of the nonphysician, salaried therapists. A major part of this treatment is provided by the nurse clinician and the social worker. More than 70 percent of this treatment must be considered supportive in view of a clinical determination that most of the patients are capable of limited insight. Because of training requirements, an attempt is made to provide more analytically oriented treatment cases to psychiatric residents and psychology externs. However, this is not always possible, and it is the author's view that trainees must learn to treat the most typical patients in the clinic setting.

Short-term, problem-focused therapy is also provided by most of the nonphysician, salaried therapists. Short-term dynamic psychotherapy is provided by psychiatric residents under the supervision of a well-known attending psychiatrist who is an experienced clinician with this modality. Applicants for treatment who are suspected of having such specific problems as alcoholism, drug dependency, phobias, and sexual dysfunctions are evaluated by voluntary attendings with subspecialty expertise in these areas.

In addition to these forms of therapy, a wide range of psychological, learning disability, and vocational testing services are administered to children and adults by the psychologists and their trainees. Psychotherapy for children and adolescents is also provided by the coordinator, chief psychologist, social worker, nurse clinician, and psychology trainees. For a long time, the clinic was deficient in the area of providing mental health services for children, adolescents, and their families. It is only in the past two years that this area has become a priority one for the Psychiatry Service. It is hoped that the addition to the voluntary attending staff of child psychiatrists and child psychologists who can provide these necessary services will be the beginning of a resurgence of pediatric psychiatry at Lenox Hill.

Lenox Hill Hospital has attracted a significant group of Spanish-speaking patients to its medical services. These patients are from various Latin American countries. Until 1980, because the language barrier is a major problem in the provision of mental health services, the clinic was not able to serve this group effectively. At that point, the author recruited a Spanish-speaking psychologist and a Spanish-speaking receptionist to serve this patient group more effectively. Since 1980, the clinic has been fortunate to have, in addition, several rotating, Spanish-speaking psychiatric residents. The result has been a significant caseload of Spanish-speaking patients in both individual and group therapy. The clinic has become well-known within the institution and the community for its ability to provide bilingual services, and the staff is very proud of this capability.

Group therapy is provided by the social worker, the nurse clinician, the bilingual psychologist, the psychiatric resident and the coordinator. Each group has a different patient profile; there is a group for Spanish-speaking patients, a group for single mothers, a group for chronic schizophrenic patients on medication, a young adult group that meets in the evening after work (also after usual clinic hours), a group of elderly patients, and a group of patients with chronic medical and psychiatric problems. This last group, led by the coordinator, is the one with the highest and most stable membership; one of its "charter members" is still attending after six years. Its patients have psychiatric problems that are predominantly chronic characterological disorders. Their medical problems include, but are not limited to, hypertension, orthopedic problems, diabetes, cardiac disease, obesity, asthma, and ulcers. They are all on numerous medications prescribed by more than one physician. It is the author's distinct impression that the frequency of medical admissions of these psychiatric-problem group members has been significantly reduced, as compared with the period of years before the group was formed. A great deal more could be said about this group alone, in view of the fact that the problems of its members are typical of urban hospital clinics.

Family therapy and couples therapy are provided by the residents, the chief psychologist, the social worker, the nurse clinician, and one additional psychologist. The residents are required to treat a family and a couple under supervision. Behavioral therapy, biofeedback, stress management and relaxation training are provided by the chief psychologist. The nurse clinician also provides stress management and relaxation training.

Many of the clinic patients receive psychotropic medications as either the primary or adjunctive mode of treatment. The psychopharmacological evaluations and follow-up visits are provided by the salaried part-time psychiatrists and a number of voluntary psychiatrists. The quality of the clinic's psychopharmacological treatment services is very high, resulting from the subspecialization of several attendings in this field.

ADMISSION CRITERIA

The clinical criteria for acceptance in the clinic treatment program are highly exclusive. Virtually all applicants are accepted for evaluation services. Patients with disorders classified in DSM–III are acceptable for admission, provided their functional condition does not require a more structured or secure treatment setting, such as a day program, acute hospitalization, a chemical dependency rehabilitation facility, or a nursing facility. Patients who are accepted for evaluation but are then found to require one of the latter facilities are appropriately referred. Of those evaluated, however, 90 percent are accepted for treatment at the clinic.

The percentage of patients who accept the clinic's offer of an evaluation or treatment is considerably less; only about 70 percent of those offered an appointment accept. The rejections are usually based on nonclinical factors, such as the clinic's restricted hours of service (9 A.M. to 5 P.M., Monday through Friday), which serve to exclude many members of the working population. The clinic's fee structure is such that lower-middle-income people are assigned relatively unaffordable fees and often need to be referred for treatment from other providers at more reasonable rates. Indeed, there are some patients for whom even our lowest fee is excessive. This situation has been for years a burdensome condition at the clinic, one for which a satisfactory solution has yet to be found. The hours of operation and fees have not been under the clinic's control, despite the staff's best efforts to change the system. If it were possible to control fee-setting and hours, the clinic would experience a much higher demand for its services.

Other factors that influence whether the clinic accepts or is accepted by an applicant include the waiting time for an evaluation appointment or for the assignment of a therapist, whether the patient lives in or near the local catchment area, and whether there is an active or prior affiliation with the institution. The latter two items are more important when there is a long (more than one week) lead time before an available evaluation appointment.

WORK FLOW

Applicants initiate their contacts with the clinic either by telephone or in person. More than 90 percent of the applications are by telephone. The applicant is asked by one of the clerical personnel to provide some basic identifying data on a brief application form. When this is completed, the applicant is ready for the first contact with a professional staff member.

The application screening, usually about 15 minutes long, is provided by a professional staff member; its purpose is to get a sense of the presenting problem and to decide whether the applicant should be offered an appointment for an evaluation or referred immediately to a more appropriate facility or practitioner. Most applicants, as noted earlier, are accepted for initial evaluation. Until recently the application screenings were provided by the nurse clinician, social worker, or the coordinator. Presently, the coordinator has taken on this clinical task to a greater degree in order to free up additional time for the other two professionals to schedule more patient visits.

When the screening is completed, the applicant is given an appointment for evaluation with one of the staff mental health professionals. The evaluation may take one or two visits, depending on the style of the evaluator and the complexity of the clinical presentation. The evaluation, in process or completed, is presented at the next scheduled diagnostic and disposition conference (D & D) for discussion, disposition, and assignment. There are three of these meetings each week, for a total of five hours. When possible, the evaluator or therapist presents the case in person. When this is not possible, the written evaluations, chart notes, and treatment plans are extremely important. The conference participants can include any clinical staff member to present cases or to join in the discussion of other cases (if the staff member does not have a patient scheduled). Attendance at the conference has been reduced recently for three professional staff members who were previously regular participants, in order to free up more of their clinical time. The conferences are now cochaired by a voluntary attending psychiatrist and the clinic coordinator.

The coordinator communicates the outcome of the conferences to the involved staff members, for example, regarding the assignments of new patients, the outcome of reviews of current patients, and quality assurance issues. Careful records are kept of each conference, with lists of patients and their dispositions. Also, in each patient's chart a note is written to document the conference outcome, the recommendations, and the date the case is to be rereviewed.

ADMINISTRATIVE PROBLEM AREAS
Missed Appointments

One of the more thorny problems resulting in lost treatment time and lost revenue is missed appointments. Initial appointments are more frequently missed than appointments made by ongoing-treatment patients. Approximately 23 percent of initial appointments are not kept; and, for many of these no-shows, no advance notice is given. This has a significantly detrimental impact in lost staff productivity. Only a small percentage of the free staff time that results from patients' failure to come to appointments can be utilized effectively for other professional activities. Medicaid and other third party payees do not permit the clinic to charge for the missed appointments, and this further exacerbates the negative impact on revenue.

Various authors have suggested ways in which attendance might be better predicted and increased. Carpenter et al. suggest that patients in the 18–24-year age group are significantly less likely to keep their initial appointments. They report that patients who have not previously received psychiatric treatment are significantly less likely to keep their first appointments than are patients who have had prior treatment. They also note that "patients who did not keep the appointment had to wait for a significantly longer period of time for the initial appointment than those who did attend the clinic."[5] In view of this finding, they suggest that, by making "crisis intake slots" available for those who need to be seen immediately, the number of "non-attenders" could be reduced.[6]

Burgoyne, Acosta, and Yamamoto attempted to replicate an earlier study by Turner and Vernon that suggested that telephone reminders to patients increased attendance at initial appointments.[7] Their conclusions, however, were different; they found that "prompting patients by telephone did not substantially alter their initial attendance; rather ascertaining whether they had a telephone identified patients more likely to keep their first appointment."[8] They noted that patients' socioeconomic levels related to their initial attendance, and that having a telephone reflected a higher socioeconomic level. They concluded that measures instituted to improve attendance must be evaluated with close scrutiny and data analysis to determine whether the results are indeed due to those measures.[9]

The Lenox Hill Psychiatric Outpatient Clinic has been struggling with this problem for many years, having already instituted the suggestion cited in the above study. None of the remedies tried has proved very successful. Given the increasing institutional pressures to become more productive and to reduce the significant financial loss attributed to the clinic, the staff have been considering instituting a system of double booking, that is, scheduling two new patients for each available evaluation slot. If both patients attend on time, both can receive evaluations but with reduced time allocated per visit; if another staff member is available at that time, one of the patients will be assigned accordingly.

In addition, a change in the roles of our staff is contemplated, giving more evaluation responsibility to nonphysician therapists. Historically, the clinic's psychiatrists have performed complete evaluations, including psychosocial history, medical history, determination of mental status, and diagnosis. It is now the staff's judgment that a nonphysician therapist can initiate an evaluation and obtain the psychosocial history. This can then be followed by a psychiatrist's interview with the patient on the same or a second visit for the detailed determination of mental status, medical history, and diagnosis. Evaluations can be initiated in either order, that is, with the physician or nonphysician therapist.

As envisioned, this plan should allow increased flexibility in assigning new evaluations, since all professional staff can participate. It will facilitate a more efficient scheduling of patients, reduce the waiting time for initial appointments, and reduce the consequences of nonattendance and lost revenue.

Recordkeeping

Recordkeeping is a problem for mental health workers in many settings, and Lenox Hill Hospital is no exception. The Lenox Hill Psychiatric Outpatient Clinic was not included in the study by Perlman et al., in which records of Medicaid patients in 29 free-standing mental health clinics and 6 hospital clinics were reviewed, but some of the findings appear pertinent to the Lenox Hill setting: "Regardless of discipline, clinical record keeping is more often than not largely incomplete. Of great concern is the fact that in the areas of mental status and medical history, in which psychiatrists would be expected to demonstrate expertise, their records were not more complete than those of their non-physician counterparts. In fact, psychiatrists have been the most deficient professional group in keeping up-to-date records."[10] Perlman et al. also note the lack of staff attention to treatment plans, which serve as valuable guidelines in determining when the goals of treatment have been accomplished.

The problem is compounded in the case of members of the Lenox Hill clinic's voluntary attending staff (psychiatrists and psychologists) who are at the clinic three hours or less per week and are nonsalaried. The deficiencies in charting are especially serious when, after medications are prescribed, the patient goes to another clinic or department (ER, or the inpatient floor of the hospital) and knowledge of this fact is important for the continued care of the patient.

Part of the difficulty with recordkeeping is the sheer volume of paperwork required for each patient visit. Proper charting includes progress notes, medication lists, treatment plans, utilization review forms, and appointment slips. Each patient who attends the Psychiatric Outpatient Clinic has both a psychiatric chart (kept in the locked files of the clinic itself) and a medical chart (kept in the Medical Records Department in another area). Both charts are prepared and made available to the therapist before each scheduled visit.

This two-chart system developed out of the concern for proper patient confidentiality; the clinic staff's view is that the many details of the psychotherapy (and much of the patient's life history) that are documented in the psychiatric chart have no appropriate application to other hospital health-care personnel, who may see the patient for other purposes. The medical chart is used by the clinic staff to review information about the patient's physical health and to document only those psychiatric data that are judged to be appropriate for other clinical care purposes, such as for medications, suicidal risks, history of drug or alcohol abuse, and so on. For example, in one case, after a patient's suicidal gesture with an overdose, it was necessary to document in the medical chart that the patient made such an attempt with her pain medication and that the drug should be prescribed with great caution, if at all. The patient was unhappy with this, but there was little question about the necessity of the documentation.

There are other aspects of a patient's treatment in a hospital psychiatric clinic that may lead to disclosure of information in the medical chart. Many medical-surgical clinic patients are referred to the clinic because of their noncompliance with treatment regimens for chronic illnesses. A therapist working with a diabetic patient who is not compliant with the prescribed diet should convey in the medical chart the progress or lack of it being made by the patient. The treating professionals in the Diabetes Clinic can then use this information in their clinical management of the patient.

From time to time, change to a one-chart system has been considered. However, this idea has been repeatedly rejected because of the detailed psychosocial information that would then be available to the many other health care personnel with access to the medical charts. The clinic continues to use the two-chart system in the absence of a more streamlined solution, and the staff are continually reminded of the importance of appropriate entries in each category of the chart.

BUDGET AND FUNDING

In 1981, Bachrach observed that, "whatever the differences between public and private general hospital psychiatric services may be, they have one thing in common: they are in trouble financially. In both cases there is competition for scarce funds both within the hospital and from outside third party sources."[11] This certainly applies to the Psychiatric Outpatient Clinic at Lenox Hill Hospital. For years the clinic staff had been hearing about the precarious financial condition of the hospital and had wondered how much the clinic contributed to that condition. There was in fact very little communication between the psychiatric staff and the financial departments of the institution; little, if any, cost-accounting information had been shared with the coordinator or with the chief of the service. Yet, the clinic staff felt that they needed more detailed information about their specific area of operation. They pressed for information on the clinic's costs and income but were warned against pushing too hard. For better or worse, however, the staff persisted, believing it preferable to work from a position of knowledge rather than ignorance.

After a number of interviews with one of the hospital's fiscal vice-presidents, the clinic's staff were presented with a report. The report was a shocker: the inclusion of indirect fixed costs put the clinic in the red by approximately $246,000 for the 1983 fiscal year. Having been unaware of the extent of the attributed indirect costs, the staff were amazed to learn that the average cost of each patient visit was $90. Clearly, Medicaid reimbursement and revenues from the large number of patients who were paying $23.10 per visit did not begin to approach this cost level.

Prior to this time, the staff's involvement with the financial aspects of the clinic operation was almost exclusively limited to direct costs for salaries and supplies. The clinic had already reduced its nonpayroll expenses by 20 percent from the previous two years. Salaries of staff members on the psychiatric outpatient budget were fixed. Each year, in the early fall, guidelines dictated the cutting of anything that could be reduced or eliminated and the justification for any essential item that required an additional appropriation. However, there was little consideration of income compared to costs, and absolutely no consideration of the extent or impact of indirect costs.

Now, with a staff that is better educated about cost accounting and indirect costs, the clinic is beginning to increase significantly the number of chargeable visits. A number of cost-cutting measures have been instituted, and others are being phased in as quickly as possible. These include:

- reducing the number of meetings and conferences to free up clinical time for patient care
- relieving some staff members of nonreimbursable duties, for example, by screening telephone applications and having all telephone screenings done by the coordinator
- closing cases of inactive patients more quickly
- developing more groups and increasing the numbers of patients per group

- identifying and capturing for the Psychiatric Outpatient Clinic the credit and income for psychiatric visits to other outpatient areas of the institution

Psychiatrists and the psychiatric nurse clinician are assigned to various medical-surgical clinics to provide on-site consultations and treatment to patients who need psychiatric intervention and who otherwise might not agree to go to the Psychiatric Outpatient Clinic. These psychiatric visits had never been considered as financial credits to the Psychiatric Outpatient Clinic. This meant that, in the cost-accounting study referred to earlier, the 400 to 500 "psychiatric visits" provided in the medical-surgical clinical locations were not credited against the costs of the Psychiatric Outpatient Clinic. It has now become apparent that all mental health services provided to outpatients, whether or not on-site at the psychiatric clinic, must be identified, appropriately billed, and credited.

Because hospital personnel policy mandates that employees cannot be charged and, further, that employees' health insurance cannot be billed, it had become apparent that, if limits were not set on the number of employee visits, the clinic would ultimately become one primarily for employees. Accordingly, the clinic reduced the number of no-fee visits available to hospital employees from an unlimited number to ten per employee per one-year period. Referrals were made to longer-term treatment facilities if the short-term intervention proved inadequate. Still, even with the ten-session limit per employee in 1983, nearly 4 percent of the total clinic patient visits were by employees. Additionally, there was difficulty in referring some employees for appropriate continuing treatment because of the relationship established with the clinic staff.

Currently, both to improve clinical service to employees and, at the same time, to reduce the number of nonchargeable visits, it is being proposed that prompt evaluation and referral be provided employees, with a limit of three visits per evaluation/crisis intervention. It is expected that employees will be easier to refer if they are not attached to the idea of ten visits to the clinic. This change is also appropriate insofar as the clinic does not have all of the confidentiality protection of an employee assistance program (EAP) that is specifically organized to counsel troubled employees. The author, however, would prefer that the hospital establish a *bona fide* EAP for its employees.

It is clear that financial departments have become increasingly critical in hospital management. Considerably more open communication must accordingly be developed between the Psychiatric Outpatient Clinic administrative staff and the hospital's fiscal managers. If all costs and credits are known, the necessary adjustments can be made so as to offer services more effectively and efficiently.

QUALITY ASSURANCE AND GOVERNMENTAL REGULATIONS

Quality assurance procedures have traditionally been part of the administrative structure at the Lenox Hill Psychiatric Outpatient Clinic. The diagnostic and disposition conferences have long been used to review both new evaluations and ongoing treatment. A policy and procedure manual is revised periodically to serve as a reference for staff and patients.

The New York State Office of Mental Health is the public regulatory health care agency that reviews and certifies the clinic on a biennial basis. Revisions in the certification requirements in recent years have required the clinic to institute additional quality control mechanisms. A Special Review Committee has been established to review untoward incidents, such as suicides, suicide attempts, and adverse drug reactions. A Utilization Review Committee has been established to ensure that patients meet admission and continued-stay criteria. And the clinic is required to participate in the local mental health planning process and to adhere to revised recordkeeping requirements.

Special Review Committee

The Special Review Committee meets a minimum of once every 90 days, but it must be convened if there has been an untoward incident. The committee consists of the clinic coordinator, one voluntary psychiatrist, a staff psychiatrist, the clinic psychiatric nurse specialist, and the director of social work. Additional staff members attend by invitation as consultants or if they are involved in the clinical care of the patient being reviewed. The committee reviews the incidents that must be reported to it under the certification regulations and takes any necessary action to limit or prevent further incidents. It can change policies and procedures and suggest or require revisions of treatment strategies. It must advise the clinic staff of such changes.

Utilization Review Committee

The Utilization Review Committee is composed of the clinic coordinator, the clinic social worker, and a voluntary attending psychiatrist. It is mandated to meet monthly and to review, or delegate the review of, all new cases within the first month of admission and all ongoing cases that have been in treatment for two years or longer and to make or hear requests for alternative-care determinations. An alternate-care determination is made when a patient is found not to meet criteria for continued stay and to be either no longer in need of treatment or in need of another type of treatment facility.

Mental Health Planning Process

The Lenox Hill Hospital Outpatient Psychiatric Clinic has for many years participated in the local mental health planning process. The coordinator is currently the cochairman of the Catchment Area Advisory Committee, which is composed of providers and consumers in the local community and which acts in an advisory capacity to the state and local (New York City) mental health agencies. This Committee provides an opportunity for cooperation and coordination among the area's various providers and also offers public relations opportunities for the clinic.

PROMOTION AND MARKETING

The promotion and marketing of mental health services have become increasingly important in maintaining the financial viability of mental health programs. Clinical programs must, increasingly, be seen from a business perspective; if a program is not profitable, its operating deficits should at least be minimized as much as possible.

The relationship between finances and the ongoing viability of the clinical program is a reality that must be faced. Reduced governmental funding has left hospitals with the responsibility of providing the funds needed to maintain their clinical programs. Hospital financial managers emphasize the importance of increasing clinic income by increasing the volume of patient services without increasing costs.

When additional clinical time is made available, new referrals must be cultivated. Referrals are stimulated through collaboration with such in-house resources as the Public Relations Department, the Community Health Education Center, and other clinical departments that may refer patients. The involvement of the clinic coordinator and other staff members in community groups and planning bodies is also essential. For example, as noted previously, the involvement of the coordinator of the Lenox Hill Psychiatric Outpatient Clinic in the local community advisory council on mental health services gives the clinic a measure of exposure to other community providers and consumer groups. Through this council, meetings have been arranged with local school guidance counselors and have yielded new contacts, referrals, and good will. The council members include local legislators and representatives from nonmental-health social service agencies and consumer groups. All of these contacts provide important potential for external referral sources.

The Public Relations Department of the hospital can assist in preparing brochures and securing media exposure for the program. The Health Education Center can assist in distributing brochures and providing referrals directly to the clinic from its community storefront and other outreach efforts. Public informational and educational programs, such as the community mental health fair, can be planned and jointly sponsored. At Lenox Hill, a recent program on stress had various exhibits and demonstrations, including a referral desk that brought in more than a dozen new referrals within the course of two weeks.

In view of the fact that it is in a geographic area of intense competition for the mental health service consumer, the Lenox Hill Psychiatric Outpatient Clinic must become more sophisticated in promotional and marketing techniques. There are many private practitioners who can provide good services at similar, if not lower, cost. Yet, in spite of this, many patients prefer the hospital setting for their psychiatric care. The availability of comprehensive health care services, and the willingness to accept Medicaid (which many private practitioners avoid) are among the reasons the clinic is preferred by many patients.

CONCLUSION

Faced with the financial realities of the 1980s, the Lenox Hill Psychiatric Outpatient Clinic must balance its fiscal requirements against the need to maintain the highest quality of care for its patients. In this situation, creative solutions have been devised to meet the problems inherent in hospital-based mental health services. The resulting management structure has evolved through trial and error but has proved to be quite workable. Some of its components may be useful and transferable to other facilities that must similarly maximize the use of modest resources. Though common to the general hospital setting, the problems described are undoubtedly shared by many facilities. It is thus hoped that problems faced and the remedies applied at the Lenox Hill Psychiatric Outpatient Clinic will be helpful to workers in other health care settings.

REFERENCES

1. L.L. Bachrach, "General Hospital Psychiatry: Overview from a Sociological Perspective," *American Journal of Psychiatry* 138 (1981).

2. Ibid., 883.

3. C.L. Rich et al., "General Psychiatry in a Subspecialty Setting," *Journal of Clinical Psychiatry* 39 (1978).

4. Ibid.

5. P.J. Carpenter et al., "Who Keeps the First Outpatient Appointment?" *American Journal of Psychiatry* 138 (1981).

6. Ibid.

7. A.J. Turner and J.C. Vernon, "Prompts to Increase Attendance in a Community Mental Health Center," *Journal of Applied Behavioral Analysis* 9 (1976).

8. R.W. Burgoyne, F.X. Acosta, and J. Yamamoto, "Telephone Prompting to Increase Attendance at a Psychiatric Outpatient Clinic," *American Journal of Psychiatry* 140 (1983): 347.

9. Ibid.

10. B.B. Perlman et al., "Psychiatric Records: Variations Based on Discipline and Patient Characteristics, with Implications for Quality of Care," *American Journal of Psychiatry* 139 (1982): 1156.

11. Bachrach, "General Hospital Psychiatry," 881.

Chapter 5

Psychiatric Emergency Care

Alice Keating, R.N., M.S.N., and Allen H. Collins, M.D., M.P.H.

INTRODUCTION

The general hospital emergency room (ER) is an area of excitement, danger, high emotions, and great activity. Crisis situations with dramatic medical interventions and unpredictable patients are an inherent part of the ER scene. The emergency room was originally organized as an "accident room" and operated for the acute medically ill and injured. However, it has now become a setting that provides care to a far more diversified patient population.[1]

There has been a tremendous increase in the numbers of patients visiting emergency rooms. A mobile society, the increase in medical specialization, and the 24-hour availability of clinical services have all contributed to the increased usage of the emergency room. Studies have shown that approximately one-third of the ER patient population presents with psychiatric needs in lieu of, or in addition to, medical needs.[2,3] In addition to patients with obvious medical needs or injuries, there is a whole array of cases that present to the staff working in an emergency room. On any given day, it may be a woman who has been raped, an elderly woman who has been found wandering in her nightclothes, an abused child, an alcoholic looking for a warm place to stay, a suicidal teenager, a young man involved in vehicular homicide, or a shopping-bag lady who has been mugged.[4] These presentations may require unique approaches, as well as a specialized mix of available psychiatric team members. The staff that faces these demanding situations on a day-to-day basis need specific educational and experiential preparation to work effectively. When patients present with some psychiatric or psychosocial need, the psychiatric clinician must possess the capacity to:

- gather facts quickly
- synthesize information from those most knowledgeable and available in the situation
- decide upon further studies and consultations
- construct a differential diagnosis
- contact possible dispositional resources
- plan treatment steps
- communicate these measures to all who are involved in the management of the case [5]

An effective emergency room provides diagnosis and treatment for medical problems and physical injuries. A more difficult situation arises in the case of a person in need of psychiatric help. Fast decisions and a crisis atmosphere can lead to overlooking the more subtle problems of such a patient.

Jacoby and Jones use a three-tier classification of behaviors as indicators of the need for psychiatric intervention:

1. psychosomatic symptoms, such as tension, nervousness, anxiety, or headache
2. assault victimizations, such as husband abuse, wife abuse, child abuse, rape, or a knife wound
3. bizarre behavior[6]

The etiology of these behaviors may be psychiatric illness, the influence of either alcohol or drugs, or a temporary environmental crisis situation. Of the three categories of clinical presentations, a psychiatric consultation is least likely to be called for with patients manifesting psychosomatic symptoms.

Very often, ER personnel demonstrate a lack of tolerance and, indeed, not infrequently express hatred when presented with cases of drug overdose or other forms of self-abuse. The same attitude extends to troublesome, disruptive patients. Such problem patients often represent an unwelcome burden on a generally overwhelmed ER staff. Their problems seem less serious than, and stand in the way of, those of "people who really need care." It is in such clinical situations that the psychiatric support team can assist and possibly effect attitudinal changes toward patients requiring mental health intervention.

THE EMERGENCY ROOM OF LENOX HILL HOSPITAL

The Physical Setting

The emergency room at Lenox Hill Hospital was established in the 1860s when the hospital was founded. Over the years, as the hospital expanded, the emergency room has changed location and size. Since 1958, it has been located in a relatively small space of 3,800 square feet on the ground-floor level. Adjoining it is the ambulance bay and patient entrance area, open 24 hours a day, seven days a week. There is also a conveniently located central nursing station, flanked by a four-litter room, a two-litter room, and a second two-litter room. A staff lounge room and x-ray room are located nearby.

Over the next 20 years, the demands on ER clinical services progressively increased. This resulted in major problems of overloading the available space. In 1982, attempts were made to alleviate the problem by the addition of patient-care rooms in a contiguous area reassigned from the Outpatient Department. The resulting spatial layout amounts to a patchwork of treatment rooms joined by hallways. Some of these rooms are at some distance from the central nursing station.

In 1982, additional space was expropriated from an underutilized conference room located near a third-floor medical clinic. The area was remodeled to include two examining rooms, a small nursing station, and a utility room and was designated as ER 2. A physician, a nurse, and a clerk staff this area Mondays through Fridays from 10 A.M. to 6 P.M. Patients with less acute medical problems are examined and treated in this area. The triage nurse in the main emergency room decides who will be seen in ER 2.

The total bed capacity of the ER (including ER 2, with 2 beds) is 16 beds. Usually, however, the actual number of patients exceeds this figure. Those patients who do not require beds are seated on chairs in the corridors.

Staffing

The Emergency Department's chief of emergency services is a full-time physician who is responsible for the planning and operations of all emergency medical services. The chief reports to an assistant vice-president of the hospital administration. Five salaried attending physicians provide the medical staffing of the emergency room. They provide direct patient care and supervise medical house staff (PGY 2 + 3), who are assigned to one-month rotations in the ER by the Department of Medicine. On-site attending physician coverage in the emergency room is available from 8 A.M. to 8 P.M., seven days a week. During the daily 8 P.M.–8 A.M. shift, the medical care is provided by medical residents. Specialists from a variety of medical-surgical disciplines, including psychiatry, are available to the ER medical-nursing staff on an on-call basis for telephone or in-person consultation.

A patient care coordinator (head nurse) and an assistant patient care coordinator (assistant head nurse) plan for and supervise nursing care on a 24-hour basis. Nursing care is provided primarily by 23 registered nurses whose work is divided into two 12-hour shifts and who are certified in both basic and advanced life support. The certification is necessary in view of the emergency room's designation as a "cardiac station" by the New York City Department of Health. Additionally, there are 8 nursing assistants, 6 full-time clerical staff, and 6 part-time clerical staff. Nursing assistants provide basic nursing care, transport patients, and do the day-to-day checking, ordering, and replenishing of supplies and equipment. Supportive clerical staff members perform registration, answer telephones, obtain medical records of patients previously treated at the hospital, follow up on lab reports, and order and stock all stationery supplies.

Clinical Services

In 1983, the Lenox Hill emergency room provided clinical services to 36,000 patients. Of these, 6,400 were hospitalized at Lenox Hill Hospital. In 1977, 26,000 patients were seen. Currently, approximately 82 percent of the ER patients are evaluated, treated, and discharged; and 18 percent are hospitalized. About 40 percent of the patients present with minor trauma to the musculoskeletal system. Another 40 percent present with a wide variety of medical-surgical problems. The remaining 20 percent are seen by other specialties, including psychiatry.

History of Lenox Hill Psychiatric ER Services

Before 1979, psychiatric coverage to the emergency room was provided by a voluntary attending on-call system. Ostensibly, this system operated as a 24-hour/day, seven-day/week emergency psychiatric coverage program. In reality, it functioned on only a nominal basis. The voluntary (nonsalaried) attending psychiatrists, who served one-week rotational periods of on-call duty to the emergency room as well as to all the in-hospital wards, were expected to cover all acute and emergency psychiatric problems that were not being privately addressed. The ER staff (or ward medical-nursing staff) was responsible for calling the psychiatrist on call directly at the psychiatrist's private office. These calls were usually followed by a delay of from one to six hours before psychiatric response occurred. During this delay, the

ER staff would become increasingly concerned about resolving the clinical problems and angry at the psychiatrist for not responding more quickly. Ultimately, when psychiatric response did occur, negative transactions usually resulted between the professionals involved. This further exacerbated the stressful aspect of the emergency consultation. Attending psychiatrists felt put upon for having the onerous responsibility of providing emergency coverage. They were quite reluctant to appear in person at the ER when requested to do so by the hospital staff and made every attempt to provide the consultation assistance by telephone. This further worsened interprofessional discussions, which frequently terminated in harsh feelings. After many years of such problems without any improvement, psychiatry became virtually *persona non grata* in the emergency room. The specialty came to be viewed as different from the other medical-surgical specialties, all of which could be relied upon to provide timely and useful emergency consultation assistance when requested.

In 1979, the appointment of a new attending-in-charge of psychiatry led to a review of all existing clinical service programs. This included the emergency on-call system, which was found to be grossly inadequate and detrimental to the growth of credible psychiatric services in the hospital. An ad hoc committee was established to delineate the psychiatric needs of the emergency room and formulate an emergency coverage program that would take into consideration the limitations of available staffing and financing, both of which imposed considerable constraints. The Department of Social Work was, of necessity, included in these deliberations as a result of its responsibility for a preexisting system of providing "psychosocial" consultations to the emergency room on a basis completely independent from psychiatry.

The ad hoc committee formulated a new system that combined elements of the older programs, took advantage of as many on-site, salaried, mental-health staff members as possible, and emphasized coordination of the various professionals involved. The mental health professionals who staffed the new program would perform specific functions but would not sacrifice the flexibility of their individual professional assets in providing interventions. This was considered an important feature of a workable system.

The new Psychiatric-Psychosocial Emergency Coverage Program entailed:

- the integration of the previous two systems with close coordination of the psychiatric and psychosocial components
- the development of a multidisciplinary team of mental-health consultants to the emergency room, including psychiatrists, psychiatric social workers, and a mental health nurse clinician

- the institution of a two-phase coverage system, consisting of the following coverage: (1) weekdays, 9 A.M. to 5 P.M., during which in-house, salaried, mental health staff would be responsible for all psychiatric emergency patients who presented to the emergency room; and (2) weekday evenings, weekends, and holidays, at which times the voluntary psychiatric attending would be responsible for providing ER emergency consultations on a more limited basis (up to 11 P.M.) and in a more responsive and substantive manner than previously.

The Two-Phase System of Psychiatric/Psychosocial ER Services

The two-phase system for providing psychiatric and psychosocial services to the emergency room involves direct consultations to patients and families, including psychiatric and psychosocial evaluations, treatment intervention, and referrals as indicated. It also involves liaison to medical and nursing staffs, including case consultation-liaison with respect to the quality of the psychiatric and psychosocial service provided and ongoing in-service training of emergency room staff in psychosocial areas of care.

The Weekday Daytime System

A psychiatric, clinic-based mental health nurse clinician is the liaison professional responsible for the smooth operation of the program of psychiatric and psychosocial coverage to the emergency room. The nurse clinician is available Monday through Friday, 9 A.M. to 5 P.M., and may be reached in the Psychiatric Clinic or by page beeper. In addition to responsibilities in the emergency room, the nurse clinician carries a psychotherapy caseload in the clinic. The nurse clinician's responsibilities to the emergency room include:

- ready availability via a page beeper for telephone or in-person triage consultation to emergency room staff concerning the appropriate mental health professional to call for the particular patient and problem
- treatment interventions and referrals as appropriate
- ongoing in-service training of emergency room staff in the areas of psychiatric and psychosocial assessment and intervention
- periodic meetings with the patient care coordinator of the emergency room to review the psychiatric program operations and any problems that may arise
- documentation of the overall program operation (number of consultations performed, presenting problems of patients and families, outcomes, and so on) and periodic presentations to the attending-in-charge

of psychiatry and the psychiatry service administrative staff (executive committee)

The mental health nurse clinician meets on a fairly regular basis with the nursing staff of the emergency room. There is no established agenda for these meetings; thus far they have been used for educational discussions, the establishment of support groups, and clinical situation problem solving. The subjects of the educational presentations have included the assessment and documentation of mental status, the management of violent behavior, psychopharmacologic agents, schizophrenia, affective disorders, psychosomatic illness, and the meaning of behavior psychodynamics. The format for the educational meetings has been that of a didactic presentation, with ample time allocated for discussion. Topics are requested by the nursing staff or are identified by the nurse clinician in light of the learning needs of the staff.

Support groups for the emergency room nursing staff have been open-ended and have generally lasted six to eight weeks. They have concentrated on such things as coping with stress, preventing burn-out, and interpersonal problems among staff members and between nursing staff and medical staff.

As the nurse clinician meets with the nursing staff, problems in the delivery of patient care or issues in working conditions are identified. The group then addresses the problems. Recently, a more efficient admission procedure was developed by the nursing group. The staff nurses had long sought a 12-hour shift (instead of the standard 8 hours) with more days off. Through the group, a proposal to this effect was prepared and presented to the nursing administration, which approved it.

In this liaison role, the nurse clinician functions as a role model, demonstrating communication skills and problem-solving abilities. Also, by demonstrating concern and a willingness to listen to nursing staff, the nurse clinician fosters a working alliance between ER staff and psychiatric staff.

The Monday-through-Friday daytime system involves an interdisciplinary team composed of a psychiatrist, a psychiatric social worker and the mental health nurse clinician. Although clinical areas are delineated for each of these three mental health professionals, there is a great deal of functional overlapping. Mutual support and assistance with treatment interventions and disposition planning also lead to a blurring of roles.

Psychiatric coverage to the emergency room is provided by two part-time salaried psychiatrists of the Psychiatric Clinic and two full-time psychiatric residents (PGY 2 and 3) who rotate through Lenox Hill Hospital from the New York Medical College Psychiatric Residency Training Consortium. In addition to being on call to the emergency room, the psychiatrists have responsibilities, either in the Psychiatric Clinic or on the medical-surgical inpatient units, as part of the Psychiatric Consultation-Liaison Service. The ER coverage is provided with the clear understanding that ER requests for intervention have priority over other activities during the period of coverage.

The psychiatric social worker, based in the Psychiatric Clinic, is on call to the emergency room Monday through Friday, 9 A.M. to 5 P.M. Like the psychiatrists and the mental health nurse clinician, the social worker has other responsibilities, including a caseload of psychotherapy outpatients and coverage for the psychiatric inpatient social worker in the latter's absence.

After a clinical evaluation has been completed and it is decided that a patient requires psychiatric hospitalization in a segregated psychiatric unit (as opposed to a scatter-bed program), arrangements must be made for the patient to be transferred from the emergency room to a local psychiatric facility. In this situation, the psychiatric social worker or the nurse clinician assists the psychiatrist in determining which psychiatric facilities are appropriate for the transfer. This can involve determining the patient's address, catchment area, insurance coverage, and the bed availability at various psychiatric facilities. The social worker or nurse clinician also assists the patient and the family in accepting the transfer and aids the ER staff in determining which mental health professional to call, based on guidelines for clinical situations as posted with the psychiatric on-call schedule. A copy of this schedule is reproduced as Exhibit 5–1.

The Weekday Evening and Weekend/Holiday System

The weekday evening (5 P.M. to 11 P.M.) and weekend/holiday (9 A.M. to 11 P.M.) system is a rotational set of procedures among approximately 40 voluntary psychiatric attendings who provide ER coverage on a rotational basis for one-week periods per rotation. Therefore, one to two weeks of such coverage is provided annually by each attending. This is one of the clinical responsibilities of the voluntary psychiatric staff members in fulfillment of the requirement to maintain active affiliations with the hospital.

The system operates as follows: When an ER staff member telephones the hospital page operator, the operator "beeps" the on-call psychiatrist, who has a long-range (50-mile) beeper. The psychiatrist, who must respond within 30 minutes, calls the page operator, who gives the telephone number and message. The psychiatrist then calls the ER staff member.

The ensuing telephone consultation involves discussion of the patient's case history and physical status; pertinent lab data; the specific clinical problem for which the staff member is requesting consultation help (for example, psychotropic medication, if any, to be given to the patient to decrease psychotic agitation); disposition arrangements; and calls, if any, to

Exhibit 5–1 The Lenox Hill Psychiatric On-Call Schedule for
ER Coverage

Psychiatric-Psychosocial Coverage to the Emergency Department
Hours: Monday–Friday, 9 A.M. to 5 P.M.
Services provided: Evaluations, treatment interventions, and referrals
Whom To Call:

Psychiatrist (see schedule)	Social Worker (Ext.)	Mental Health Nurse Clinician (page)
Suicide attempt	Alcoholism & drug abuse	Patients needing counseling or referral for:
Acute psychosis	Victims of rape and crime and battered spouses	—depression
Violent behavior	Suspected child abuse/ neglect	—anxiety disorders
Homicidal ideation	Undomiciled individuals	—conversion reactions
OMS	Patients and/or families requiring psychosocial assessment relative to:	—psychosomatic disorders
Severe depression	—isolation	—sudden death
	—malnutrition	
	—poor living situations	
	—need for community resources	
	—need for health care follow-up	
	—(How will patient manage at home?)	

Call the mental health nurse clinician for (1) problems with the daytime system and (2) triage questions.

---

a local psychiatric receiving hospital for admission. It is also determined if there are any important clinical issues involving disposition that require the psychiatrist to provide in-person attendance in the ER. If there are differences of opinion as to whether in-person consultation is necessary, they must be negotiated between the ER physician and the attending psychiatrist. Major discrepancies and problems with the system are referred to the chief of the Psychiatric Consultation-Liaison Service, who also carries a long-distance beeper.

Certain problems with the weekday evening and weekend/holiday system have been ameliorated by (1) designating the chief of the consultation-liaison service as the coordinator of the program; (2) modifying the method of contacting the on-call psychiatrist, by providing long-range beepers and making the hospital telephone operators, rather than the ER staff, responsible for the paging; and (3) providing ongoing education of emergency-room staff in relation to the use and practice of psychiatric consultation.

Problems with the Two-Phase System

The weekday daytime system is staffed 60 percent of the time by psychiatric residents in training with varying amounts of experience in emergency psychiatry. There is great variability in the kinds of consultations requested, and clinical judgment varies from one resident to another. Immediate access to back-up supervision is not always available, and sometimes inappropriate dispositions are made.

Problems also arise from the fact that staff members assigned to provide psychiatric and psychosocial coverage to the emergency room are based primarily in other areas of the hospital, and generally their loyalties are to the primary area, for example, the clinic and the consultation-liaison service. Staff assigned to cover the emergency room are consistently asked to interrupt their customarily scheduled activities to provide service in the emergency room. This can lead to stress for the psychiatric staff member and difficulties for the ER patient and staff.

Psychiatric dispositions from the emergency room are problematic, in that Lenox Hill Hospital does not have a segregated inpatient unit, nor does it have adequate in-hospital facilities for the difficult-to-manage psychiatric patient. Also, there are no facilities for partial hospitalization or other alternative treatments.

The weekday evening and weekend/holiday system presents greater problems than the weekday daytime system, because the majority of attending psychiatrists still resent having to provide ER coverage, and they attempt to provide such service with minimum disruption to their personal lives and private practices. This exacerbates problems with ER staff, who feel they are not getting the same kind of in-person service from psychiatry that they are getting from other medical specialties. Lenox Hill Hospital is one of the few voluntary teaching hospitals in the New York City area that requires voluntary attending psychiatrists to take ER calls. In most area hospitals, paid residents provide this coverage. In particular, Lenox Hill Hospital's many senior, board-certified psychiatrists find the ER requirement odious and foreign. The requirement is especially trying when the psychiatric attending on-call has a busy week with nine or ten patients needing ER evaluation. Indeed, the reason that the 11 P.M.–9 A.M. shift was not included in the psychiatric-attending-on-call coverage was that it was considered excessive and might have precipitated resignations of many voluntary attendings.

The existing two-phase system is thus workable but not very successful. The Psychiatry Service is currently working on the allocation of ER space as a designated interview room that would be soundproof and ensure privacy. Ultimately, the Psychiatric Service would like sufficient staff on the premises on a 24-hour basis so that in-person consultation would be possible all the time.

CASE STUDIES: LENOX HILL PSYCHIATRIC EMERGENCY CARE

The following case studies reveal various aspects of the Lenox Hill psychiatry emergency care service in operation.

Case 1: Collaboration between the Psychiatric Resident and Nurse Clinician

The mental health nurse clinician was paged by a staff nurse from the Prenatal Clinic. A 35-year-old woman, four months pregnant, came to the clinic for her first prenatal visit. She had alcohol on her breath and expressed suicidal ideation to the obstetrical resident. The nurse clinician decided that, since hospitalization was a possibility, the evaluation would best be conducted in the emergency room. The clinician called the emergency room staff to alert them to the situation and also paged the psychiatric resident on call to the emergency room.

After escorting the patient from the Prenatal Clinic to the emergency room, the nurse clinician did a psychosocial assessment. It was learned that the patient had been raped by her father when she was 14 and by her father's friend when she was 15. She became pregnant by the second rape and had the child. The child currently lives with the patient's mother in the South. Following the birth of the child, the patient took an overdose and was hospitalized psychiatrically. She did not follow through on outpatient treatment. There followed years of alcohol abuse. After trying to stop drinking for about eight years, the patient finally entered an alcoholism treatment program, and she had been sober for two years prior to marrying her alcoholism counselor three months before the present incident. Following her marriage, she had not wished to have sexual intercourse with her husband and had started drinking. She stated that, though her husband was happy about having a child, she was ambivalent: "I can't even take care of myself; how can I take care of a baby?" One month prior to her prenatal visit, not knowing she was pregnant, the patient took an overdose of Sinequan, which she had been given in the outpatient department of another hospital. She stated that she was very depressed at the time and wanted to die. She was hospitalized at this other hospital for one week, but again did not follow through on the referral for postdischarge outpatient care.

The nurse clinician called the patient's husband to apprise him of the situation. The psychiatric resident further interviewed the patient to establish a diagnosis and to initiate a disposition. The patient was diagnosed as having a major depression and being in need of hospitalization because of the presence of the significant suicidal risk.

In view of the fact that Lenox Hill Hospital does not have a segregated (closed) unit, the patient had to be hospitalized elsewhere. Trying to locate an available psychiatric bed can sometimes be an arduous and time-consuming task. It involves calling various local hospitals and waiting for admitting physicians to return calls. In this case, arranging a disposition took one hour. Transportation was arranged by the nurse clinician, who contacted the city ambulance transport service. The nurse clinician also advised the emergency room staff that a security guard would have to remain with the patient because she was suicidal.

Case 2: Multidisciplinary and Community Involvement

The mental health nurse clinician was called by the emergency room to talk with an 84-year-old woman who was refusing hospitalization despite the fact that the ER attending felt it was imperative to admit her. The woman appeared frightened and confused, gesturing that she wanted to get off the stretcher and leave. The reason for the plan to admit was the discovery that the patient had a serum hemoglobin of 5 (nl = $12 - 14$).

Adding to everyone's difficulty was a language barrier. The patient's language was Hungarian, and she seemed unable to speak or understand much English. The Administration Department of Lenox Hill Hospital keeps a list of employees who speak languages in addition to English and who might be available to translate. As luck would have it, none of the Hungarian-speaking people were on duty that day. The nurse clinician learned that the patient attended a local church that had a large Hungarian-speaking population. The church was contacted, and one of the priests who knew the patient quite well agreed to come to the emergency room to attempt to address the patient's concerns about hospitalization and to persuade her to stay. The patient still refused to stay, expressing to the priest her fear that if she came into the hospital she would die. The ER attending, using the priest as translator, explained why admission was necessary; the patient still refused and did not seem to understand the gravity of the situation. The nurse clinician called the psychiatric resident on call to evaluate the patient. The resident attempted to explain again the reason for hospitalization and offered reassurance, but the patient remained confused and anxious, refusing to stay.

Given the patient's age, low hemoglobin, and confused state, the issue of competence was raised. The psychiatric resident's supervisor and the hospital's legal department were contacted. All agreed that the patient did not understand the nature of her illness and was currently not competent to decide about hospitalization. When the patient was told by the psychiatric resident and the priest that she had to stay, she became tearful but offered no protest. Since the woman had no living relatives, the priest promised to visit regularly and to mobilize the patient's acquaintances from the church to do so also. As it turned out, the patient was operated on successfully for a perforated ulcer.

Case 3: The Nurse Clinician as Role Model for an ER Staff Nurse

The mental health nurse clinician was contacted by an ER staff nurse to talk with a patient about a referral for outpatient psychiatric services. The patient was a 31-year-old truck driver who had been brought by police to the emergency room after he had collapsed at the scene of an accident. The patient was in his delivery truck and had pulled out of the intersection when the traffic light changed. He heard one voice screaming and then many people yelling. The patient stopped the truck, realizing he had struck someone. He looked out the window and saw an elderly woman pinned under the wheel. The police arrived on the scene in minutes, as did medical service ambulance personnel, and the woman was pronounced dead at the scene.

The staff nurse who had contacted the nurse clinician asked if she could sit in on the interview because she wanted to improve her therapeutic skills in helping patients in crisis. The nurse clinician met with the patient and encouraged him to talk about what had happened. The patient tearfully described the shock, horror, and remorse he felt at having "killed someone." He also expressed his fears for the future, specifically the fears that he would be charged with a crime and/or would lose his job. The patient was a married man with one young child and a pregnant wife due to deliver in five days. In these circumstances, the patient felt he could not burden his wife with the current crisis and was therefore lacking his usual support system.

The nurse clinician suggested that the patient might need someone on an ongoing basis to talk to about his feelings and ability to cope with the crisis. In exploring this, the patient stated that he did not want to see a psychiatrist or mental health worker but that he had a family physician who had been helpful in past crises. The patient decided to call this physician. At this time, the patient mentioned that his father was also a truck driver and decided that his father could also be counted on for understanding and support.

The nurse clinician spoke to the police, learned that no charges were being pressed, and relayed this information to the patient. The patient regained some emotional equilibrium and was discharged from the emergency room. The nurse clinician then reviewed with the staff nurse the paradigm of crisis intervention that she had used:

- helping the individual to gain an intellectual understanding of his crisis
- reducing tension by helping the individual bring into the open his present feelings to which he may not have access
- exploring coping mechanisms[7]

DISCUSSION

The above case studies illustrate the collaboration between the members of the emergency psychiatric team and demonstrate the interplay between the team and the emergency room medical-nursing staff. The majority of cases that require psychosocial interventions in the emergency room are managed by the mental health team member who is first contacted to see the patient, whether it is the psychiatrist, psychiatric social worker, or mental health nurse clinician.

Psychiatric Services at Lenox Hill Hospital: Current Service Levels

The number of psychiatric consultations—that is, those in which the psychiatrist was the primary provider of clinical care—performed annually at Lenox Hill has risen to over 300 compared with less than 100 in the years prior to 1979. In addition to these services, there are approximately five to seven psychosocial interventions per week (280 per year) in which the psychiatric social worker or the mental health nurse clinician is the primary provider.

In 1984, the age categories of the patients seen in psychiatric consultation at Lenox Hill Hospital were as follows:

- Less than 25 years: 22 percent
- 25–44 years: 33 percent
- 45–64 years: 28 percent
- Over 65 years: 17 percent

Of these patients, 60 percent were Caucasian, 25 percent were black, and 15 percent were Hispanic. With respect to catchment area, 52 percent of the patients were local upper eastside Manhattan residents, and 48 percent came to the hospital from other areas.

Of the average 300 psychiatric consultation cases per year, 38 percent required psychiatric hospitalization. The remaining 62 percent were discharged from the emergency room with other dispositions, including:

- outpatient treatment: 60 percent
- alcoholism treatment programs: 15 percent
- drug treatment programs: 10 percent
- referral back to current therapist: 15 percent

The psychiatric diagnoses of the two dispositional categories of patients seen in consultation in the ER are as follows:

1. Hospitalized patients
   - major depression: 29.8 percent
   - suicide attempts: 13.2 percent
   - bipolar affective disorder: 10.5 percent
   - chronic schizophrenia: 10.5 percent
   - atypical psychosis: 18.4 percent
   - substance abuse: 10.5 percent
   - acute adjustment disorder: 1.8 percent
   - schizoaffective disorder: 5.3 percent
2. Discharged patients
   - personality disorders: 9.7 percent
   - anxiety disorders: 15.1 percent
   - schizophrenia: 5.7 percent
   - alcoholism: 15.1 percent
   - substance abuse: 9.1 percent
   - depressive disorders: 30.2 percent
   - psychosomatic disorder: 15.1 percent

As noted earlier, studies have found that approximately one-third of all patients who present to a general hospital emergency room have significant clinical problem areas for which psychiatric intervention is required. The fact that only 580 psychiatric-psychosocial consultations were performed among the more than 38,000 patients who presented annually to the Lenox

Hill emergency room in 1984 indicates clearly that many of these patients' psychiatric needs were not addressed. This is noted, not necessarily to point up Lenox Hill's particular deficiencies, but rather to suggest the clinical problems involved in the provision of psychiatric services by many community general hospitals today, given their limited resources.

Problems in the Provision of Psychiatric Emergency Service

The problems inherent in the provision of psychiatric emergency services in the general hospital can be categorized in terms of the nonpsychiatric ER milieu, psychiatric staffing, patient characteristics, the medical network, and financial and legal factors.

Nonpsychiatric ER Milieu

The problems stemming from the ER milieu have to do, in physical terms, with the adequacy of interview rooms to ensure privacy and calm interaction and the availability of 24-hour holding beds. In a psychological context, the negative attitudes in the medical nursing staff subculture toward psychiatric patients and staff can also have an important problematic impact. Finally, the ER environment may present difficulties in ensuring adequate security arrangements for hostile or violent patients.

Psychiatric Staffing

Psychiatrists, particularly in initial stages of training, are often out of their depth when confronted by the wide range of severe problems in the time-pressured ER setting. Added to this is the low status that emergency psychiatry often is accorded by senior psychiatric staff. The "on-call" nature of ER service results in primary loyalty and identification remaining with the clinical service to which they are principally assigned, and most psychiatrists desire to return to that service as soon as possible after ER duty. Finally, for many psychiatrists, problems may arise from the fact that the clinical model of orientation of the on-call staff is one of triage to ER patients rather than crisis intervention.

Patient Characteristics

ER patients present a variety of problems for the on-call attending psychiatrist:

- life-threatening behavior or symptoms
- deteriorated states, resulting from waiting until they are no longer able to tolerate their problems

- difficulty or inability to care for self
- helplessness and/or fear of losing control
- long-standing and complex psychosocial problems
- involuntary presentations, resulting in poor motivation for treatment, uncooperativeness, or belligerence
- multiple medical problems that are poorly or inadequately treated
- poor familial-social support structures, accompanied by the inadequate capacities of many patients to use those that are available

The Medical Network

Poor relations between neighboring health care institutions often result in a lack of cooperation and coordination of care for patients who may need to be transferred from one institution to the other.[8] Also, in the medical network, there may be conceptually ambiguous or poorly implemented mental health agency policies and procedures pertaining to catchment area responsibilities and interinstitutional patient transfer arrangements. There may also be inadequate system definitions of the acute, intermediate, and long-term psychiatric inpatient care responsibilities of the providers in the network. Poor or overburdened emergency medical transportation systems may result in long delays for necessary transfers.

Added to these problems, there may not be enough acute care, intermediate care, and long-term care psychiatric beds in the area. For the beds that are available, stringent medical insurance admitting criteria may limit real accessibility for many patients. Finally, long waiting lists in local outpatient clinics might preclude their serving as viable alternatives to hospitalization. The medical network that lacks residential treatment facilities for chronic patients, crisis intervention (mobile and static) programs, and day hospital services as alternatives to hospitalization poses major problems for ER staff in need of dispositional resources.

Financial Factors

In general, the reimbursement rates currently applied to emergency psychiatric services are grossly inadequate. The problems manifested by many, if not most, patients who are referred for these services in the emergency room are complex and multifaceted; and lengthy, multiprofessional interventions are often necessary for assessment, crisis intervention, and disposition. Existing charges, whether self-pay or third party reimbursed, simply do not meet the institutional costs of such services. This basic fact underlies the significant staffing problems, particularly the resort to "on-call" solutions, of the great majority of general hospitals in efforts to provide psychiatric emergency care. Permanent, on-site staff can be provided only in institutions which have a great many residency lines, designated grant support for emergency psychiatry service, and/or a strong ideological commitment to such services.

Legal Factors

The statutes and procedures documenting the professional responsibilities (and adjunctive malpractice litigation risks) of medical personnel in the ER treatment of psychiatrically impaired patients must be carefully weighed against the laws and regulations (and the litigation risks) pertaining to the civil rights of those patients. As legal and other patient rights groups have organized to champion the protection of psychiatric patients, it has become essential that emergency psychiatric staff pay careful attention to the often conflicting sets of concerns involved in the emergency crisis scene.

Dispositional Alternatives and Problems

A variety of dispositions can be made for patients who present with psychiatric-psychosocial problems. Indeed, the disposition is a significant part of the clinical task in the resolution of psychiatric emergencies. There is palpable pressure to arrive quickly at an appropriate disposition. Space is always needed in the emergency room for other patients, and the on-call psychiatric team members have pressing problems in other areas of the hospital.

The attitude and activity of the evaluator must be geared toward the nature and implementation of the disposition. Should the patient return home? Should the patient receive further treatment in or out of the hospital? What are the available family and community resources that can be called upon to help resolve the crisis?

The crisis resolution that can be effected in the emergency room is partial, at best. Much of the time, the patient remains in crisis, with the presenting problems persisting. Still, the patient may have gained hope for future resolution by virtue of having formulated a treatment plan with a psychiatric professional. In effect, the patient does not feel as alone or out of control as before.[9] Indeed, patients can often be helped to grow and cope through their crisis experience in a manner that did not seem possible prior to the intervention.

When the decision is made to pursue outpatient care, a community mental health resource book can be extremely helpful to members of the psychiatric team. In the Lenox Hill experience, the psychiatric social worker usually has the most comprehensive and up-to-date information about the relevant community services and can be an invaluable, time-saving resource for other members of the team.

At Lenox Hill Hospital, the disposition decision to hospitalize a patient is a complicated one. Since the hospital has no segregated psychiatric inpatient unit, patients can be considered for admission only to the scatter-bed program (see Chapter 2). In these cases, the admission must be voluntary, the patient's behavior must be such as to be manageable in a semiprivate room situation on an open, medical-surgical unit, a bed must be available, and appropriate financial coverage must be available. Given these requirements, only a small percentage of patients requiring hospitalization have been admitted to the Lenox Hill scatter-bed program. For the great majority of patients for whom the decision to hospitalize has been made, the decision as to which facility the patient should be transferred to is based on the answers to the following questions:

- Is the admission voluntary or involuntary?
- What is the patient's (family's) preference?
- What is the patient's residential address?
- Which facility has catchment area responsibility for the patient?
- What is the nature of the patient's financial coverage for psychiatric hospitalization?
- Who is the patient's current therapist? What is that therapist's institutional affiliation? What is the current status of the therapeutic relationship? What is the judgment of the therapist regarding the decision to hospitalize and, if indicated, where to hospitalize?

By and large, if unwilling to be hospitalized, the patient must be transferred to the acute care institution designated by the New York City Department of Mental Health, Mental Retardation and Alcoholism Services, as having catchment area responsibility for such admissions. If the patient is voluntary and does not have medical insurance coverage for psychiatric hospitalization, the patient also must be transferred to the designated appropriate catchment-area hospital. Voluntary status patients who have third party coverage for inpatient services can be referred to other hospitals, provided psychiatric beds are available, the other institution accepts the transfer, and the patient agrees to the disposition.

Regardless of the particular circumstances, the process of arranging the transfer of a patient to another facility for psychiatric admission is often a tedious, frustrating, and time-consuming task. It involves waiting for admitting psychiatrists and administrators to evaluate their situations, returning telephone calls, reviewing the case, and finally approving the transfer. At Lenox Hill Hospital, the practice of sharing these various aspects of the disposition process among the psychiatric team members has significantly helped to alleviate the pressures of time and the frustration that inevitably accompany the process and has facilitated the flexibility of the team members in returning to their other clinical responsibilities.

The psychiatric residents who rotate through Lenox Hill Hospital find the disposition process especially difficult and burdensome. Normally, their previous clinical rotations were at institutions with segregated inpatient units and ready bed availability. In such institutions, few or no clinical or financial constraints hampered admission. Yet, their experience on emergency call at Lenox Hill, with its many obstacles to easy admission, not infrequently has resulted in creative disposition solutions, especially among those residents with high frustration tolerance levels.

In general, the lack of an on-site inpatient unit to which a majority of psychiatrically hospitalizable emergency patients can be admitted and the considerable logistical effort that must be expended to transfer patients to other facilities have served to motivate Lenox Hill team members to explore alternative treatment avenues. Considerable time is spent interviewing patients, their families, their friends, and involved others in order to assess the feasibility of referring the patient to the Lenox Hill Psychiatric Clinic, to private attendings, or to other community mental health resources. Disposition, as opposed to crisis intervention, is still the principal focus of Lenox Hill ER transactions, but alternatives to hospitalization are thoroughly considered.

CONCLUSION

The utilization of psychiatric emergency services in the United States has increased significantly over the past 20 years.[10] However, growth of adequate programs to meet the increased demand has not kept pace. The inadequacies of the Lenox Hill program are representative of many acute care community hospitals. The staff at Lenox Hill Hospital have attempted to cope with the psychiatric clinical demands of its emergency room by maximizing the utilization of existing salaried staff and recognizing the limitations on involvement of the voluntary attending staff. In considering further programmatic improvements, the four guidelines proposed by Gerson and Bassuk are clearly relevant:

1. Psychiatric emergency services should be organizationally unique treatment facilities, with quiet and comfortable interviewing rooms, their own permanent staff, and distinctive intervention procedures.
2. "Holding units" should be available on a 24-hour basis for more extensive assessment and rapid treatment.
3. Senior attending and salaried staff should be available for teaching and supervision.

4. The principal treatment philosophy should be based on crisis intervention rather than triage.[11]

In the context of these guidelines, but given the inherent fiscal limitations
that impact on psychiatric ER staffing and physical milieu, the following
modest recommendations for improving the psychiatric emergency service
at Lenox Hill and other similarly situated hospitals seem appropriate:

First, a mental health nurse clinician or psychiatric social worker should
be assigned to the emergency room on an exclusive, full-time basis. Sheridan and Teplin found that housing a psychiatry department staff member in
the emergency room produced significant improvements in the recognition
of psychiatric symptoms and referrals for mental health interventions. This
staffing change also significantly reduced the tension and disruption caused
by the entrance of a psychotic patient into the ER milieu.[12]

Second, the process of selecting emergency room clinicians should take
into account the personality attributes (in addition to requisite professional
education and experience) that are important in being able to function
adequately in the ER setting. These attributes include high stress tolerance,
empathy and sensitivity, flexibility, openness to other persons' views, a
good sense of humor, good decision-making skills, emotional control, and
an adaptability to new situations.[13]

Third, liaison support and the education of the emergency room medical
and nursing staff should be emphasized. This includes, but should not be
limited to, participation in a weekly teaching conference, open to all ER
staff, that focuses on the interplay among biological, psychological, and
social factors in the presentations of patients who have been treated
recently. In addition, a core course for new clinicians and continuing
education for veterans should be developed in appropriate aspects of emergency psychiatry, including crisis intervention principles and techniques.
Slaby suggests that an interdisciplinary and intertheoretical approach be
employed to help break down territorial barriers in delivering emergency
psychiatric care.[14] In these educational efforts, Slaby has listed the clinical
areas in which proficiency by ER clinicians should be required. They
include diagnosis and differential diagnosis of behavioral disorders, focused
interviewing under stressful circumstances, mental status testing techniques,
crisis management, and knowledge of mental health resources for provision
of appropriate aftercare by the family, hospital, and community.

Fourth, guidelines must be developed to delineate clearly the clinical
situations for which psychiatric consultation should be requested. An effective emergency room must have access to a competent psychosocial support
system, not only for the needs of the patient population, but also for its own
needs.

In sum, the emergency room of a general hospital is a busy, stressful, and fascinating place. All manner of situations present, and many lifetimes of psychiatric education are available, if one can tolerate the pace and the pressure. Indeed, if mental health clinicians can learn to interview with sensitivity and tact in this milieu, other therapeutic contacts will seem easy by comparison. If mental health professionals can, in such a situation, manage to keep their coolness of thought, remain able to formulate clearly the dimensions of the clinical problems, and develop appropriate intervention and dispositional strategies, all manner of other psychiatric emergencies they may encounter subsequently, no matter what the setting, will surely be grasped with a firmer hand.

REFERENCES

1. L.L. Walker, "Why Do Patients Use the Emergency Room?" *Hospital Topics* 53 (1975).

2. S. Jones, P. Jones, and B. Meisner, "Identification of Patients in Need of Psychiatric Intervention," *Medical Care* 16 (1978).

3. G. Bartolucci and C.S. Prayers, "An Overview of Crisis Intervention in the Emergency Rooms of General Hospitals," *American Journal of Psychiatry* 130 (1973).

4. G. Barton, "Psychiatric Staff and the Emergency Department: Roles, Responsibilities, and Reciprocation," *Psychiatric Clinics of North America* 6 (1983).

5. Ibid., 317.

6. L. Jacoby and S. Jones, "The Psychiatric Clinical Specialist in the Emergency Room," *Journal of Psychosocial Nursing* 22 (1984).

7. D. Aguilera and J. Messick, *Crisis Intervention-Theory and Methodology* (St. Louis, Mo.: C.V. Mosby, 1974).

8. L.R. Marcos and R.M. Gil, "Psychiatry Catchment Areas in an Urban Center: A Policy in Disarray," *American Journal of Psychiatry,* 140 (1984): 876.

9. E. McCarthy, "Resolution of the Psychiatric Emergency in the Emergency Department," *Psychiatric Clinics of North America* 6 (1983).

10. S. Gerson and E. Bassuk, "Psychiatric Emergencies: An Overview," *American Journal of Psychiatry* 137 (January 1980) 1.

11. Ibid., 4.

12. E. Sheridan and L. Teplin, "Evolution of an Emergency Room Psychiatric Staffing," *American Journal of Orthopsychiatry* 52 (1982).

13. M. Elstun and M. Faas, "Psychiatric Emergency Service: A Growing Speciality," *Journal of Psychiatric Nursing and Mental Health Services* (August 1979).

14. A. Slaby, "Emergency Psychiatry in the General Hospital: Staffing, Training, and Leadership Issues," *General Hospital Psychiatry* 3 (1981).

Chapter 6

Teaching Psychiatry in a General Medical Hospital

Loren Skeist, M.D.

INTRODUCTION

Psychiatric training programs have moved steadily into medical settings over the past 75 years. Once predominantly placed in separate "institutes" or "psychopathic" hospitals and state mental institutions, psychiatric training now resides largely in general hospitals, which are often affiliated with community mental health centers.

It is important that psychiatric training programs be located in medical hospitals, in that medical students and medical and psychiatric house staff can thereby learn to combine biological and psychosocial approaches in patient care.[1] This type of close collaboration between psychiatric and medical specialties is particularly important because of the increased sophistication of psychotrophic medications, advances in behavioral and short-term psychotherapies, greater understanding of mind-body interactions, and the increased efforts directed toward primary prevention of diseases. However, most hospitals with psychiatric training programs have segregated psychiatric inpatient units, which causes difficulties for collaborative work between psychiatric and medical-surgical house staff. For example, specialized psychiatric units do not readily accept transfers from general medical floors; and, when they do, continued liaison involvement of the medical house staff is limited (see Chapter 2). Medical house staff are often reluctant to provide consultations to psychiatric patients, and they find it difficult to utilize psychosocial factors in the care of their own patients.[2] Indeed, many psychiatric house staff feel isolated from their medical colleagues and anticipate their consultation-liaison rotation as if they were being dispatched to a hostile country.

Both conceptual and attitudinal differences contribute to the isolation of psychiatric house staff from their medical colleagues. Conceptually, the relationship of mind to body still remains an ambiguous area. Yet, in order to make clinical decisions, data on that relationship must be simplified. For instance, a question that often must be answered is whether a disorder is organic or functional. This of course is a useful clinical question, but its theoretical meaning becomes blurred as evidence indicates organic predispositions for the anxiety, somatoform, and personality disorders as well as for the potentially psychotic mental disorders. Conversely, the view that application of the term *psychosomatic* should be limited to a few specific illnesses has given way to one that accepts the influence of stressful life events and patterns of living on most physical illnesses.

To intervene effectively in clinical situations involving complex mind-body interactions, the clinician must be able to utilize different conceptual levels. For example, the clinician must understand a patient undergoing a psychotic process from several viewpoints: (1) a neurophysiological viewpoint, which considers effective pharmacological agents; (2) a phenomenological approach, which considers the structure of psychotic symptoms as an aid in diagnosis; (3) a psychodynamic approach, which examines the content of the psychotic symptoms to guide the therapist to a deeper understanding of the patient's unconscious mental life; (4) a social viewpoint which can clarify stressful interpersonal events; and (5) a cultural understanding, to help place the patient's model of the world, value systems, and self-expectations in a broader perspective. In most cases, if a comprehensive evaluation approach is adopted, clinicians can intervene effectively on all or most of these levels. (For a description of a theoretical framework that can encompass multilevel evaluations, see the discussions of general systems theory by Von Bertalanffy and Gray, Duhl, and Rizzo.)[3,4]

Attitudinal differences between psychiatry and other medical specialties also present communication barriers in hospitals. Psychiatric house staff may be defensive about the gradual atrophy of their medical skills and knowledge, and they may react by subtly impugning the medical house staffs' presumed lack of humanistic concerns. On the other hand, medical house staff may have little patience for time-consuming interactions with anxious, depressed, or noncooperative patients because they may be unsure of their psychiatric expertise and afraid of making wrong decisions. The constant strain of dealing with patients facing morbidity or mortality often leads to emotional distancing by house staff physicians in order to avoid an intense sharing of emotional pain.[5] Yet the ability to identify temporarily with one's patients is the foundation of empathy.

One way in which medical house staff cope with these problems is to develop interpersonal styles that either downgrade their role or overemphasize their knowledge and authority. However, exaggerating one's knowledge and authority can lead to further self-doubts and fears of being exposed, resulting in increased rigidity and condescension. In any case, the choice of an appropriate interpersonal style is a particularly hazardous undertaking for psychiatric house staff who are unsure of their own clinical effectiveness and skills.

The development of an accurate empathic capability is essential for intervening effectively with a wide range of patients' personalities,[6] as well as for overcoming conceptual and attitudinal barriers among specialists in hospitals. One way in which house staff can enhance their empathic capacity is through increased self-awareness.[7,8] Paradoxically, increased self-awareness involves accepting one's limitations. To the extent that trainees accept having only partial awareness and control over their own psyches, they will better be able to acknowledge uncertainty, mistakes, and feelings that embarrass them.[9] Humane treatment begins with oneself.

Clinicians' realistic expectations of themselves can result in a more accurate appreciation of the limits of their power to change their patients' lives. Accepting these limits will better enable trainees to see themselves as only one component of a medical care team, and as only a subcomponent of the patient's social environment. This awareness will motivate trainees to attempt to extend their therapeutic leverage by recruiting staff, and the patient's family and friends into the treatment plan, instead of feeling threatened by them.

In the following sections, specific techniques for utilizing self-awareness are discussed in the context of:

- introducing third-year medical students to clinical psychiatry
- helping medical house staff to respond to psychiatric illnesses and the intrapsychic and interpersonal needs of their patients
- training psychiatric house staff to treat the biopsychosocial needs of patients on medical floors

THE THIRD-YEAR MEDICAL STUDENT CLERKSHIP

The general hospital offers exceptional opportunities for medical students to learn psychiatry in the setting where they are most likely to use such knowledge in the future. This kind of "state dependent" learning is a powerful aide for both retention and recall of information. For instance, if a student learns to evaluate and treat on a medical floor a depressed diabetic patient who was initially admitted in ketoacidosis because of failure to eat adequately, the student will be more likely to consider depression as a possible contributing cause of poor control over blood sugar in future patients.

Unfortunately, most clerkships are based almost exclusively on segregated psychiatric units. As a result, the students have little or no exposure to psychiatric consultation services on medical floors; the students' most intensive experiences are with major primary psychiatric disorders, such as schizophrenia. Yet, while some exposure to these disorders is necessary, they are the least relevant to the students' future responsibilities as medical clinicians. Clerkships in which the students' primary clinical assignment is to the psychiatric care of medically ill patients have in fact been found to develop better attitudes toward psychiatry while teaching comparable amounts of general psychiatric subjects, as compared with clerkships in which students are assigned to segregated inpatient units.[10-12]

Goals

The educational goals of a psychiatric clerkship can be subdivided into three categories: factual knowledge, skills, and attitudes. (For a detailed description of carefully conceived goals, see Rosen and Blackwell.)[13]

Factual Knowledge

The subjects taught during the four-to-eight week clerkship should be oriented to the needs of the general medical practitioner. They should include both facts relating to the diagnosis and treatment of mental diseases and facts about human personality, the area that is most difficult to objectify. Medical practitioners must understand basic psychiatric phenomenology and the spectrum of mental illness if they are to include psychiatric disorders in the differential diagnoses of their medically ill patients. They must also gain sufficient knowledge of the range of major treatment modalities to make appropriate referrals. Both of these requirements fit well in the medical model of disease, which implies that diseases are linearly caused by specific etiologies. However, dynamic and interpersonal models—utilizing the concepts of intrapsychic conflict, self and object representations, and defensive styles, among others—are needed to understand and describe personality.

Skills

The essential skills to be gained during the psychiatric clerkship include the ability to be tactful with patients and colleagues and to use the resulting professional rapport to elicit systematic psychiatric histories and perform mental status examinations. The history gathering must include both a focused search for diagnostically relevant facts, and a more open-ended, associative search for dynamically relevant biographical information. Associative interviewing allows the patient greater latitude to determine the sequence of topics, and it requires an attitude of active listening rather than probing on the part of the interviewer. Students need to be able to organize the information they have gathered into differential diagnoses, multiaxial diagnostic systems, and dynamic formulations. They must then be able to use that information to propose and implement treatment plans. Finally, they should be able to utilize basic ego-supportive psychotherapy.

Attitudes

Of utmost importance is the cultivation of certain attitudes that prepare the students to address throughout their medical careers the psychosocial aspects of their patients' illnesses. The most desirable such attitude is curiosity about mental phenomena and the subjective experiences of the individual who is ill. This reinforces the second most desirable attitude: a disposition to treat the person who is ill, not just the illness. A third desirable attitude is the acceptance of a constant interaction between mind and body, which implies that emotional factors and psychiatric illnesses should be included in the differential diagnosis of almost all physical symptoms. A final desirable attitude is the view that, while psychiatric symptoms often have meaning and purpose, psychiatric disorders are not consciously chosen and therefore do not result from moral weakness.

Training Techniques

Medical educators rely primarily on their own past experiences in medical school to understand and evaluate students and to provide guidance in what their students need to learn. But how accurately does the medical educator's past experience mirror the experiences of students today? The medical school experience has evolved significantly from what it was a scant five years ago. For example, physicians now are often perceived as members of a self-serving elite rather than of a self-sacrificing profession. Stable, high physician incomes, coupled with an increasing proportion of patients' incomes going toward medical care, contribute to this perception. Moreover, someone attending medical school is now more envied than admired. Gaining entry into medical school has become a goal that students pursue single-mindedly, concentrating on achieving a cumulative college grade point average as close to 4.0 as possible. By the time these students begin medical school, they feel they have just completed a race, and they expect to be welcomed to the winner's circle. Instead they are confronted by two years of basic science courses that primarily tax their ability to memorize.[14] In fact, the explosion in medical knowledge makes a teachable and learnable curriculum more difficult to develop. By the end of the first year, most students have abandoned the ideal of trying to learn everything, or even what they imagine will be most relevant to their medical practices. Instead, they adopt a strategy of learning what they think will be asked on examinations.

While professors often frown on test-oriented learning, a glance at how the basic sciences are taught induces more sympathetic feelings toward such a learning mode. For instance, lectures are apportioned among subspecialized members of a department so that few faculty members are responsible for more than one or two topics. Students quickly realize that they are not their medical school lecturers' first priority. Indeed, the lecturers are often junior faculty who must concentrate instead on producing valid research or risk losing the increasingly scarce grants that support their positions. The result is often an actual decline in empathic capacity during medical school.[15] In fact, interpersonal skills can even regress as the opportunity for social life becomes limited; old friendships are difficult to maintain and new friends difficult to cultivate when so much of a student's time is occupied by studying. Compounding all this, the withdrawal of government support has contributed dramatically to increased tuitions, and payments on student loans must now begin much earlier.

An awareness of the changes in medical school and of the nature of students' expectations enables the educator to bridge potential empathic lapses that may arise when students approach the clerkship with a burden of accumulated frustrations and resentments. Providing students with opportunities to ventilate their frustrations and to gain insight into their own needs and behavior patterns is perhaps the most powerful technique for conveying the importance of responding to patients' emotional frustrations and needs.

The Clinical Setting

A crucial question in the design of the clerkship is where to assign students to do their clinical work. Segregated inpatient units provide students with an ample supply of patients and the support of a highly trained and cohesive team. But every effort should be made to provide the students in such units with additional direct clinical responsibility in the Psychiatric Consultation-Liaison Service and the Psychiatric Outpatient Clinic. These settings provide students with the kinds of patients and problems that they will eventually encounter in their clinical practices.

The consultation-liaison service provides exposure to depressed, anxious, somatoform, organic, and substance-abusing patients, as well as patients with adjustment and personality disorders. Further, the students have the opportunity of focusing on the emotional factors of being in the hospital, undergoing tests, being told a serious diagnosis, and experiencing staff and patient reactions to frightening situations, such as AIDS. The Psychiatric Outpatient Clinic gives students the opportunity to evaluate patients, with the knowledge that, at the conclusion of the evaluation session, the patient will return to an unprotected environment. Having to complete the evaluation in the allotted time sharpens students' interviewing skills and forces them to formulate their impressions and plans quickly. For both clinical and legal reasons, a supervisor must observe the evaluation interview and intervene when indicated. The students must receive substantial clinical and emotional support if they are to assume active roles in treating psychiatrically ill patients in settings where the extensive support structure of the segregated psychiatric unit is absent.

The Case History

Obtaining a psychiatric history challenges students with vital didactic issues. To obtain a history, the students must first establish rapport. Motivating patients to reveal details of their personal lives requires a much greater degree of tact than getting permission to do a physical exam. It is particularly difficult for students to grasp the notion that what a patient reports may be a defensively motivated reweaving of events that must be unraveled to obtain an objective picture of what actually occurred. Thus, tact in a psychiatric interview does not mean routinely respecting a patient's avoidance of painful topics; rather it means making it clear that the interviewer is interested and will be supportive if the patient is willing to share painful topics. In such situations, the most sensitive students often have the most difficulty in obtaining the necessary objectivity. The positive aspects of students' overidentifications should thus be underscored, since empathy is developed through identification.

Supervisors can help students structure their history taking by providing specific strategies and tasks. A key task is to obtain histories with enough detail in order to be able to reconstruct sequences of events in the patients' lives with all their attendant effects. To determine which events need to be reconstructed in detail, students should be instructed to look for significant changes in a patient's life. If a symptom occurs concurrently with a life stress, a causal linkage is suggested.

As students search for the causes and effects of life changes, they will be confronted with patients' inabilities to discuss their motivations and reactions. Patients' inabilities to relate important aspects of painful events reveal the existence of resistances and defenses, which should alert students to attend to both what the patients are willing to relate and what they are not able to describe. A helpful strategy is for the students to utilize verbal and nonverbal cues to make a trial identification, that is, to temporarily "walk in the patients' shoes." The more students are able to experience events in a patient's life from the patient's point of view, the more "three-dimensional" their histories of patients will become. To aid in making trial identifications, the students can be instructed to ask themselves such questions as, "How would I have felt if that had happened to me?" or "What would I have done in that situation?" and then to compare their own reactions to what the patient reports feeling or doing. This comparison can help the student gain insight into hidden aspects of the patient's life events, which can then guide the student to inquire about particular feelings the patient may not have reported.

Multiaxial Diagnosis

The next step is to develop a DSM III multiaxial diagnosis. A differential diagnosis (Axis I) is similar to a differential diagnosis for medically ill patients, with one important difference: The lack of definitive diagnostic tests makes psychiatric diagnoses less certain than medical diagnoses. Thus, students need to make diagnostic and treatment decisions with an open mind regarding alternative diagnoses.[16] To formulate a personality diagnosis (Axis II), students must learn to recognize recurrent patterns of behavior and to distinguish pathological degrees of variation from the norm. Careful review of past and present object relations, including the relationship of the patient to the student, usually enables the students to see both the similarities and the differences between their own personality traits and those of their patients. Medical conditions (Axis III) must be carefully considered, both as contributing stresses and as factors affecting treatment. Evaluating the degree of the patient's current life stress (Axis IV) and best level of functioning in the past year (Axis V) depends upon having elicited a clear history of present illness.

Dynamic Formulation

Finally, the dynamic formulation should try to describe the current intrapsychic and interpersonal conflict in terms of precipitating events and predisposing personality factors. The student should be instructed on how to pull together many disparate observations into a coherent statement regarding the patient's overall mental functioning, and to answer the question "Why did this patient with this personality become ill in this manner at this time?"

Educators must frequently evaluate their students' progress and also provide opportunities for them to evaluate the quality of the educators' teaching. Students are better able to learn and accept criticism if they feel that their needs and criticisms of the program are respected. It is especially useful to supplement weekly in-house reviews of the program with mid-clerkship evaluation sessions in which students are asked to express criticism of the rotation to someone who is not personally involved in the program's administration. Evaluation of the students should be sought from nonmedical as well as medical staff. In this way, a better sense of the students' ability to work with nonauthority figures can be obtained and respect for nonphysician staff can be fostered. Students' deficits should be clearly communicated as early as possible during the clerkship; poor performance is often a disguised request for help, and considerable growth can occur when students feel the criticisms are accurate.

In sum, a consistent approach to evaluation and treatment, one that relies on the development of curiosity and empathy, is needed in the clinical setting.

PSYCHIATRIC TRAINING FOR MEDICAL-SURGICAL HOUSE STAFF

Goals

In a review of the literature, Houpt et al. found that 20–80 percent of medically ill patients have significant emotional symptoms.[17] In this context, several attempts have been made to delineate psychiatric educational goals for primary care physicians.[18-20] The guiding principle in these efforts is relevance to primary medical practice.

Factual Knowledge

The relevant information includes a working knowledge of the panoply of psychiatric phenomenology and illness and detailed knowledge of the syndromes that present with physical symptoms,[21] have physical side effects, or are seen in reaction to physical illness. Primary care physicians should be aware of the main therapeutic modalities in order to make individualized referrals. They should have detailed knowledge of the classes of psychotropic medications, of their side effects and interactions, and of indications and contraindications. Finally, they should be aware of personality issues that can complicate medical care.[22,23]

The establishment of clear standards or psychiatric normality is essential in order to detect subtle degrees of pathology. In psychiatry, the establishment of a normal standard is particularly difficult because of the vagueness of the symptoms and the intrusion of personal reactions and values. House staff must be helped to develop a standard of normality if they are to avoid the most common type of error in medicine: failure to recognize that a problem exists.[24] Failure to recognize a problem is particularly common when the problem is regarded as, in itself, anxiety producing, or when the intervention is unfamiliar, emotionally draining, and time-consuming. A good example of this is the task of exploring for suicidal intent. A patient who has overdosed obviously needs to be evaluated regarding continued suicidal potential. On the other hand, a patient with chronic hypertension whose blood pressure has increased markedly might not be suspected of intentionally violating dietary restrictions.

Cohen-Cole et al. conducted a needs assessment on medical outpatients and cited the following areas in which increased educational effort is needed:

- recognition and treatment of emotional disorders
- evaluation and management of negative life events
- communication with patients concerning their diagnoses and treatment
- elicitation and recording of psychosocial history and mental status[25]

Skills

The ability to obtain a psychosocial history depends upon skillful, tactful interviewing.[26,27] House staff must be able to appreciate the patient's point of view in order to ask questions that are relevant, nonjudgmental, and caring. They should be able to obtain a chronological history of present illness that integrates life events, disturbances of interpersonal relationships, and symptom development.

Of particular importance is the ability to recognize and elicit patients' reactions to illness and treatment and to utilize these reactions to develop individualized treatment plans. Ego-supportive therapeutic techniques are helpful in exploring these issues, since patients are unlikely to share painful effects unless the interviewer is able to help place them in a comprehensible, reality-oriented context. In responding to patients' sadness or fear, untrained house staff may deal with their own anxiety by offering premature and superficial reassurance. When this occurs, the patient's sense of isolation can unwittingly be intensified.

Finally, it is important that physicians be able to motivate their patients' to explore their own affective lives. This serves to foster optimal therapeutic alliances with the patients. It also increases the physicians' ability to influence the patients' maladaptive habits, noncompliance, and general mental health.

Korsch has summarized certain practical approaches in communicating interest in one's patients:

- Find out what the patient's worries are. Do not confine yourself merely to gathering medical information.
- Determine what the patient's expectations are. If they cannot be met, explain why.
- Provide information about the diagnosis and the cause of the illness.
- Adopt a friendly rather than a business-like attitude.
- Avoid medical jargon.
- Spend some time on nonmedical topics.[28]

Attitudes

As noted earlier, an underlying attitude that house staff need to develop is that their role is to treat patients, not just illnesses. House staff can benefit considerably if they are able to accept their reactions to patients as important signals of crucial interpersonal events, influenced by the transference needs of their patients. If house staff are unable to accept their reactions to their patients' transference needs in this way, they risk acting out their patients' early, often sadomasochistic, transference relationships. When detected in a timely manner, however, these same reactions provide the opportunity for a deep appreciation of the patient's interpersonal needs and point the way toward individualized treatment plans.

The following case points up the importance of developing sensitive interpersonal attitudes toward patients. A medical resident was trying to help a 28-year-old woman who suffered from chronic pain. He extended himself considerably, even arranging to spend extra time talking with her during his outpatient clinic time. Referral to psychiatry was resisted by the patient. A crisis developed when the patient called in acute distress and the resident recommended that she come to the emergency room. When she arrived, the emergency staff paged the resident, who then left a major teaching conference. Before the resident got to the emergency room, the patient had abruptly left with the message that "I've waited long enough." Embarrassed and insulted, the resident looked for ways to terminate their relationship. In a subsequent discussion with a psychiatric consultant, the resident had an opportunity to express his resentment and was then able to recognize how his desire to be liked and admired by this patient had led to his own failure to set appropriate limits. As a result, the resident was subsequently able to establish a more effective therapeutic relationship with the patient.

Training Techniques

The teaching of psychiatry can occur most effectively when actual patient care is involved, as in psychiatric consultations.[29] All too often, psychiatric consultants limit their involvement with house staff to communications through progress notes in the medical charts. This tendency must be counteracted by redefining the consultant's role to include both the training of house staff and their enlistment in the treatment process.[30] Consultants should make a special effort to communicate in person with the house staff. Under supervision, house staff are usually eager to examine mental status, discuss procedures and test results, obtain histories from relatives and friends, and follow the side effects of medications. They usually welcome the opportunity to hear the consultant's impressions and to contribute their own observations.

Conversely, consultants can benefit from the house staff's more current medical knowledge. One danger here is that the psychiatric consultant may adopt a critical role toward house staff and ward personnel. This may occur because the consultant is not personally involved in managing a provocative patient. By appearing to be reasonable and empathic toward the patient, the consultant may represent an unattainable ego ideal and thus increase house staff's guilt and defensiveness.

The challenge is to help the house staff gain a perspective on their own affective responses, which may help them appreciate their patients' motivations. Another useful way of understanding motivations is to view the current relationships of patients as attempts to re-create crucial aspects of previous relationships. Often a brief description of a patient's childhood suffices to undo a medical house staff judgmental response to a provocative patient; it is difficult to be angry at a provocative patient after one has discovered how the patient suffered as a child.

Formal psychiatric teaching can be arranged in lectures or conferences. House staff's interest in liaison conferences can be maintained by interviews with patients that explore affectively charged areas and thus enable house staff to understand their patients in a more three-dimensional way. Issues of personal relevance—such as reactions to patients or dissatisfactions with the hospital—can also be actively solicited by the psychiatric consultant.

Another very useful approach is for a medical attending to join a psychiatrist for joint medical-psychiatric case conferences. Seeing interspecialty collaboration carries much more weight than just hearing about it.[31]

The Clinical Setting

The outpatient medical clinic setting provides medical residents the opportunity to follow patients for two to three years. When residents have such long-term relationships with their patients, diagnostic and acute management issues become less prominent and other issues become important: the patients' attitudes toward illness, their medications, and their physicians; compliance; and the relationship of medical illnesses to life stress. The residents are confronted with both their patients' and their own personality limitations as they work to establish collaborative relationships. An excellent model for psychiatric training in this setting is described by an attending psychiatrist observing residents' ongoing treatment of their patients and intervening when necessary. After the patient is seen, the attending psychiatrist discusses both the patient and the interview style of the resident. In the clinic setting, the enthusiastic support of medical attending is critical.

The emergency room offers exposure to more acute psychiatric disorders, such as panic states, acute conversion disorders, suicidal and homicidal states, confusional states, drug intoxication and withdrawal, psychotic states, and many others. However, a major problem in most emergency rooms is the inordinate time pressure and the need to give lower priority to the assessment of nonlife-threatening conditions. Still, even with these constraints, vital learning can occur if the staff is provided with techniques for rapid psychiatric assessment. The techniques must be simple, effective, and broadly applicable if they are going to be assimilated by preoccupied house staff. For example, the following questions would quickly screen for major psychosocial changes and stresses:

- Who are the most important people in the patient's life?
- What has happened to these relationships over the past six months?
- How has the patient's work status and living situation changed recently?

These questions should be supplemented by a simple but comprehensive mental status exam that screens for organicity, affective state (including suicidal and homicidal potential), psychosis, and judgment. Any history of serious loss (including loss of health) or self-destructive behavior (including noncompliance) demands a careful exploration for suicidal ideation.

Impulsive, destructive acts raise suspicions of homicidal ideation. With the same priority as learning cardiac pulmonary resuscitation (CPR), medical house staff should be motivated to learn about managing psychotic, violent, acting-out, and suicidal patients. Patients' potential for violence is a major preoccupation of emergency personnel, despite the relative infrequency of its occurrence. Training emergency personnel to deal with the potentially violent patient reduces anxiety and minimizes the chance of someone being injured while trying to be a "hero." Also, managing a violent patient provides a useful opportunity to direct residents' attention to their own reactions to fear and to being provoked. When fear is equated with cowardice, the fear may have to be denied through unnecessary risk-taking. By emphasizing that fear is a sensitive signal of the presence of danger, house staff are enabled to use anxiety adaptively, to indicate a situation that must be approached cautiously. As house staff become more comfortable in sharing their fears, they can be helped to see that violent patients are themselves usually afraid of losing control and of being hurt. This will minimize overly punitive reactions.

Another appropriate clinical area in which to concentrate psychiatric teaching is the neurology service.[32] Especially for the more medically oriented house staff, demonstrating the subtle behavioral effects of brain lesions can stimulate interest in behavior and cognition that might not have been elicited if these states were seen merely as the result of functional (that is, "not real") disorders. Frontal lobe syndromes, complex partial seizures, hemi-inattention, the "aprosodies" (inability to sense or express effect), reactions to brain injury, and conversion symptoms are but some of the fascinating entities that lend themselves to psychiatric teaching. A video library is particularly important when teaching neurology, since cognitive and movement abnormalities are complex, difficult to describe, and extremely varied. The sodium-amylobarbitone interview is also pertinent to the neurology service setting,[33] as are hypnotic techniques. Since almost all house staff value highly their own cognitive functioning, they tend to react strongly to neurological disability and to be willing to consider psychiatric aspects.

Psychiatric educators are more effective when they are attentive to and show respect for the house staff, even when the latter come late to conferences or make derogatory comments about "shrinks." The manner in which medical house staff treat psychiatrists reveals much about how they feel they themselves are being treated. Educators should keep in mind that extensive service requirements limit house staffs' normal social and physical outlets. Monthly changes in assignment decrease the satisfaction inherent in treating patients and working with colleagues. Little opportunity for socialization is available during the long days; lunch hours give way to luncheon conferences. House staff autonomy is further infringed upon by what seem to be arbitrary abuses of attending and bureaucratic power. Inefficiencies seem difficult to correct. Even the house staff's desire to learn may conflict with their own sense of fairness and altruism as they compete to do procedures and admit unusual cases. Yet, psychiatric educators can utilize these frustrations to deepen house staff's awareness of how psychosocial factors can impact on their own lives.[34] The staffs' own self-awareness can then be applied to deepen their appreciation of psychosocial factors in their patients' lives.

CONSULTATION-LIAISON TRAINING FOR PSYCHIATRIC RESIDENTS

Almost all psychiatric residency training programs in general or psychiatric hospitals begin with a 6- to 12-month rotation on a segregated psychiatric inpatient unit. This arrangement is beneficial for residents despite the apparent incongruity of assigning the least experienced staff to treat the most severely ill patients. Inpatient units are one of the few settings in which experienced mental health staff can work intensively with residents and supervise them on a daily basis. Experience with psychotic states and the major affective disorders enhances the residents' judgment and therefore their ability to handle psychiatric emergencies. Also, treating severe psychiatric disorders helps consolidate the residents' professional identities, since dramatic results are often possible and the boundaries between physician and patient are clear.

The situation changes when residents are assigned to the consultation-liaison service. Psychiatric residents and supervisors experience their greatest difficulties in working on medical-surgical floors with physically ill patients and nonpsychiatrically trained or oriented staff.[35] These difficulties stem both from the nature of the medical setting and the problems for which consultations are requested. Psychiatric house staff feel isolated and vulnerable on medical floors, yet are expected to produce rapid solutions to complex problems. The problems themselves are more often seen by the medical staff as obstacles to treatment of medical illness than as illnesses worthy of treatment in their own right. Medical staff also may be unfamiliar with the terminology used by mental health professionals. And they may resent treatment recommendations that require additional time or special treatment or reveal nontherapeutic actions that have been taken by staff.

Often, psychotic patients exhibit provocative behavior that invites retaliation and requires unusually mature staff to respond in a nonpunitive way. The following case illustrates such a situation. A 26-year-old man with schizotypal and narcissistic personality traits was bedridden from back injuries received during an attempted suicide. The patient demanded more pain medication. His grandiose, demanding attitude contributed to the staff's passive resistance to suggestions that they approach him at frequent, regularly scheduled intervals. One nurse justified her attitude by saying "He caused his own pain; I don't have to take care of him for that."

The clinical problems for which psychiatric consultations are requested differ from the problems the residents have previously managed. While medically ill patients often have definable psychiatric conditions, the immediate problem is often management of aberrant behavior rather than diagnosis and treatment of the underlying illness. In these situations, the resident is asked to function as an agent of social control—albeit usually for "the patient's own good." Despite the best of intentions, the resident is placed in a dilemma. How can the resident develop a therapeutic alliance when the primary task is to convince the patient to do something that the patient does not want to do? To complicate matters further, either for medical or insurance reasons, an atmosphere of emergency usually envelopes the evaluation process. A sudden breakdown in the disposition plan, noncompliance with urgent diagnostic and treatment procedures, or bizarre behavior that is upsetting to other patients and staff—all demand quick resolutions. In the resident's previous assignment to a segregated inpatient service, emergencies were generally handled by either heavy sedation or physical restraint.

In contrast, a patient's refusal of treatment for an acute medical illness or refusal to abide by the strict behavioral limitations placed on medical inpatients create parameters in a consultation emergency that are quite novel for the psychiatric trainee. Nurses on medical floors often ask for advice on how to gain a patient's cooperation in such tasks as eating or hygiene or how to limit screaming or frequent calling for the staff. In these situations, residents may feel they are stretching the limits of both their training and ingenuity. While they have been trained to utilize behavior as a guide to diagnosis and treatment, they have also been trained to minimize manipulation of patients' behavior in order to preserve the treatment alliance and encourage the patients' autonomy. In response to a request to evaluate a noncompliant patient, the resident typically approaches the patient hoping that the problem will be resolved when a specific psychiatric illness is discovered and treated. Unfortunately, in such a case, an excellent diagnostic work-up with specific treatment suggestions may fail to address the immediate management issue on the ward.

In addition to the difficulties of social enforcement, the psychiatric consultant faces many patients who are seriously medically ill. Residents have been trained to help patients distinguish fantasy from reality, and even to explore distortions of reality induced by intrapsychic conflict or affective swings, but this training does not adequately prepare residents to help patients cope with a major, "quality-of-life"-threatening illness. When working with such patients, the residents may easily develop a sense of futility and inadequacy. Helping a patient prepare for death requires both a nonresentful view of one's own death and the maintenance of a caring relationship with the patient while simultaneously preparing for the patient's death.

Goals

Several descriptions of comprehensive educational goals for psychiatric residencies have been advanced.[36,37] Other, more specific, goals have been suggested for consultation-liaison training and, recently, a list of basic readings addressing these specific goals has been prepared.[38–40] These goals are reflected in the following discussion of factual knowledge, skills, and attitudes in the consultation-liaison training of psychiatric residents.

Factual Knowledge

Effective consultation-liaison work is based upon a thorough knowledge of psychiatric symptoms, syndromes, and treatment modalities. Beyond that, a consideration of the many different factors that may affect a patient's condition (biologic, phenomenologic, dynamic, cultural) may yield a more comprehensive diagnosis.[41,42] Finally, a probability approach to differential diagnosis will help the resident avoid premature closure and commitment to an initial impression.[43]

In using the latter technique, the clinician first decides on the range of possible diagnoses. An approximate probability that it is the correct one is then assigned to each diagnosis. The diagnosis with the highest probability becomes the working hypothesis, and treatment based on that diagnosis may be initiated. Additional history, test results, and response to treatment are used to modify the original probabilities. This approach encourages residents to remain open-minded about alternative diagnoses and discourages them from becoming narcissistically attached to their first impressions.

Multilevel evaluations require sufficient medical knowledge to review medical charts and to evaluate laboratory tests. Expertise is also required to utilize specialized diagnostic procedures, such as general psychological and neuropsychological tests,[44] endocrine tests, neurological tests, and the sodium-amylobarbitone interview. Certain syndromes need to be mastered in great depth because their presenting symptoms may be atypical and the underlying disorder may be masked by concurrent somatic conditions. For example, affective disorders may present with back pain or anxiety symptoms. Organic disorders, both diffuse (dementias and deliria) and focal (frontal lobe, partial complex seizures, aprosodies, aphasias, learning disabilities, postconcussion syndromes, and so on), often present with complex mixtures of personality, affective, and cognitive changes.

The resident should be able to distinguish the major types of dementia and be particularly alert to reversible etiologies. Familiarity with the varied presentations and etiologies of delirious states is essential, since delirium can be an unrecognized medical emergency if the patient's disordered behavior has been ascribed to a functional cause. Substance abuse is common, yet difficult to detect without an intimate knowledge of the subtypes and the clinical course of the addictions. Somatoform disorders must also be included in many differentials, together with the factitious disorders and malingering. The anxiety disorders, which frequently present with physical symptoms, may both exacerbate and be exacerbated by physical illnesses. Subtle, low-grade paranoid disorders are common in patients with poor compliance and accusatory, litigious behavior. While the DSM III multiaxial diagnostic and formulation system represents a major step forward and is useful for certain psychiatric disorders, Leigh et al. have proposed an alternative "comprehensive medical model of the patient," the patient evaluation grid, which may be more suited to most clinical situations seen by residents on consultation-liaison rotations.[45]

Skills

A wide range of evaluation and intervention skills should be made available to the resident. The resident's first priority is to develop and maintain a therapeutic alliance with the person who requested the consultation. When that person is the patient or the patient's family, the task does not differ from that of the usual psychiatric evaluation. When medical staff initiate the psychiatric intervention, the maintenance of a therapeutic alliance with the patient may be more difficult, especially if the patient is not informed of the consultation request. The latter case is an exception to usual medical practice but is often justified by staff due to their concern that the patient would feel insulted or frightened and would refuse the consultation if given the option. In such situations, it is helpful to utilize the concept of "identified patient" to help the resident maintain an open mind concerning the source and nature of the problem. The resident must enquire about the nature of the staff's reluctance to inform the patient but must also be aware that unconscious factors that operate in everyone at all times might have colored the staff's perception of the patient. The staff may be correct in anticipating that the patient would be insulted. However, their judgment that the patient would be insulted may just as likely have resulted from a displacement of the staff members' fears that their own insensitivity or inadequacy would be exposed.

In such circumstances, without an effective working alliance with medical colleagues, the resident's efforts to help the patient will be severely hampered. How many times has a psychiatric consultant returned for a necessary follow-up visit only to find the patient was prematurely discharged? Premature discharges cannot be dismissed simply as the inevitable consequences of medical colleagues' hostilities toward psychosocial issues. They may reflect the psychiatric resident's failure to address the difficult issue of the interaction between a patient and the patient's medical treatment team. In such a situation, given the fact that, in a hospital psychiatric and medical house staff develop personal and professional relationships with one another, confronting a colleague's behavior toward a patient is often like trying to do family therapy on one's own family.

Having established an alliance with the person who referred the patient, the resident must then try to develop a therapeutic alliance with the identified patient. Here, when exploring sensitive issues like substance abuse, the resident may seem more like an interrogator than a therapist. The educator must point out any judgmental trends displayed by the resident and any tendency by the resident to minimize or oversimplify the patient's self-destructive and manipulative behavior. Patients who have developed physical symptoms because they are unable to express their feelings verbally may view any attempt to uncover psychosocial stresses as an accusation that they are not really sick. The educator must underline the importance of not depriving the patient of a necessary symptom until a firm relationship is established and the context of the symptom is understood.

The mental status examination may be perceived as a threat by certain patients with impaired cognitive function and thus must be performed flexibly, with unusual tact and active reassurance. Setting aside sufficient time for terminating the interview will decrease anxiety and help to establish trust, since unresolved issues tend to become distorted and exaggerated when the patient is once again alone. Major themes should be summarized, subsequent steps discussed, time for questions allowed, and fears eased as much as possible. Residents should be encouraged to supplement individual sessions with family sessions to obtain further history and first-hand experience with the patient's support system. The resident should also be alerted to delicate issues of confidentiality.

Attitudes

The challenges of consultation-liaison work demand concern, optimism, and a sense that one can positively affect one's environment and oneself. A resident should be able to look at the positive side, noting what a patient has lost but focusing on what the patient still has and can enjoy. Consistent efforts to deal openly with major losses and disappointments helps to sustain a sense of meaning to the cycle of life and death. A resident's interest in the current priorities in a patient's life, no matter how trivial they seem, may help to restore the patient's self-respect while the patient spends long hours to accomplish basic tasks of self-care. For example, a resident's willingness to become involved in such unappealing issues as bowel care may be the most effective way of communicating concern and boosting the patient's morale. A full appreciation of the extent of a patient's loss, bitterness, and fear helps the resident to maintain a positive attitude, even when faced with provocative or accusatory behavior by the patient.

Training Techniques

The opportunity to function both as a consultant and as a liaison psychiatrist should be provided. The basic liaison experience is most often with a general medical service. However, a specialized liaison assignment to neurology can provide particularly rich and relevant exposure to issues of brain function and conversion symptoms.[46] The resident should also have the opportunity to provide consultations in varied settings, for example, critical care settings, such as the intensive or cardiac care units; chronic-care services, such as renal dialysis; oncology; and surgery. To ensure exposure to a variety of case material, the maintenance of a patient list and regular review of it with the training director are suggested.

Continuing to work with patients after they are discharged is worthwhile, but it is seldom used as an opportunity to deepen the educational experience afforded by the consultation rotation. The rapid turnover of patients on medical floors limits both the therapeutic goals and the chance to evaluate the efficacy of one's interventions. However, individual or group therapy for discharged patients in the psychiatric outpatient clinic should be encouraged. Home visits and follow-up visits to nursing homes are also useful adjuncts to the training experience.

The Clinical Setting

Supervision

The optimal balance between autonomy and supervision will vary with the resident and the setting. Particularly in consultation-liaison services, the potential for isolation from one's psychiatric support system must be countered by the provision of peer interaction and adequate supervision. A clinical load of five to ten patients permits sufficient diversity and provides opportunity for in-depth work.

A variety of supervisory experiences should be made available to residents. The resident should have one primary supervisor scheduled for at least two to three sessions each week for the purpose of exploring the resident's reactions to patients. This should be done in the context of intensive, short-term psychotherapy with selected patients. Daily walking rounds with an attending can provide the resident with immediate clinical back-up and can give the supervisor ongoing feedback regarding the resident's performance. Subspecialty supervision in psychopharmacology is highly beneficial, since the use of psychopharmacological agents in medically ill patients is particularly complex. Similarly, behaviorally oriented supervision is relevant to patient management, compliance, and habit modification.

Supervising staff should be alert to the potential for avoidance to be used as a defensive response. Escaping observation is much easier on consultation than it is on an inpatient unit. Such avoidance may be global, as in a failure to answer any calls or provide follow-up, in which case detection is immediate and confrontation swift. Or it may be subtle, as in limiting interventions to medication advice.

A variety of supervisory techniques can enhance residents' learning. Supervision should include some direct observation of the resident's work with patients. Videotaping sessions can give visual feedback about nonverbal as well as verbal communications. Audiotapes are less absorbing and informative, but they are more convenient to obtain and less intrusive on the interview. The more traditional use of process notes remains a worthwhile technique, but it requires the same amount of time as the interview. An often overlooked source of material for supervision is the actual written consultation and subsequent progress notes. They have immediate clinical relevance, and the trainee will likely view them more as a help than as an additional burden. In addition, use of progress notes challenges the supervisor to confront the complex diagnostic and management issues that might be overlooked in supervision based on five minutes of an audiotape.

The writing of effective psychiatric consultation reports is comparable to condensing a novel to a short story. A clear sense of the purpose of the consultation will determine what information should be included. The differential diagnosis requires the recording of pertinent historical and phenomenological data, and effective management requires noting important aspects of the individual's personality, social environment, and recent life events. The formulation of the case demonstrates the resident's ability to use the information in a thoughtful and logical manner.

In reviewing consultations, the supervisor should evaluate whether the resident has understood and responded to the initial reason for the consultation request.[47] Has the chronological development of the clinical picture been elicited? Has its relationship to events in the patient's life been established? Have relevant alternative diagnoses been considered and recommendations for further evaluation made? Has the resident obtained sufficient premorbid history to derive a sense of the patient's personality? Finally, have specific treatment suggestions been made? Medication suggestions should be appropriately tailored but should rarely be the only modality employed. Psychotherapy should be directed toward a particular area of conflict; and its methodology, duration, and frequency should be specified. Environmental strategies should also be considered.

The review of progress notes is often helpful. However, progress notes are rarely reviewed because the notes are not copied and the original notes remain on the chart. Other drawbacks to such review are the uncertainty regarding the amount of detail to be included in the progress notes, the difficulty of organizing historical data as they emerge each day, and problems of dealing with issues of confidentiality and liability.

Concern about confidentiality should be encouraged, since many people have access to medical charts. A useful initial guideline is for residents to write their notes on the assumption that their patients are going to read them. In this way, because the residents view their communications from the vantage of their patients, tactless statements can be minimized and empathy can be developed. Concern about liability should also be encouraged. When supervisors are reminded that they are legally responsible for their trainees' actions, they become more motivated to ensure that clinical problems are accurately noted and that relevant interventions are undertaken and justified.

Evaluation of Residents

Several innovative approaches to the evaluation of residents have been suggested.[48,49] A readily available, informal source of information regarding residents' performance is the nonmedical staff. For many reasons, nursing staff are ideally situated to recognize patients' psychosocial needs and to evaluate whether psychiatric consultants are responding effectively. Patients usually develop good rapport with floor nurses, and residents can gain useful feedback from such nurses to evaluate themselves and their patients.

Psychiatric residents must be helped to take criticism seriously, but they should not be scapegoated for internal ward or hospital political struggles. Once criticism has surfaced, it should be discussed openly with the resident. This should usually be followed by discussions between the resident and the source of the criticism. Such discussions must be approached nondefensively if they are to lead to the residents' professional growth and flexibility. In such situations, the residents will tend to be less defensive if their supervisors make it clear they appreciate the complexity of the task facing the residents and are trying to help them achieve their full potential.

SUMMARY

In efforts by psychiatric educators to enhance the abilities of medical students and residents to evaluate and treat the psychosocial needs of their patients in a general hospital setting, techniques must be developed to reinforce humanistic approaches to patient care. The general hospital is the ideal setting in which to develop such approaches. Trainees' intrapsychic resources and interpersonal skills should be challenged by focusing on treating the patient who is ill, not just the illness itself. Access to the emotional lives of one's patients depends crucially upon empathy, which requires an awareness of one's own emotional responses. A difficulty in maintaining empathy, overly intense identifications with or reactions to patients, and a lack of curiosity about the patients' lives are all sensitive indicators of intrapsychic rigidity and defensiveness. To counteract trainees' emotional distancing, personality limitations, and weaknesses, humanistic approaches to patients and patients' caretakers are essential.

The training director's responsibility is to help trainees achieve their potential as people, not just as medical technicians. Supervisors must address, not just what a trainee is failing to grasp, but why the trainee is having such difficulty. In-depth evaluations are a natural extension of the educators' efforts to encourage trainees' interest in and awareness of their reactions to patients. As long as the supervisor and trainee understand that confidentiality is limited and that the supervisor is responsible for evaluating the trainee, open discussion of strengths and difficulties offers the best chance for trainees to increase their emotional and behavioral repertoire.

The role of psychiatry in addressing the psychosocial environment of the general hospital itself should also be emphasized. Psychiatric educators should be active in creating support groups for house staff, developing effective programs for impaired physicians and staff burn-out, and designing preventive approaches to mental health. The concern demonstrated by psychiatric staff for the mental health of trainees will help to establish a receptive environment for increasing trainees' motivation to intervene effectively in the psychosocial spheres of their patients' lives.

REFERENCES

1. G.L. Engel, "The Biopsychosocial Model and the Education of Health Professionals," *General Hospital Psychiatry* 1 (1979).

2. D. Goldberg, "Mental Health Priorities in a Primary Care Setting," *Annals of the New York Academy of Science* 310 (1978).

3. L. Von Bertalanffy, "General System Theory and Psychiatry," in *American Handbook of Psychiatry*, vol. 3, ed. S. Arieti (New York: Basic Books, 1966).

4. W. Gray, F.J. Duhl, and N.D. Rizzo, *General Systems Theory and Psychiatry* (Boston: Little, Brown & Co., 1969).

5. A.S. Trillin, "Of Dragons and Garden Peas: A Cancer Patient Talks to Doctors," *New England Journal of Medicine* 304 (19 March 1981): 12.

6. G. Bibring and R. Kahana, *Lectures in Medical Psychology* (New York: 1968).

7. R. Gorlin and H.D. Zucker, "Physicians' Reactions to Patients: A Key to Teaching Humanistic Medicine," *New England Journal of Medicine* 308 (1983).

8. A. Margulies, "Toward Empathy: The Uses of Wonder," *American Journal of Psychiatry* 141 (September 1984).

9. D. Hilfiker, "Sounding Board: Facing Our Mistakes," *New England Journal of Medicine* 310 (12 January 1984).

10. F.P. McKegney and S. Weiner, "A Consultation-Liaison Psychiatry Clinical Clerkship," *Pyschosomatic Medicine* 38 (1976).

11. W.W. Weddington et al., "Consultation-Liaison versus Other Psychiatry Clerkships: A Comparison of Learning Outcomes and Student Reactions," *American Journal of Psychiatry* 135 (1978).

12. C.S. Orleans et al., "Traditional vs. Consultation-Liaison Psychiatry Clerkships: A Closer Look," *Journal of Psychiatric Education* 5 (1981).

13. D.H. Rosen and B. Blackwell, "Teaching Psychiatry in Medicine." *Archives of Internal Medicine* 142 (1982).

14. T.J. Gaensbauer and G.L. Mizner, "Developmental Stresses in Medical Education," *Psychiatry* 43 (February 1980).

15. R.A. Diseker and R. Michielutte, "An Analysis of Empathy in Medical Students Before and Following Clinical Experience," *Journal of Medical Education* 56 (December 1981).

16. R.C. Fox, "Training for Uncertainty," in *The Student-Physician,* ed. R.K. Merton, G.G. Reader, and P.L. Kendall (Cambridge, Mass.: Harvard University Press, 1957).

17. J. Houpt et al., "The Role of Psychiatric and Behavioral Factors in the Practice of Medicine," *American Journal of Psychiatry* 137 (1980).

18. U.S. Department of Health and Human Services, *Report to the NIMH Work Group on Mental Health Training of Primary Care Providers* (Washington, D.C.: U.S. Government Printing Office, 1977).

19. Z.J. Lipowski, "Consultation-Liaison Psychiatry: Past Failures and New Opportunities," *General Hospital Psychiatry* 1 (1979).

20. J.P. Schemo et al., "Psychiatry as an Internal Medicine Subspecialty: An Educational Mode," *Journal of Medical Education* 55 (April 1980).

21. D. Lipsitt, "Medical and Psychological Characteristics of 'Crocks,' " *Psychiatry in Medicine* 1 (1970).

22. J. Groves, "Taking Care of the Hateful Patient," *New England Journal of Medicine* 298 (1978).

23. D.A. Drossman, "The Problem Patient: Evaluation and Care of Medical Patients with Psychosocial Disturbances," *Annals of Internal Medicine* 88 (1978).

24. J. Marks, D. Goldberg, and V. Hillier, "Determinants of the Ability of General Practitioners To Detect Psychiatric Illness," *Psychological Medicine* 9 (1979).

25. S.A. Cohen-Cole et al., "Psychiatric Education for Primary Care: A Pilot Study of Needs of Residents," *Journal of Medical Education* 57 (December 1982).

26. F.W. Platt and J.C. McMata, "Clinical Hypocompetence: The Interview," *Annals of Internal Medicine* 91 (1979).

27. E. Schildkrout, "Medical Residents' Difficulty in Learning and Utilizing a Psychosocial Perspective," *Journal of Medical Education* 55 (November 1980).

28. B. Korsch, B. Freeman, and V. Negrete, "Practical Implications of Doctor/Patient Interactions," 121 (1971).

29. C.P. Kimball, "The Clinical Case Method in Teaching Comprehensive Approaches to Illness Behavior," *Psychosomatic Medicine* 37 (1975).

30. H.A. Pincus et al., "Models of Mental Health Training in Primary Care," *Journal of the American Medical Association* 249 (10 June 1983).

31. S. Rosenblum and B. Frankel, "Teaching the Biopsychosocial Model to Medical Residents in an Outpatient Clinic," *Psychosomatics* 25 (October 1984).

32. R.S. Stewart and M. Stewart, "Psychiatric Interface with Neurology: Conflicts and Cooperation," *General Hospital Psychiatry* 4 (1982).

33. N.G. Ward, D.B. Rowlett, and P. Burke, "Sodium Amylobarbitone in the Differential Diagnosis of Confusion," *American Journal of Psychiatry* 135 (January 1978).

34. Schildkrout, "Medical Residents' Difficulty."

35. S. Perry and M. Viederman, "Adaptation of Residents to Consultation-Liaison Psychiatry. II. Working with the Nonpsychiatric Staff," *General Hospital Psychiatry* 3 (1981).

36. J. Yager and R.O. Pasnau, "The Educational Objectives of a Psychiatric Residency Program," *American Journal of Psychiatry* 133 (February 1976).

37. M.G.G. Thompson, *A Resident's Guide to Psychiatric Education* (New York: Plenum Publishing Corp., 1979).

38. J.L. Houpt, H.M. Weinstein, and M.L. Russell, "The Application of Competency Based Education to Consultation Liaison Psychiatry," *International Journal of Psychiatry Medicine* 7 (1976–1977).

39. J.S. Eaton, "The Educational Challenge of Consultation-Liaison Psychiatry," *American Journal of Psychiatry* 134 (March 1977).

40. P.C. Mohl and S.A. Cohen-Cole, "Basic Readings in Consultation Psychiatry," *Psychosomatics* 26:5 (May 1985): 431–440.

41. Z.J. Lipowski, "Consultation-Liaison Psychiatry: An Overview," *American Journal of Psychiatry* 131 (June 1974).

42. G.L. Engel, "The Clinical Application of the Biopsychosocial Model," *American Journal of Psychiatry* 137 (May 1980): 5.

43. Fox, "Training for Uncertainty."

44. R. Lovitt, "Psychological Testing and Consultation-Liaison Psychiatry," *General Hospital Psychiatry* 4 (1982).

45. H. Leigh et al., "DSM III and Consultation-Liaison Psychiatry: Toward a Comprehensive Medical Model of the Patient," *General Hospital Psychiatry* 4 (1982).

46. Stewart and Stewart, "Psychiatric Interface."

47. S.J. Kantor, I. Chiarandini, and S.S. Heller, "The Use of the Psychiatric Consultation Record for Residency Training," *General Hospital Psychiatry* (1979).

48. T.B. Mackenzie, M.K. Popkin, and A.L. Callies, "Consultation-Liaison Outcome Evaluation System, Part 1, Teaching Applications " 109 (1981).

49. S.A. Cohen-Cole, "Training Outcome in Liaison Psychiatry: Literature Review and Methodologic Proposals," *General Hospital Psychiatry* 2 (1980).

Chapter 7

Psychiatric Services from the Internist's Perspective

Ira R. Hoffman, M.D., and Allen H. Collins, M.D., M.P.H.

INTRODUCTION

The internist has come to have a rather comfortable relationship with the psychiatrist over the past two decades. In spite of the intraspecialty chauvinism of many medical disciplines, with its attending propensity to demean and avoid the clinical dimensions offered by other disciplines, the internist now recognizes a closer kinship to the psychiatrist than ever before. This is especially true in the general hospital setting. The reasons for this striking change are varied, but many of them relate to the psychiatric aspects of the demands on medical clinicians in the provision of clinical care to their patients, for example:

- the significant emotional overlay in many patients with somatic disease
- the anxious and depressive reactions of patients' families as the reality of the illness comes to be understood
- the increased number of pharmacologic agents that can be utilized to help manage emotional problems in medical patients

The interspecialty collaboration between internist and psychiatrist has been further facilitated by the use of a common medical model approach in treating patients, including a working understanding of, and a common language to discuss, clinical issues in each other's specialty; and the increased need and willingness of psychiatrists to utilize internists for the diagnostic and treatment needs of the patients whom they admit to the general hospital. These developments have injected a greater reciprocity and collegiality into the mutual referral process.

In the general hospital setting, the internist-psychiatrist relationship is usually more complicated than in office practice. In the hospital, the two physicians operate within the confines of the same physical space and share a common institutional staff. Treatment instructions ("orders"), consultation notes, and progress notes in the patient's medical chart serve as a common cooperative or confrontational ground on which the diverse physicians who attend the patient can interact.

This is in marked contrast to the situation in office practice. In this setting, the two physicians operate on their own individual turfs, in relative isolation from the activities of other care providers. This has often fostered the illusion that professional contact with other health care professionals could be avoided. In the past, this illusion was especially prominent in the relationship between the internist and the psychiatrist. It was rationalized on the assumptions that (1) the psychotherapeutic relationship between patient and psychiatrist is more confidential than the relationship between patient and internist, thus precluding the psychiatrist's willingness to discuss any aspect of psychiatric care of the patient with the internist; and (2) the internist's difficulty in relating the "magic" of psychiatric procedures to the professional efforts of the internist. Thus, the internist-psychiatrist relationship in the private setting though more subtle and considerably less confrontational than in the hospital, frequently became infused with avoidance and noncollaboration.

In contrast, the general hospital setting is becoming increasingly a meeting place for internists and psychiatrists. This development has been facilitated by improved communication and increased understanding between the two disciplines and by increased acceptance by the patient of a team concept of inpatient management. Today, the better educated house staff of a general hospital has generally had considerable exposure to psychiatry in undergraduate medical and residency training. As these physicians emerge as fully trained practitioners, this exposure leads to a more comfortable manner and involvement with psychiatric colleagues.

At the same time, the psychiatrist is now more readily recognized and understood by the attending internist and medical house staff officer. The psychiatrist now speaks a similar language, knows more medicine, and is more easily integrated in the consultation-liaison role. General hospital practice now frequently requires the internist's use of specialty consultants, both within the broad field of internal medicine and with other specialties like surgery, ophthalmology, and, increasingly, psychiatry. In the case of psychiatry, the need for consultation may arise in an emergency situation, for example, when a patient becomes acutely psychotic, demands to leave the hospital (against medical advice), pulls out intravenous lines, and accuses the staff of trying to kill the patient. This kind of clinical situation can become critically similar to one in which the internist turns to the surgeon for aid in the interpretation of the acute abdomen. In the comparable acute psychiatric situation, the internist may need consultation to interpret and help resolve the progressive and unexplained development of agitated, irrational behavior in a formerly rational and cooperative patient. In such circumstances, without psychiatric consultation-liaison and other related services, the general hospital is clearly inadequate as an acute care center serving the comprehensive medical needs of a community. Indeed, today psychiatric consultation coverage, 24 hours a day, seven days a week, is as necessary in the work of the general hospital internist as roentgen and laboratory services.

PSYCHIATRIC CONSULTATION-LIAISON SERVICES

The practice of medicine has matured considerably over the past two decades. With the maturation has come greater complexity. Most practitioners have learned the limitations of assuming simple linear causality in the etiology of medical disease, though some may still cling to simplistic notions, for example, that "the *Treponema pallidum* causes syphilis." We now have some appreciation of the psychological stresses and patterns of living—involving nutrition, exercise, familial tranquillity, and social-vocational gratification—that impact substantially on our patients' health.

Still the psychological systems on which compliance with medical regimen depends have not received the full appreciation they require from medical practitioners. This is true in spite of their day-to-day experiences with patients who have problems cooperating with the therapeutic plans devised for them.

The development over the past decade of consultation-liaison services in general hospital departments of psychiatry has the potential to alleviate this situation. The model that underlies these services transcends the old model of specialist consultation dating back to the 19th century. The consultation-liaison psychiatrist now becomes a full-fledged member of the patient management group, thereby bringing a more sophisticated psychosocial appreciation to patient care.

Psychiatrists can highlight for the medical team the many emotional factors involved in the etiology of the disease process, the patient's experience of illness, and the patient's interpersonal relationships with physicians and others who provide health care services that impact on the therapeutic process. The psychiatrists who provide this kind of service, in effect see both sides of the fence: They *liaison* with providers to understand their problems with patients, and they *consult* with patients to comprehend the difficulties experienced from the patients' perspective.

Internists who still view all obstacles that block implementation of their diagnostic-therapeutic plans as intrinsic patient "crockiness" are at considerable disadvantage in their relations with this new breed of psychiatrist. They must endure alone the inevitable frustrations and disappointments attending the failure to achieve immediate clinical success. These frustrations and disappointments are compounded by the multiplicity of hospital requirements for utilization review, quality assurance, and other patient care monitoring mechanisms. These requirements impose serious time constraints on lengths of stay and the evaluation of the appropriateness of care provided in the general hospital setting.

To alleviate this situation, in the context of the ever-increasing involvement of nonclinical personnel in hospital-based medical care, the psychiatrist is destined to play an increasingly important role. For physicians, nurses, other health care providers involved in the increasingly coupled management and disposition decisions for "difficult" patients who do not seem to get better, do not die, but for a variety of reasons, are unable to be cared for at home, the liaison psychiatrist is now found to be the negotiating link among the various factions.

The growing importance of disease chronicity and the demand that medicine provide more effective and humanistic care are emerging as significant issues in the delivery of medical services. Well-educated, dispassionate, yet caring professional personnel are needed to cool heated feelings and find more workable solutions.

An important aspect of this situation is the rising average age of patients under the care of the internist. We are seeing increasing numbers of patients in their 80s and 90s. Many of these patients are alone and have finally come to the end of the line because of their inability to manage living, no matter what medical regimen is applied. Others require long and complicated therapy by several disciplines before rehabilitation is successful. Such patients—at death's door one day and fully alert and ambulatory the next— are a source of great pride for many physicians. Other patients, not so fortunate, pose profound problems to the treatment team and to families unable to handle the burden.

The value of psychiatric consultation-liaison help in this area has long been recognized but is perhaps still not fully appreciated. Newer and more effective psychoactive drugs have radically altered the options available in the treatment of agitation, depression, anxiety, and disorientation in the geriatric patient. They have at the same time increased the potential for negative drug interactions and side effects, both subtle and detrimental. Against this backdrop, the internist turns to the psychiatric colleague for help in choosing a particular agent and in interpreting the therapeutic response. The psychiatrist must respond with a thorough knowledge of what is available, of the potential side effects of the drugs, and of the way the drugs can be integrated with the rest of the armamentarium of agents provided to the patient.

The following case illustrates the various issues involved in this kind of collaboration. Dr. C was requested by Dr. H to see a 72-year-old housewife in psychiatric evaluation of multiple somatic complaints and depression. For many years, the patient had a history of polydrug abuse for "sleep problems." The drugs included barbiturates, Valium, Librium, Quaalude, and other sedative hypnotics. Six months prior to admission, the patient sustained a fracture of the left hip and was subsequently hospitalized for surgical pinning. Several additional hospitalizations ensued for pain and other less specific somatic complaints. The patient was seen in psychiatric consultation and evaluated to be clinically depressed. Her long-standing precarious living equilibrium had been markedly disturbed by the fracture and resulting problems with ambulation, which were judged to be among the principal causes of the depression. A course of antidepressants and supportive individual psychotherapy with family involvement was undertaken. Considerable improvement occurred over the following three weeks of stay. Continued care was recommended on an outpatient basis, to be closely coordinated with the follow-up care provided by the internist.

EMERGENCY CONSULTATION SERVICES

Emergency medical-surgical care in an ER milieu is now considered to be an essential service in any community acute care general hospital. Among the many medical emergency care patients brought to the ER, psychiatric patients are now being brought or are being self-referred regularly to ER departments. These cases include:

- suicide overdoses
- emotionally based somatic presentations, for example, pain syndromes and headaches
- anxiety disorders and panic states
- confusional states
- drug and alcohol abuse/withdrawal
- psychotic conditions
- depressive disorders

These psychiatric conditions require specialty consultation for the medical house staff officer or attending internist who provides the initial clinical evaluation. Diagnostic and treatment decisions hinge on the vital input of the psychiatrist called upon to participate in the process. Without the ready availability of this type of psychiatric consultation service, the medical physician is seriously handicapped, clinically and legally, in the evaluation of the patient. Following diagnostic assessment and treatment interventions that can be quickly applied in the emergency room, the disposition decisions also frequently require the input and often the in-person attendance of a psychiatrist.

The following case illustrates this clinical situation. A 28-year-old, single unemployed man was brought to the emergency room by the police. He was found in an acute confusional state in Central Park, unable to give his name, address, or next of kin. The medical resident, who was responsible for providing the initial medical evaluation of the patient, tried to take a history from the man but could not obtain any coherent story. Not only was the patient incoherent, he was also found to be actively hallucinating and probably delusional. The patient was passive, but seemingly cooperative. The physical examination—including neurological assessment, chest x-ray, toxicologies, and other blood screening tests—was unremarkable. The attending psychiatrist on emergency duty was called to see the patient to determine if admission to a psychiatric inpatient service was necessary or whether another treatment approach was indicated. Admission to the hospital's psychiatric scatter-bed program was to be considered against the alternative of transferring the patient to the local city psychiatric acute care receiving hospital. It was established procedure with that hospital that a psychiatric evaluation had to be performed by a psychiatric attending or resident at the requesting institution, and specific clinical indications for hospitalization had to be found before transfer could be accepted and effected.

This type of extension of the emergency medical evaluation gives the hospital the capability of handling what is predominantly a psychiatric problem, confirmed by psychiatric consultation. For the internist or medical house staff officer who calls the consultant, the ability to maintain the patient in the same hospital provides a distinct advantage. Because the underlying factors responsible for the presenting problems requiring admission may not yet be elucidated, much less resolved, the medical and psychiatric diagnostic work-up initiated in the emergency room can be more closely followed by a detailed assessment on an in-hospital basis. In this way, the continuity of care is preserved, and more effective medical education is available for the physicians who are responsible for managing the patient. In this context, a psychiatric inpatient service, either on a scatter-bed basis or as a segregated unit on the premises, affords the internist and the patient's family desirable accessibility and involvement in the ongoing treatment process.

PSYCHIATRIC INPATIENT SERVICES

At Lenox Hill Hospital, the development in recent years of a psychiatric inpatient scatter-bed service has, in conjunction with clinical internal medical practice, greatly facilitated access to patients who require dual professional support. Medical and psychiatric house staffs now can meet and consult with each other. Educational services prosper, and more comprehensive nursing care can be provided. There is no need for professional boundary warfare; the predominant clinical problem area toward which clinical management is directed dictates whether the patient is identified as a "medical" or a "psychiatric" patient. This identification is important for a variety of administrative reasons—including third party insurance reimbursement, utilization review, and departmental census statistics—however, the issue of which physician "controls" the case is rarely a point of contention.

In the Lenox Hill system of collaboration and mutual consultation, the number of patients admitted by internists to "medical" beds and then subsequently "converted" to the psychiatry service is comparable to the number admitted to the scatter-bed service and then transferred to "medicine" during the course of their stay. There is no actual physical change of bed or ward for any of these patients. This easy transfer process between medicine and psychiatry is a direct manifestation of the openness that exists between the two specialty disciplines at Lenox Hill.

Another such manifestation is the relative lack of resistance encountered by physicians of the two specialties when they request consultations from each other; informal ward and telephone conversations on cases of mutual involvement are daily occurrences.

The following case illustrates the system of collaboration at Lenox Hill. A 52-year-old married insurance man was admitted by the internist to the general medical ward of the hospital. The man had experienced a grand mal seizure at home in the presence of his wife and was brought to the emergency room by ambulance. He was poorly hydrated on admission, with enlarged liver and multiple hemangiomata. The history was noteworthy in that the patient admitted to chronic alcohol ingestion over at least 15 years, with recent poor appetite, increasing weakness, and lethargy. The man abruptly stopped drinking six days prior to admission, with the culmination of a grand mal seizure in the morning before coming to the hospital.

A routine lab work-up revealed elevated liver function studies, iron-deficiency anemia, and normal CAT scan. A psychiatric consultation following neurological evaluation was unremarkable. The attending psychiatrist recommended standard detoxification protocol with concurrent assessment of a suspected depressive disorder. Clinical evaluation, with confirmatory psychological testing (no cognitive defect elicited), yielded the affective diagnosis with anxiety. Conversion to the psychiatric scatter-bed service was recommended after acute medical intervention efforts were concluded. The patient was so transferred and was treated with antidepressants, individual psychotherapy, and the available milieu modalities of the scatter-bed program. He was discharged 17 days after admission in a much improved condition and was followed coordinately by both the psychiatrist and internist on an outpatient basis.

ADMINISTRATIVE RELATIONSHIP BETWEEN THE MEDICAL DEPARTMENT AND THE PSYCHIATRY SERVICE

At Lenox Hill Hospital, the Psychiatry Service was organized as a section of the Department of Medicine. As a short-term measure, this provided an adequate launching pad. Today, however, this kind of organizational structure must be considered an anomaly in the acute care setting of a moderate-sized general hospital like Lenox Hill, located in the heart of a major metropolitan center.

The administrative location of psychiatry as an adjunct to a department of medicine often is found in smaller, exurban or rural hospitals that do not have adequate consumer demands for specialized psychiatric services or sufficient professional mental health resources to establish an independent department of psychiatry. At Lenox Hill, this kind of organizational relationship resulted from an unusual confluence of historical events. Subsequent developments in psychiatric clinical services and training programs at the hospital have now dramatically altered the initial administrative structure. From this experience, we can draw some useful conclusions about the relative advantages and strengths, the disadvantages and limitations, of various administrative arrangements between the medical department and the Psychiatry Service.

Advantages and Strengths

The paternalism implied in the relationship of a strong department of medicine with a weak psychiatry service was an invaluable underpinning for the survival and eventual revitalization of the psychiatry service at Lenox Hill. The medical department's protective and supportive attitude enabled the psychiatric section to make continued attempts to recruit able clinical psychiatrists and to cope with the repeated disappointments resulting from the failures of the recruited physicians to make necessary changes in the psychiatry section. The view of the medical department was that psychiatric services were an essential specialty component in the array of patient care services available at the hospital. This constructive attitude has facilitated the many programmatic changes in psychiatry that have occurred at Lenox Hill Hospital over the past decade:

- the development of a close working alliance between the medical director, associate medical director, and the psychiatric attending-in-charge on strategic planning and, when necessary, day-to-day operations

- political and financial support for the professional salaried positions necessary to provide administrative direction for new programs

- support for allocations of requisite space for new services

- the provision of general care beds on medical floors for use by psychiatric scatter-bed inpatients

- development of a policy to have medical house staff provide admission work-ups and back-up medical care for psychiatric inpatients

- the support of the medical director in facilitating the process of bringing new psychiatrists onto the hospital voluntary attending staff

- the active involvement of the medical director in the negotiating process with the medical college to include psychiatry into the teaching affiliation agreement

These administrative collaborations enabled the Psychiatry Service to improve greatly the quality of its clinical services and to initiate training programs at the undergraduate medical school and residency levels.

Probably the most important result of this collaboration relationship was the unusually close working clinical cooperation that evolved between the attending and house staff physicians of the two specialties. This is attested to by the high level of activity of the Psychiatric Consultation-Liaison Service on the medical floors of the hospital, the frequent cross-consultations requested by private medical attendings of both areas for their private patients (in-hospital and office), the involvement of internists in psychiatric teaching conferences, and the corresponding involvement of psychiatrists in medical conferences. Today, the Psychiatry Service has electives in psychiatry for the medical house staff and is recognized by the medical college as a service that emphasizes humanistic training in medicine and medically oriented training in psychiatry.

Disadvantages and Weaknesses

In the long developmental process of the Psychiatry Service under the aegis of the Department of Medicine, there were, not surprisingly, frequent disagreements between the leaders of the two disciplines. These sometimes involved a lack of knowledge in one of the areas due to the pressure of time or emergency circumstances. For example, in the period 1974-1976, the difficulty of providing adequate psychiatric emergency coverage to the in-hospital wards of the hospital resulted in untoward occurrences. This severely tested the patience and tolerance of the medical department, which had come to expect responsive, quality clinical care from its sections and whose director was providing active support for the psychiatric staff.

Problems also resulted from the administrative representation of the Psy-chiatry Service—still an area of relative unfamiliarity and professional non-identity—by the director of medicine on the medical board. In one instance, the high degree of turnover of members of the voluntary psychiatric attend-ing staff was criticized by members of the medical board and the board of trustees. This embarrassed the medical director, whose lack of knowledge of the reasons for the high turnover made a defense of the situation at the board level quite difficult and seemingly untenable. Other problems resulted from the inevitable competition for hospital space and financial resources as new programs required increasing support from a limited pool.

On the other hand, problems of personality have played a remarkably minor role over the years. In spite of the ego gratifications and the need for recognition that are inevitable for hard-pressed medical administrators, the personality conflicts between the two disciplines, proved to be limited and controllable. Indeed, certain personality factors came to play an important role in the operational collaboration between the leaders of the two disci-plines. The genuine respect and affection, which developed slowly and painfully, ultimately proved to be important mitigating factors in later conflicts of interest and provided a solid foundation for the evolution of the organizational relationship in a mutually constructive manner.

The growth and development of the Lenox Hill Psychiatry Service has resulted currently in a full array of psychiatric patient care services. These services are well-integrated with the other medical-surgical programs and are responsive to the needs of both the hospital and the community of patients and physicians. Psychiatric training programs have taken a respected place alongside the teaching activities of the other medical disci-plines.

Today, to achieve continued growth—most notably, the development of a segregated psychiatric inpatient unit with a comprehensive, free-standing residency training program—it is necessary that the Psychiatry Service be given full clinical departmental status. This will afford it the administrative autonomy and professional quality it needs for full productivity and growth. It will permit creative leadership and facilitate the requisite respect from other clinical disciplines in the hospital community.

Psychiatry today is recognized as an independent specialty in the national subculture of American medicine, with a distinct data base and clinical procedures, a separate specialty board (with neurology), and its own unique national, state, and local administrative regulations. We have no doubt that the unique relationship enjoyed by psychiatry and medicine at Lenox Hill Hospital will continue to grow through any future organizational restructurings. Beyond the Lenox Hill experience, the two disciplines are destined to share many patients and duties in future general hospital settings. Because this prospect is increasingly accepted by physicians and patients alike the future of medicine appears measurably brighter.

BIBLIOGRAPHY

Allen, J.R. "Psychiatry and Medicine, 1980." *Journal of the Oklahoma State Medical Association* 74 (February 1981): 35–42.

Billig, N. "Liaison Psychiatry: A Role on the Medical Intensive Care Unit." *International Journal of Psychiatry* 11 (1981–1982): 379–386.

Cohen-Cole, S.A. "An Oral Examination of the Psychiatric Knowledge of Medical House Staff: Assessment of Needs and Evaluation Baseline." *General Hospital Psychiatry* 4 (July 1982): 103–111.

Dorfman, W. "Closing the Gap between Medicine and Psychiatry—Revisited." *Psychosomatics* 22 (February 1981): 143, 164–150.

Fauman, N.A. "Psychiatric Components of Medical and Surgical Practice, II: Referral and Treatment of Psychiatric Disorders." *American Journal of Psychiatry* 140 (June 1983): 760–763.

Hales, R.E. "Teaching Psychosocial Issues to Medical House Staff: A Liaison Program on an Oncology Service." *General Hospital Psychiatry* 4 (April 1982): 1–6.

Hashimoto, M. "The Role of the Psychiatrist in the General Hospital. I: Investigation and Analysis Pertaining to the Status of the Psychiatrist in the General Hospital." *Tokai Journal of Experimental and Clinical Medicine* 7 (March 1981): 181–186.

Joyce, P.R. "The Medical Model—Why Psychiatry Is a Branch of Medicine." *Australian and New Zealand Journal of Psychiatry* 14 (December 1980): 269–278.

Steinberg, H. "An Analysis of Physician Resistance to Psychiatric Consultations." *Archives of General Psychiatry* 37 (September 1980): 1007–1012.

Chapter 8

Specialized Psychiatric Services to the Intensive Care Unit

Thomas Sedlock, M.D., and Karen Ann Burns, R.N., B.A.

INTRODUCTION

Psychiatric consultation is the foundation of mental health services to the intensive care unit (ICU). The consultation process begins when a physician requests that a psychiatrist evaluate a medically ill patient who is suspected of having a concomitant emotional disorder. The liaison concept involved in this process developed in the 1930s and 1940s with the interest in teaching of psychiatric principles of patient care to medical doctors. According to Strain, "what makes the liaison model particularly appropriate to psychiatry is the fact that psychosocial issues arise in the context of any speciality, and the biopsychosocial model dictates that every illness and every patient requires the inclusion of psychological and social considerations in assessment, treatment, and follow-up."[1] The philosophy of liaison psychiatry underlying the discussion in this chapter derives from principles developed and outlined by Caplan and Strain.[2,3]

Liaison psychiatrists enhance the quality of the psychological care the medically ill receive by anticipating and preventing the development of psychological symptoms (primary prevention), by treating such symptoms after they have developed (secondary prevention), and by rehabilitating patients in order to prevent the symptoms' recurrence (tertiary prevention). In the medical setting, case detection is a major skill of the liaison psychiatrist. The liaison psychiatrist also helps the physician make a diagnosis and formulate a treatment strategy by providing additional information about the relationship between physiological, psychological, and social factors that influence the patient's condition.

This model of liaison psychiatry posits that the responsibility for the psychological care of the medically ill hospitalized patient is not the sole

169

responsibility of the psychiatrist but is shared by the physician, nurse, social workers, important family members, and others who determine the psychological climate of the ward. In this model, a crucial function of the liaison psychiatrist is to assess the degree of stress experienced, and the adaptive capacity possessed by, the patient, family, and the medical care providers. Further, the psychiatrist must evaluate the capacity of these persons for the proposed psychological treatment.

The liaison psychiatrist teaches the medical and nursing staff to "become more skillful in eliciting, interpreting, and applying psychosocial data to biopsychosocial management plans."[4] The opportunity to do so occurs at morning rounds, nurses conferences, ward-staff meetings, staff-run patient groups, and grand rounds presentations and in the evaluation of patients in the presence of house staff and nurses. The liaison psychiatrist attempts to give the nonpsychiatric staff a theoretical foundation that incorporates psychosocial considerations in patient care. The psychiatrist helps the staff apply knowledge of human behavior, psychobiology, and psychiatric treatment to an understanding of the psychiatric aspects of the medically ill patient.

Liaison psychiatry also attempts to make changes in the management of psychiatric conditions throughout the hospital that will endure beyond the stay of a particular mental health professional. For example,"after it became apparent at one teaching hospital that psychological factors were responsible for a failure to maintain patients in the 'life island' (the complete isolation technique for immunosuppressant therapy of leukemia and aplastic anemia), psychiatric clearance became mandatory for all life island candidates."[5]

At Lenox Hill Hospital, structural changes have included the establishment of a requirement of a psychiatric clearance for all drug overdose patients admitted to the ICU. Another such change was the requirement for psychiatric evaluation of all candidates for open heart surgery after it became known that mortality is higher among depressed patients who undergo this kind of operation. Rather than depend upon the whim of a patient, physician, or a department, mandatory psychiatric evaluations should be the policy for patients who have repeated hospital admissions and those whose need for surgery is in doubt. Indeed, "psychological assessment of these patient groups—and other groups yet to be identified—should be regarded as an intrinsic part of patient evaluation and management in the contemporary teaching hospital."[6]

According to Strain, "structural changes in patient-care systems may be brought about by the efforts of the liaison psychiatrist who must decide what to do, where to do it, and with whom to do it."[7] On some services and wards, only consultation service is possible; the attending physicians and house staff on these services are not able to become sufficiently involved with the psychological aspects of patient care to make liaison services possible. Unless an explicit contract with overall goals and objectives can be negotiated with a chief of service, it may be better to offer only consultation services. If such a contract can be negotiated, it should specifically include the goal that the liaison services will demonstrate how to provide psychological care for patients if the medical and nursing staff agree ultimately to take over this function themselves. The liaison services should be provided only if there is adequate teaching time and cooperation by attending physicians; if mandatory attendance, as at any medical conference, is ensured; and if the psychiatrist has access to medical patients for teaching purposes. In Strain's words, "liaison psychiatry should occur when the conditions prevail or can be created that allow it to take place."[8] Since there is plenty of liaison service to be done on medical services where it is desired, it is not necessary to try to convert the skeptical. Missionary zeal undercuts the value of mutual collaboration of needs and desires and ignores an essential aspect of effective teaching—a positive working alliance.

THE CONSULTATIVE AND TREATMENT PROCESS

The Setting and Organization of the Intensive Care Unit

The evolution of the Lenox Hill ICU has closely paralleled the historical development of critical care in the United States. In the mid-1950s, Lenox Hill Hospital was faced with the dilemma of providing care for an increasing number of acutely ill patients. The average number of hours of nursing care needed for these patients exceeded the amount provided by the nursing staff on the general nursing units. The concept of a special care unit was presented to the medical board as a viable solution to this problem. In 1968, the concept became a reality with the creation of the hospital's first medical-surgical ICU. As the trend toward specialization in medicine and nursing accelerated, the hospital's concept of critical care expanded to include a cardiac care unit (CCU), a postoperative cardiac unit, and a progressive coronary care unit.

At the time of its inception, the Lenox Hill ICU was the first of its kind in Manhattan; as such, it was the forerunner of the hospital's present system of critical care units. It was created to provide a separate, self-sufficient area for the concentration of seriously ill patients who required constant and intensive nursing and professional care. Its specialized equipment, situated in a central area, made it possible to deal more effectively with skilled personnel to improve patient care. Although its technological equipment has since changed radically, the underlying philosophy remains the same.

Physical Setting

The original ICU was located on the site of a former male surgical ward. The unit had a 20-bed complement divided between a male and female ward. In 1968, the ICU was moved to its present location on the 8th floor of a building constructed in 1966. The unit was composed of an open "ward" area with six beds plus six individual rooms, for a total of 13 ICU beds. A three-bed hemodialysis unit was located at the northeast corner of the unit. In 1977, the unit's bed capacity was increased to 15 beds when the hemodialysis unit was moved to another building. The renovations to the ICU included the installation of sliding glass walls in two of the single rooms and the remodeling of the unit's pantry. An additional patient bathroom with a bathtub was also installed. The most recent renovations included the installation of four additional sinks in order to provide better facilities for proper handwashing between patient contacts. Also, a new air-conditioning system was installed to provide a more comfortable environment.

However, in the years since 1968, the expansion of the ICU and the accompanying physical renovations have lagged behind technical advancements and the changes in patient population. The increases in the size and amount of equipment needed for monitoring and support systems continually encroach on available space. Open beds are separated only by curtains, and the single rooms are surrounded by partial glass walls. The patients are all within view of each other and have little privacy. Because the patients are exposed to the sounds and sights of emergency situations, they develop a distorted perception of the environment. The increase in isolation cases places additional restrictions on available space, since the unit was not originally designed with proper areas for the storage and disposal of supplies and with anterooms for gowning and disrobing. In fact, the spatial limitations of the ICU environment produce feelings of frustration in the staff, who feel they are competing with equipment for unhindered access to the patient lying in the bed. Also, the poor isolation facilities increase the staff's fear of cross-contamination.

Space for family and staff members is severely limited. The medical and nursing staff must share a small conference/locker room that is easily accessible to visitors. The staff has no other area in which they can relax or unwind without constant interruptions. There are no facilities for private consultation or discussions with families. Bereaved families are often forced to wait in the visitors' lounge surrounded by the family members of other patients.

Nursing and Medical Staff

A patient care coordinator (PCC/head nurse) and assistant patient care coordinator (APCC) are responsible for the 24-hour development and management of the professional nursing staff, nursing aides, and ward clerks. Educational programs are coordinated with the educational specialist. All new staff nurses must complete a basic critical care course during their probation period. Their initial clinical training on the unit is monitored by an assigned senior staff nurse, the APCC, and the educational specialist. The unit is staffed with a minimum of seven nurses on each tour. Staffing patterns provide a maximum nurse patient ratio of 1:3, with an optimum ratio of 1:2 when there is a full staff complement and no absences. Each tour has an assigned charge nurse to coordinate patient care and provide a direct channel of communication with the PCC, APCC, and assistant directors of nursing (supervisors). Each tour has one nurse's aide, and the day and evening tours have a ward clerk on duty Monday through Friday. On weekends, a part-time clerk is assigned to the day tour. The PCC coordinates support services for the patient and family with the mental health nurse specialist and the social worker assigned to the unit. Both the PCC and APCC rotate to the evening and night tours to evaluate and monitor the quality of patient care.

Medical and surgical house staff physicians are assigned to the unit on a rotational basis. The medical department assigns a PGY-3 resident and two PGY-1 residents to the unit on a monthly basis. The surgical department assigns one PGY-2 resident to the unit for a two-month rotation. The medical PGY-1 residents alternate 24-hour coverage. Both the PGY-3 and PGY-2 residents are on duty during the week from 8:00 A.M. to 5:00 P.M. and are assigned to on-call coverage at night on a rotational basis. The Departments of Medicine and Surgery are responsible for their respective medical staffs. Rounds are made daily during the week with the attending physician designated by the respective services.

Administration

Administrative policies and decisions are the responsibility of the ICU-CCU Committee. This committee is composed of members from the Medical, Surgical, Nursing, Radiology, Respiratory Therapy, and Psychiatric Departments and the hospital administration. The representatives from the Nursing Department include the PCCs from the ICU and CCU and the nursing director of the Critical Care Division. Quality assurance monitoring, the formulation of medical policies, and the utilization of critical care beds on the ICU and CCU are reviewed bimonthly by committee members.

Admission to the ICU is based on patient acuity level and the availability of beds. Patients are transferred from the unit at the direction of the resident and/or the patient's private physician in collaboration with the PCC. On admission, the patient and family are oriented to the ICU by the bedside nurse.

Patient Population

Medical patients account for 60 percent of the total admissions to the ICU. Their clinical problems include severe to moderate gastrointestinal bleeding, respiratory insufficiency or failure from pneumonia or chronic lung disease, *Pneumocystis carinii* pneumonia (AIDS), acute myocardial infarctions, pulmonary edema or congestive heart failure, metabolic crisis, substance overdose and abuse, and severe hematologic disorders. The majority of the medical patients (68%) are admitted directly from the emergency room and are transferred from the unit to regional medical units. The surgical population includes cases of multiple trauma, major gastrointestinal revisions, neurosurgical cases, pulmonary resections, cases of severe gastrointestinal bleeding, and cardiovascular cases. The recovery room accounts for 73 percent of all surgical admissions.

The average length of stay on the ICU is 7 days. Approximately 17 percent of the patient population has an ICU course over 9 days; their length of stay ranges from 10 days to 3 months, with an average length of stay of 20 days. The rate of expirations for the chronic ICU patient population is high, 39 percent, and this group of patients provides the most stress for the ICU staff. These patients are generally respirator dependent and require an inordinate amount of nursing care and intervention. Extraordinary measures and effort are expended on these patients, and the staff frequently perceives the patient's death as a personal failure.

Only about 5 percent of the total number of ICU patients, or about 25 patients a year, are seen routinely in psychiatric consultation. These are patients who have overdosed (hospital policy), are grossly psychotic, or pose extremely difficult behavioral problems. In the authors' opinion, an additional 25 percent of the patients admitted to the Lenox Hill ICU would benefit from psychiatric evaluation and intervention.

The Psychosocial Aspects of the ICU Environment

Patient and Family

The technological nature of the ICU environment is often not conducive to fostering the role of psychological support in the management of the critically ill. With advances in medical technology, the ICU environment has become more frenetic and chaotic. Patients are surrounded by cables and tubing from pressure and ECG monitors, defibrillators, pacemakers, pulmonary artery catheters, drainage tubes, and respirators. The visual impact of electronic monitors flashing constantly at each bedside is superimposed on the background sounds of humming and hissing respirators, gurgling suction machines, and beeping monitoring systems. Over time, the ICU staff become inured to the auditory and visual stimuli that are part of the environment. However, because they come to accept the environment as a routine work setting, they are often unaware that it can be a terrifying experience for the patient and the patient's family.

Patients attempting to cope with major illnesses find themselves in a frightening and alien environment. The implied limitation of motion from cables and catheters further increases the stress. Overhead lights remain on 24 hours a day, and the patients are exposed to the sights and sounds of emergency situations in other areas of the unit. Uninterrupted sleep is impossible. The sensory overload and monotony are compounded by the effects of sleep deprivation. Disorientation as to person, time, and place can occur.

Stress for the patient is not addressed in the flurry of activity surrounding the delivery of patient care. In emergencies, the call for help brings a stampede of nurses, physicians, and respiratory therapists. Even during "normal" periods in the ICU, the busy medical and nursing staff can become so involved with the monitoring devices and the evaluation of laboratory data that they lose sight of the patient lying in the bed.

The families of critically ill patients also experience a tremendous amount of stress. They too must cope with the impact of a serious illness. They may experience feelings of helplessness, isolation, and frustration. Families are banished to a waiting room filled with other visitors who are strangers to them. They are usually excluded from active participation in the care of their loved one. Information concerning sudden acute changes in the patient's condition is frequently delayed or overlooked. Families may even receive insufficient or unrealistic information while the staff focuses all their attention on the patient. All of this creates an environment of heightened anxiety and confusion.

Professional Staff

The environmental stimuli of the ICU can also be stressful for the medical and nursing staff. They are continually bombarded by data from monitoring systems and laboratory tests. Patients must be transported to radiology and other areas of the hospital for diagnostic studies. The physical workload can be overwhelming. Patient care is complicated by the life support systems, tubes, and drains attached to the patient. Quick assessments and therapeutic interventions must be conducted constantly. Accurate patient records must be continually updated. The staff are exposed to daily environmental hazards from x-rays, cross-contamination, infection, needle punctures, and back injuries from lifting obtunded patients.

Volatile changes in patients' conditions, the introduction of new types of monitoring equipment, and rapid changes in medical procedures place additional stress on the professional staff. Unfamiliarity with the specialized technical equipment in the ICU can pose significant problems for physicians rotating through the unit, as well as for new staff nurses. The insecurity that this produces, along with the ever-present potential for life-threatening clinical situations, creates an emotionally charged situation.

The continuous turnover of medical and surgical staff through assigned rotations, combined with the turnover of nursing staff because of resignations, places additional stress on senior staff nurses. New staff members must be oriented to policies and procedures, equipment, and supplies without interrupting the delivery of patient care. Each month, the nursing staff must adjust to the personalities and varying levels of clinical expertise and experience of new professional staff. The ensuing disruption of normal routines and patient care created by inexperienced medical and nursing staff increases the frustration of senior staff nurses.

In the ICU, a succession of crisis interventions appears to be the norm, rather than a more carefully planned treatment approach utilizing the expertise of all members of the physician-nurse team. Orders are written by the physicians while the nurse implements the treatment process. The nurse is expected to obtain and report laboratory data, coordinate prescribed treatments, monitor vital signs, calculate intake and output, and titrate multiple intravenous infusions as ordered. The nurse's direct input into the proposed treatment process is in fact often overlooked until an emergency situation arises. In an emergency situation, the nurse may be the only professional person with the training and experience to deal with the problem, especially if it involves technical equipment. At this time, the inexperienced physician may actively seek the nurse's opinion or delegate responsibility for decision making. This is in direct conflict with the nurse's role to act only on written physician orders. Ultimately, the lack of recognition of the nurse's proven clinical judgment and skills and the resulting inconsistency of the nurse's active participation in the planning of the patient's treatment process lead to increased tension between the medical and nursing staff.

Staffing of ICU Mental Health Services

Psychiatrists

At the inception of the ICU in 1968, its physicians would either ask an attending psychiatrist whom they knew to see one of their private patients or they would leave a request for a psychiatric consultation with the psychiatry service secretary, who would then try to find an attending psychiatrist for the referral. When a psychiatrist could not be found, which occurred most of the time, the medical staff would prescribe medication and use restraints to control psychotic and unmanageable behavior. There were no salaried mental health professionals and no formal system of providing psychiatric services. Only psychiatric emergencies were seen, and then only on a haphazard basis. No psychiatric services were provided to the nonprivate patients on the ICU. Psychotic behavior was labelled "ICUitis," and the attitude was, "It'll go away after the patient is transferred." Until such transfer, the patient would be restrained in bed. In those early years, only about 2 percent of the ICU patients, or about ten patients a year, would be seen in the ICU by a psychiatrist. Almost all of these were overdose patients, for whom consultation was required by hospital policy.

In 1974, a Psychiatric Consultation-Liaison Service was initiated, headed by a part-time salaried attending psychiatrist. The consultation-liaison psychiatrist spent five to six hours a week on the ICU, meeting with the nursing staff and providing psychiatric consultations for private and nonprivate patients. Subsequently, the number of patients seen for psychiatric problems tripled. For about a year, a nursing support group was co-led by the attending psychiatrist and the social worker assigned to the ICU. This was a closed group in which clinical problems and interpersonal issues were discussed. The attending psychiatrist also gave conferences for the nursing staff on mental health topics.

Although consultation-liaison services have since expanded greatly in other ward areas of the hospital, the number of such services performed by attending psychiatrists has remained about the same on the ICU. A few of the attending psychiatrists have elected to spend their required time on the ICU, giving occasional conferences and leading support groups. Some of the attending psychiatrists who consult for private patients on the ICU include, as an important part of their evaluation and management of the patients' emotional problems, interviews with the patients' families and talks with the nursing staff about the patients' difficulties. This type of collaborative practice has increased the value of psychiatry in the eyes of the nursing and medical staff.

Over the years, newly appointed attending psychiatrists, because of their availability, have provided most of the private consultations. However, as the office practices of these psychiatrists increase, their places are filled by newer attendings eager for referrals. In recent years, another group of psychiatrists has become regularly active in seeing ICU patients. The group consists of the salaried psychiatrists and a small number of attending psychiatrists who devote their private practice exclusively to psychopharmacotherapy.

When the Psychiatry Service's teaching program began in 1979, a PGY-2 psychiatric resident became available for a four-month rotation on the consultation-liaison service. During weekdays, this psychiatry resident is responsible for all of the hospitals nonprivate psychiatric consultations, including those in the ICU. At night and on weekends, the voluntary psychiatric attending staff provide emergency psychiatric consultations on an on-call basis. The psychiatric resident does about 25 percent of the consultations on the ICU each year. Because it is often a few days before the consultation-liaison resident responds to a request for a consultation, the patient is often transferred before being seen on the ICU. The psychiatry resident is supervised weekly by two voluntary attending psychiatrists; didactics are taught by the chief of consultation liaison, also on a weekly basis.

Mental Health Nurse Clinician

The mental health nurse clinician (MHNC) is a full-time psychiatric nurse working on the Psychiatry Service. This position was created in 1979. The MHNC's duties consist of providing direct service for the psychiatric inpatients and of collaborating with nursing staff on the medical wards about the care of the psychiatric patients in the scatter-bed system. The only direct service performed by the MHNC on the ICU is to evaluate, with the psychiatric resident or private attending psychiatrist, all overdose patients. The MHNC is called about once per month to perform this service. In addition, the ICU staff usually calls upon the MHNC for help when a member of the patient's family becomes hysterical or hostility breaks out among family members or against the staff.

Social Services

Social services on the ICU are provided by a part-time social worker who is a member of the Department of Social Services and whose primary responsibilities are to other wards. The social worker assigned to the unit routinely visits and evaluates the projected discharge needs of the elderly patients. Communication with the nursing staff is handled informally and through progress notes in the patient's chart. The social worker is available, but in actuality has very little time, for consultative assistance when problems arise with patient management or with the family.

Staffing Problems

Because no mental health professionals are directly assigned to the ICU, only a small number of its patients receive mental health services. The time of the hospital's mental health professionals is consumed by their responsibilities on other medical services. Also, there are no evening or week-end mental health professionals in the hospital. In these circumstances, the ICU nursing staff have learned to get by and to ask for psychiatric help only when situations become unmanageable.

The Consultation Process

A request for psychiatric consultation generally begins when a staff nurse recognizes the early signs of emotional difficulties. Initially, the problems and possible solutions for nursing intervention are coordinated with the MHNC and the social worker. When medical intervention becomes necessary for what appears to be potentially destructive behavior—for example, the patient is pulling at intravenous and arterial lines and constantly attempting to climb out of bed—the resident is notified of the problem. Initially, the physician may assume the problem is merely the nursing staff's intolerance of the behavior and expect the difficulty to pass. Restraints may be ordered to prevent the patient from self-harm. Sedation may be added when the problem accelerates. When an unmanageable situation develops, a psychiatric consultation is requested.

If it is a private patient, unless the private attending physician requests direct assistance, the MHNC may be asked to help the staff cope with the problem. In accordance with hospital policy, all overdose patients are seen by the MHNC and a psychiatric resident or attending psychiatrist for evaluation and indicated treatment before the patient is transferred from the unit.

Private psychiatric consultations are requested primarily by the house staff physicians with the agreement of the patient's private attending physician. Because the house staff physician tends to focus on the biological disorder and is likely to be skeptical or apprehensive about psychiatric treatment, that physician usually does not raise the issue of asking for a consultation until an emotional crisis occurs.

The psychiatry resident on the consultation-liaison service is called to see nonprivate patients when it is clear that the ICU medical and nursing staff cannot manage the patient's emotional difficulties. Because, most of the time, the psychiatry resident is on other services and because the house staff is on the ICU for only two months, at the most, the availability of psychiatry is generally only dimly realized.

In doing a psychiatric consultation, the resident reads the chart and interviews the patient. Unfortunately, the psychiatric resident often misses the chance to obtain potentially valuable information by talking with the ICU staff and the patient's family. This may occur because the ICU is seen as an unfamiliar and intimidating environment or because the staff appear harried and involved in their work and therefore unapproachable. Also, the family may not be on the unit when the resident sees the patient and thus must be located.

Communication between the resident and the staff is primarily by chart notes, and often psychiatric terminology is used that is unfamiliar or not meaningful to the medical and nursing staff. Supervision time with an attending psychiatrist who is experienced in ICU consultations would provide the necessary training for and attention to these issues. However, currently the consultation-liaison service does not encourage a broader use of psychiatric services. The medical and surgical house staff on the ICU are more likely to attempt to manage most psychiatric situations by medicating the patients than by asking for psychosocial management.

The Liaison Process

Limitations

Because current medical insurance reimburses psychiatric consultation but not liaison services, very little liaison work is possible in the ICU. The little that does take place is done by the voluntary attending psychiatrists.

With the development of the position of the MHNC, some additional liaison service has become available in the ICU. The MHNC has taken an active part in meeting with the PCC on the ICU about mental health issues. Over time, the MHNC has become a valued resource in helping the nursing staff deal with emotional issues and in providing occasional in-service programs and conferences about mental health issues of interest to the staff. The combined medical-surgical nursing and psychiatric experience of the MHNC has helped to foster a credibility that has enhanced as well as promoted the concept of total care for the ICU patient. The major problem has been the little time, outside of other psychiatric responsibilities, that the MHNC can devote to this kind of service.

For a short period of time, an interested social worker co-led, with the mental health nurse clinician and PCC, a group of families of ICU patients. As time passed, however, their other duties crowded out this service. Also, professional staff were not available during the time when families were most likely to be in the hospital.

Only a limited amount of other aspects of liaison psychiatry have been available on the ICU. Attending psychiatrists have sporadically attended medical rounds but have spent little time in educational activities and conducted virtually no research. Though they have spent some time with the

PCC in assisting with organizational issues, their major influence has been in promoting and running support groups on the ICU.

Staff Support Groups

As noted earlier, the chaotic and technically frenetic ICU environment exposes the staff to the same type of stress-related situations that patients experience. In addition to environmental stress factors, the staff is burdened with observing, preserving, and integrating the vital functions of critically ill patients. The ability to manage a clinical situation is often affected by external factors over which they have little or no control. These factors include the limitations of the physical environment in which they work, staffing and budgetary restrictions, societal attitudes toward death, and rapid turnover in the medical and nursing staff.

Support groups play an important role in alleviating these stress factors in that they afford the staff the opportunity to share their feelings, perceptions, and insecurities. These groups can be structured or open-ended, but to be effective they should be designed by the nurses and the group leader, who may be a mental health professional or the ICU nursing manager.

Lenox Hill's experiences with support groups in the ICU confirms the value of sharing experiences and feelings. These support groups were instituted to provide the staff members with the opportunity to express their anxieties and opinions and to work through their conflicts away from the distractions of the clinical environment. Although the ICU support groups did not follow the classic phases of group development, they were nevertheless effective in achieving conflict resolution and extending support for staff members.

Initially, the support groups were co-led by the liaison psychiatrist and MHNC. Group process was reviewed with the PCC and APCC on a regular basis following the weekly morning and afternoon group sessions. When it became evident that separate meetings, with the unit's nursing managers were creating a rift between leadership and staff, the nursing managers joined the groups to facilitate direct communication about issues important to the nursing staff and their leaders.

Later, the Unit PCC and APCC led the groups under the supervision of the liaison psychiatrist and the mental health nurse clinician who taught principles of group process and leadership. Since the role of the mental health professional on the ICU was historically transient in nature, it made sense for the more permanent nursing leadership to learn how to do it on their own. Subsequent experience supported this view. When the voluntary attending psychiatrist and MHNC became unavailable, the principles learned were used by the nursing managers to meet with the nursing staff on an as-needed basis to talk about emotional issues.

CLINICAL PSYCHIATRIC PROBLEMS IN THE INTENSIVE CARE UNIT

Certain types of patients in the ICU pose predictable problems because of the nature of their psychiatric conditions, while others manifest particular emotional symptoms or behaviors that are directly related to the patients' psychological make-up and coping mechanisms.

Delirium and Psychosis

A 76-year-old man was doing well, following a right upper lobectomy for carcinoma of the lung, until the fourth postop day when he angrily and fearfully told his nurse to get rid of the visitor at the foot of the bed who was bothering him. Pointing out that no one was there and attempting to have him talk about his fears relieved this state for a short time, but psychiatric consultation was finally requested after numerous similar episodes and when other patients complained about being disturbed by the patient loudly arguing with a nonexistent person.

Delirium can be conceptualized as a process with several stages. The symptom frequently seen first is hypervigilance. Lights seem brighter and sounds are sharper. Irritability also occurs in this early period. This stage is brief and is followed by mild confusion with some impairment in orientation, attention, and recent memory. Lethargy with yawning and sighing may be seen. Later, increased confusion occurs, along with impaired judgment and abstraction. The final stage is delirium. At this time, the patient is active and agitated. Delusions and hallucinations are manifest. If not treated, this state either resolves or progresses to a more somnolent state and ultimately coma.

In evaluating delirium, the possibility of an acute brain syndrome should be considered first. The specific points of the patient's history, physical examination, and laboratory tests necessary to identify the cause of the delirious condition are listed in Table 8–1.

When the patient becomes delusional, irrational, hallucinates, and is agitated to the point of becoming combative, antipsychotic medication is required. Minor tranquilizers can make the condition worse, since sedation often makes the patient feel more frightened, suspicious, confused, and hostile.

Haldol is an excellent drug for patients with impaired respiratory status, since its effect on blood pressure, pulmonary artery pressure, heart rate, and respiration is even milder than that of the benzodiazepines. The recom-

Table 8-1 Laboratory and Assorted Checkpoints in Screening Causes
of Delirium

Prior psychiatric history
Withdrawal: alcohol, barbiturates, benzodiazepines, meprobamate
Drugs: steroids, levodopa, amphetamines, psychotropics, digitalis, lidocaine,
  anticholinergics
Temperature
Blood pressure
Hematocrit, mean corpuscular volume greater than 96, vitamin B_{12}, folic acid
Erythrocyte sedimentation rate, lupus erythematosus preparation
Electrolytes, magnesium, calcium, phosphates, tetraiodothyronine
Blood urea nitrogen
Fasting blood sugar
Oxygen pressure (arterial)
Carbon dioxide pressure (arterial)
Ammonia, liver function tests
Venereal disease report
Electrocardiogram
Skull roentgenograms
Electroencephalogram
Brain scan
Cerebrospinal fluid proteins, cells
Computerized tomography scan

Source: Reprinted from *The Massachusetts General Hospital Handbook of General Hospital Psychiatry,*
p. 325, by N.H. Cassem and T.P. Hackett, with permission, © 1978.

---

mended dosage is two to ten milligrams administered parenterally (I M)
every half hour, beginning with 2 mg, then increasing the dose to 5 and 10
mg , as necessary. Once sedated, it is important to maintain the adequate
blood level of the medication. The medication should be reduced to the
minimum dose necessary to keep the patient calm. If agitation is absent,
Haldol may be given orally, although this route decreases the absorption
rate to approximately half the effective dose of the parenteral route.

A common mistake is to order regular repetitive doses, such as 5 mg of
Haldol every six hours; this may produce hazardous excessive sedation.
Delirium in the ICU is usually transient. After the acute stages have
completely subsided, a small nighttime dose of 1 to 3 mg should be given
to prevent recurrence, which usually occurs nocturnally. Rarely, a patient
may remain agitated even after 60 mg has been given. If this occurs, an
acute brain syndrome secondary to anticholinergic drugs should be considered. This syndrome is immediately responsive to a 1 ml IV dose of
physostigmine.

Occasional paradoxical responses to haloperidol may be seen. In this situation, Haldol should be discontinued and a thiothixene or a piperazine phenothiazine, like trifluoperazine, substituted.

Confusion and Agitation

> An elderly woman with a documented history of hypertension and organic mental syndrome was admitted for eye surgery. Postoperatively, she was admitted to the ICU for treatment of malignant hypertension. After this was controlled, the patient, although in a continuing good mood, confabulated, did not know the month or year, and had a poor memory for recent events. Psychiatric consultation was requested when she became agitated, began taking off the monitoring electrodes and pulling out her Foley catheter, continued trying to regulate her intravenous lines, and kept climbing out of bed.

An organic basis for confusion and agitation should be considered when there is an impaired sensorium. This should be strongly suspected in patients who are not alert, do not know the date or name of the hospital, are unable to remember three objects after a few minutes, and cannot follow a three-stage command or draw the face of a clock.

Haldol is the drug of choice and is given as described above in treating delirium. The administration of Haldol should be accompanied by a search for a treatable cause of the organic problem, among which are electrolyte imbalance, drug reactions, metabolic disturbances, and decreased cerebral oxygenation.

Reliance on sedation and restraints is unsatisfactory. Oversedation can cause increased confusion, hypotension, and insufficient ventilation. Restraints can lead to increased belligerence, suspicion, uncooperativeness, and excessive exertion by the patient.

Awareness of the limitations of a restraint and sedation regimen encourages the staff to use psychological management to influence the confused and agitated patient. Because confusion, not inherent hostility, leads to the defiant and uncooperative behavior of the organic patient, the goal is to decrease the confusion by helping the patient to clarify and understand the environment and to correct misconceptions. Comments must be simple and repeated over and over again because of poor memory organization. Since this is so time-consuming, relatives should be encouraged to share the task. They can be instructed to treat the patient as a young child awakening from a nightmare who needs to be reassured, comforted, touched, and to have misperceptions corrected. This also provides helpless family members with the opportunity to participate in the patient's care. The family can also be instructed to bring in a calendar, a clock, or other items familiar to the patient to help maintain the patient's orientation.

Fear, Anxiety, and Panic

A 46-year-old male business executive was admitted with upper gastrointestinal bleeding. He was seen to be sitting in bed, nervously looking cross-eyed at the nasogastric tube. He was fearful about how much he was bleeding, about further discomfort, and about the findings from an upcoming endoscopy.

At the outset of their ICU admission, patients can experience a significant level of fear and anxiety, related to their perceptions of impending death or disability. Verbosity or silent withdrawal are common manifestations of these feelings.

If they have the time to spend with the patient, nurses have more success in managing this clinical problem than do physicians. Explanations and reassurance can be very soothing. The patient's perceptions should be explored and the findings used as the basis for correcting misconceptions and for providing realistic reassurance. At this point, the course of the illness and treatment should also be explored, and the condition's positive aspects should be emphasized. The more grave the prognosis, the more important it is to identify the fear, so that valid reassurances can be given. False reassurances by the staff at this point will reduce the credibility and effectiveness of reassurances given the patient later in the course of the illness.

The simplest and shortest acting benzodiazepine derivatives oxazepam, (serax) should be utilized as necessary, with the dosage adjusted to the patient's clinical response. Since chlordiazepoxide (Librium) and diazepam (Valium) might cause paradoxical rage or hostility, oxazepam (serax), 15 mg q.i.d., should be used if the patient shows signs of hostility.

Treatment of panic states utilizes emotional support and medication. Emotional support is provided by eliciting the specific fears of the patient and tailoring an authentic response of hope and reassurance to these concerns. If the anxiety that accompanies severe illness increases to the point where reassurance and explanations are ineffective, medication is necessary.

On occasion, anxiety may build to a panic state, requiring that medication be given before emotional support can be experienced. Unless the patient is psychotic, benzodiazepines are given orally or IV, since IM absorption rates of these drugs are unpredictable. Initially this medication is given in divided doses; but, after a few days, when adequate tissue saturation has been reached, only a bedtime dose is necessary. Daytime doses are ordered as needed.

The patient should be told that the medication will alleviate the anxiety. Also, former coping methods, such as thinking positively, and using religious support, should be encouraged by the physician. Sole reliance on medication may foster patient helplessness.

Denial and Noncompliance

A middle-aged woman was admitted with intracerebral bleeding. Despite being placed on aneurysm precautions, the patient insisted upon walking around the room and climbing out of bed. The patient denied that she had a serious problem, despite the fact that she had been admitted semicomatose from the emergency room. Repeated explanations about the severity of possible complications if she continued to disregard restrictions on her activity were ignored.

There are many adaptive mechanisms to handle the fear that goes with acknowledging illness: minimizing the seriousness of the problem; attributing it to a minor cause; realizing intellectually what the illness is, while remaining emotionally detached; or keeping awareness of what has happened suppressed until reminded that there is a problem. Studies have shown that patients who are able to diminish their anxiety in these ways have a better prognosis.

Global denial unconsciously defends against the threat of illness by disregarding aspects of reality. Confrontations about the seriousness of the illness usually increase the fear and need for denial. If a patient threatens to leave the hospital, denying that anything is wrong, and is then told that there is a danger of getting worse or dying, the patient will probably become more fearful and therefore even more insistent on leaving the hospital. To reduce this fear and elicit cooperation, the patient should be told that the worst is over. Convalescence should occur in a place where the patient can be closely observed, so that unexpected complications can be prevented or treated. Ensuing panic and fear can be prevented and treated with medication and the management techniques for panic reactions, as described above.

When the patient refuses to have diagnostic tests done or to follow such therapeutic regimens as deep breathing and coughing, the staff may first attempt to cajole the patient into cooperating. If this is not effective, they may assume responsibility for decision making by obtaining administrative consent to administer the refused test or medication physically. Too often, reasons for noncompliance are not investigated and the patient's fear and anxiety are not recognized or explored. The patient is then labeled as "difficult" and a "trouble maker."

There are many reasons why patients are reluctant to give up control and place themselves in the position of depending on others. Management must be suited to the specific underlying psychodynamic reason for noncompliance. Noncompliant behavior can be a defense against such feelings as humiliation, helplessness, fear of emasculation, mistrust of others, or the sense of a threat to the integrity of the self.

If patients refuse treatment because they have delirium tremens or are delirious, psychotic, demented, or combative, they should be protected by using treatment methods for the particular symptom, including the use of restraints. Detailed mental status reports in the charts should include quotes from the patients, showing that they do not understand the nature of their illness and are incompetent to make informed decisions regarding their care.

Dependency

> An elderly woman was admitted from the recovery room following an above-the-knee amputation. The patient would not make attempts to feed herself or participate in activities of daily living. The staff had to lift the patient physically out of bed when she refused to bear weight on her good leg.

The patient who pleads to be fed and comforted, requesting constant attention and reassurance, is frequently viewed by the overworked medical and nursing staff as disruptive and intrusive. This type of patient constantly insists upon input from the staff and interferes with their activities. Staff members, in their frustration, may retreat from the situation by hesitating to set limits or be firm with the patient, thereby often increasing the regression.

The principles of dealing with fear and anxiety, as previously described, can be useful in these situations. It is important to learn what the illness means to the patient and why the patient is frightened. Reinforcement of limits and steady mobilization are essential, along with reassuring words aimed at dispelling the fear of illness, without encouraging further dependency. For example, the patient may be told, "It is important at this point that you begin getting out of bed. I know how frightening it must be to try and take a few steps, but this is necessary for you to get better."

Refusal to comply with limitations on eating, smoking, and getting out of bed is typical of patients who have long-standing conflicts about dependency. When forced to be dependent, many people react by making an issue of being independent. The consultant's aim in such instances is to help to restore control of the situation and to avert fights between the patient and the staff over limit setting.

Hostility

A man in his early 20s was admitted to the ICU following his third laminectomy for spinal cord injuries suffered in a fall. The injuries resulted in limited movement of his legs and was accompanied by a neurogenic bladder. During the first two admissions, he was quiet and cooperative. This time he became very angry and berated the nurses for lousy care and for not bringing him the kind of food that he wanted. He never talked about his handicaps.

Hostility is difficult to manage and sometimes can lead to volatile clinical situations. Angry persons feel threatened; they fight because they feel endangered or demeaned. Hostility can also protect the person from despondency.

Anger and resentment about being sick is common. Gripes about the hospital, food, and nursing care should be listened to patiently and taken seriously. Sympathy, expressed as feeling sorry that the patient is having such a hard time and realizing that being sick is unfair, can also be helpful. Past experiences of the patient with hospitals and illness can be explored insofar as they relate to the patient's expectations about the current situation.

Hostility is also encountered frequently in family members who are experiencing feelings of isolation and helplessness. Families often become angry in response to being relegated to roles of observers, waiting for infrequent reports on changes in the patient's condition.

It is important to acknowledge to the staff that coping with hostile behavior is infuriating. This emotional support can reduce the potential for an explosion between the staff and the patient or family. Attention is directed toward determining the basis of the hostility. Is it related to the patient's fear of dying if left alone, a feeling of entitlement because of the illness, or a fear of being neglected as experienced in the past? After empathically exploring the situation with the patient or family member, the patient should be confronted tactfully and told that the hostile behavior is in fact producing the opposite of the desired effect. It is necessary to point out that, if this behavior continues, it will lead to increased resentment by the staff and their subsequently paying less attention to the patient. An agreement should be reached among everyone involved about reasonable expectations and the limits of care. These limits should be explicit, and a certain amount of testing of them should be expected.

Substance Overdose

A single 26-year-old woman, living alone, was found at home after she overdosed on meprobamate and aspirin. She was admitted comatose with salicylate toxicity. Her mother quickly came to the ICU to be with her daughter. The mother was cooperative with the nursing staff. Upon awakening, the patient was quiet and contrite.

A 25-year-old single man was admitted to the ICU for treatment of a Quaalude overdose. When he awakened, he was verbally abusive and threw a food tray at the nurse. He then jumped out of bed, backed the nurse up to a wall, and cursed and screamed at her for giving him soup and jello when he was hungry and wanted "real food." He was confronted and told that this behavior was not acceptable and that he had the choice of being cooperative or he would be restrained. He was cooperative for the rest of his stay on the ICU.

Treatment of the overdosed patient presents a complicated clinical situation in the ICU. The patient is perceived as requiring minimal attention once the presenting problem has been treated and attention is shifted to patients with more acute physical problems.

If the patient appears contrite, the staff are more likely to be responsive to the patient's underlying emotional distress. However, the patient who is a repeater or who becomes verbally abusive or physically combative is perceived as disruptive and engenders staff anger. The patient is then viewed as "monopolizing valuable time" that could have been spent treating sicker patients.

A psychiatric consultation should be requested as soon as possible after such a patient is admitted to the unit. This allows the consultant to prepare the staff for the possible psychological responses the patient may exhibit. Since the staff's expertise lies in the area of physiologic responses, they are often ill-equipped to handle the patient's psychological needs. In this clinical situation, early recognition of psychological problems is necessary to provide the appropriate treatment for the patient and to provide support for the staff.

Chronic Illness

A 54-year-old woman with a history of vascular disease was admitted to the ICU following the second revision of extensive arterial bypass surgery. During the third week of admission, following vascular occlusion, her right leg was amputated below her knee. After two months on the ICU, because of an extension of the arterial occlusion, an amputation was done above the knee of the same leg. In the following month, her course was downhill; the wound became infected and would not heal. She was placed on life support systems and became respirator dependent. Her husband, who was very dependent upon her, was continually critical of the medical and nursing care. She died after three months on the ICU.

Work with chronically ill patients creates considerable stress for the ICU staff. Many of these patients have a long and painful ICU course in which the staff see little or no improvement in the patient's condition. The staff may view their role as accessories in prolonging the patient's suffering and regard themselves as imperfect in respect to the expectations of the patient, family, and physician.

Initially, the staff assume the role of provider and curer. As the patient's prognosis becomes bleak, the staff's role begins to shift toward the role of carer, in an attempt to protect the patient from "painful" and "unnecessary" treatments. They continue to invest more and more emotion in a situation that seems to have no hope. This is especially true with the patient who is respirator dependent. Clinical improvement in the patient's condition may be so subtle that neither the staff nor the patient perceive any self-reinforcement.

The patient's emotional status is frequently overlooked until overt symptoms of withdrawal, confusion and agitation, or self-destructive behavior become unmanageable. Restraints are often mistakenly used in place of sedation.

Psychiatric consultation is valuable in helping the patient, family, and staff cope with the stress of chronic illness. Consultation with the psychiatrist or MHNC during patient rounds provides the medical and nursing staff the opportunity to discuss the psychological management of the patient and to share their feelings.

Respirator Dependency

A 74-year-old, thin, cachectic woman with chronic obstructive pulmonary disease was admitted numerous times over several years to the ICU when pulmonary infections compromised her respiratory functioning. On the current admission, she was treated for pneumonia. When she failed to respond to this treatment and her respiratory distress became worse, she was intubated and put on a respirator. When she was unable to be extubated, a tracheostomy was done. She died of cardiovascular collapse during the third month of treatment on the ICU.

Patients requiring mechanical respiratory ventilation for long periods of time may become so anxious when weaning begins that a psychiatrist must be consulted. Anxiety may so increase metabolic demands and cardiac work that, at least temporarily, the patients are physically incapable of further weaning. In addition, relaxation induced by taking slow deep breaths cannot be performed by patients with respiratory problems.

Because of the complexity of respiratory therapy, the psychiatrist must accept the judgment of the referring physician that the patient is physiologically ready for weaning. Prior to seeing the patient, the psychiatrist who has to deal with this problem will find it helpful to review with the physician how weaning is to be accomplished.

Although the decision by the primary physician concerning when to wean the patient has to be accepted, it is well to rule out any existing condition, such as hypoxemia and hypercapnia, that precludes weaning. Blood gases can change unexpectedly; and, if they are not within normal limits, the patient will not be weaned successfully. If the arterial oxygen content has not changed, the pH should be checked to make sure it is not less than 7.35.

A number of different treatment methods may be necessary to deal with the inability to wean a patient from a respirator. Prior to weaning, benzodiazepines can be administered to treat moderate anxiety; or an antipsychotic drug, such as haloperidol, can be given if the patient is near panic. Patients are usually cooperative in indicating whether a drug is helpful and whether some are more beneficial than others. Hypnosis and relaxation techniques may also help reduce the anxiety associated with the weaning process. Explaining to the patient that the weaning process itself can be expected to produce some anxiety may also be helpful.

Isolation

A 37-year-old man with acquired immune deficiency syndrome (AIDS) was admitted for treatment of *Pneumocystis carinii* pneumonia and placed in an isolation room. All contacts with staff, friends, and family were made with the contacting person gowned, gloved, and masked. Food was served with paper and plastic utensils, and everything used in the room was disposable. The patient was demanding and frightened. When alarms of other machines sounded, he would think, "This is it." At night, he would frequently hallucinate. This would clear up when he talked with another person.

The patient who is isolated is usually desperately ill and, from an emotional standpoint, is poorly prepared to cope with the additional stress of sensory deprivation that occurs in isolation. Personal interaction between the patient and the staff and family is disrupted by masks that block facial expressions. Tactile sensation is diminished by the use of gloves. Auditory contact is limited to the monotony of sounds of the monitoring equipment and support systems within the room. Entry into the room, in full isolation garb, is usually planned around the tasks involved with routine patient care. Spontaneous visits to chat with the patient are discouraged by the need to gown and mask.

These environmental stressors frequently result in confusion and agitation, in demanding or dependent behavior, and in heightened feelings of fear, panic, and anxiety on the part of the patient. A significant stress factor for the staff is their frequent exposure to active hepatitis, tuberculosis, meningitis, or AIDS and their fear that they will contract a toxic organism from the patient. The patient senses the staff's apprehension and frequently experiences this as rejection. Psychological support under these circumstances should emphasize the sharing of feelings and emotions. Irrational fears need to be elicited, and realistic information concerning the nature of the patient's illness should be available for the patient, the family, and the staff.

The Elderly

A widowed, 78-year-old woman was admitted to the ICU for treatment of congestive heart failure. During the day, she knew that she was in a hospital, knew the correct month and year, and recognized familiar staff members. As night approached, she did not recognize any of the staff, interpreted the sound of alarms on monitors as her doorbell ringing, and insisted that she had to go to the kitchen and check the food she had left cooking on the stove. She also insisted that certain things on the unit belonged to her, and she continued to try to climb out of bed at night.

The elderly patient with multisystem disease is now seen with increasing frequency on the ICU. These patients often respond to stress by becoming confused and agitated. The lights and noise of the ICU promote "sundowner's syndrome," which is notable for its increasing disorientation and agitation during the night. The disorientation may be a normal concomitant of an elderly patient being in an unfamiliar environment. The family and staff can be advised that the condition usually reverses when the patient is back in a familiar setting. A psychological rather than biological approach is needed on the ICU to help the patient become familiar with the setting.

Confusion, agitation, and disorientation in the elderly may be mistakenly labeled as "senility" and managed by the use of restraints and oversedation. More appropriate treatment modalities—including frequent contacts with the patient, the removal of unduly stressful stimuli, and the use of reality orientation programs—are often inconsistently used or overlooked. The medical and nursing staff's awareness of the potential for psychiatric and cognitive disorders in the elderly is an integral component of restorative mental health services.

RECOMMENDATIONS FOR CHANGE

Liaison Services

The development of liaison programs is often discouraged by the fact that insurance reimbursement schedules pay for psychiatric consultation but not for liaison services. Until the value of liaison services is recognized by their inclusion for reimbursement, the ICU consultation-liaison service is best provided by part-time or full-time, salaried, attending psychiatrists and MHNCs. The salaried attending liaison psychiatrist can provide and help coordinate mental health services concerned with treatment, education, support groups, and organizational development.

The MHNC can be a useful resource in helping the nursing staff cope with emotional issues on the ICU. The nurse clinician's experience establishes a credibility and basis for trust that other health professionals do not possess. Ideally, ICU nurses should not be in this role, because they tend to be more physiologically and technically oriented and are not accustomed to dealing regularly with emotional issues.

The MHNC can meet with the social worker and nursing staff on a regular basis to discuss patient and family problems and recommendations for appropriate referrals. Such meetings can reduce the stress that the staff experiences when handling these issues alone and also reinforce the role of mental health in the care of the critically ill.

A team approach to the provision of health services can be effective. The attending psychiatrist can coordinate liaison services provided by the MHNC, social worker, and psychiatric resident. These individuals can provide part-time service on a flexible basis. In addition to working with patients and staff, they can provide emotional support for the families of patients and arrange for support services for the patient after discharge. Such support services can include skilled nursing facilities, hospice care, visiting nurse service, and psychiatric aftercare.

The attending liaison psychiatrist can also meet with the leadership of the ICU as a consultant on organizational issues. In this capacity, the liaison psychiatrist may be of help in the management of personnel issues related to job dissatisfaction, absenteeism, and other staff behavior problems and may also be able to help in efforts to cope with structural changes relevant to the ICU.

Treatment

During patient care rounds, by serving as a resource for the psychiatric issues raised by the medical staff and surgical staff, the attending liaison psychiatrist can have an immediate impact on the psychosocial aspects of patient care. At such times, mental health issues can be identified and discussed.

Through participation in regularly scheduled multidisciplinary treatment planning conferences, the attending liaison psychiatrist can be useful in anticipating problems with specific patients and families, in managing identified emotional issues, and in planning the mental health aspects of transfer and discharge from the unit. In such contacts, the importance of providing accurate, detailed, and honest information to the patient and family should be stressed.

Family Services

The liaison psychiatrist can develop with the head nurse, social worker, and MHNC services to help families manage the stress of dealing with a family member who has a life-threatening illness.

In treatment conferences and patient rounds, the liaison psychiatrist can make the medical staff aware of the need to provide reassuring, but realistic, information to the families. The tendency to be overly optimistic and to keep hopes alive unrealistically is confusing to family members, can increase their subsequent disappointment, and keep them from the important process of dealing appropriately with a dying member of their family.

Attention should be directed toward the family's relationship with the patient, especially with regard to the ways in which the situation is stressful for the family members, how the staff can be helpful in caring for the family members, and the means for family interaction with the medical and nursing staff.

Open channels of communication between the staff and family members must be maintained. The charge nurse can make a point of being available to families for this purpose, or the mental health clinician and liaison psychiatrist can support the nursing staff and help them overcome their anxieties about being involved with families. Whether communication is provided by the nurse or the physician, the channels must be kept open.

A detailed routine for orienting the families to the ICU is essential. The orientation should include information on hospital and neighborhood services and unit policies, a brief description of the equipment needed for the care of their family member, and reassurance that the unit staff will provide them with daily reports of the patient's status, with additional reports as the patient's condition changes. This information can be included in a pamphlet that the family can use as a reference.

Family group meetings can be held at regular times to provide the opportunity to ventilate family members' concerns and fears. These meetings help reduce family stress and alleviate some of the pressure the staff experiences from the family during patient care. The group can be led by the liaison psychiatrist, head nurse, MHNC, or social worker or by a staff nurse who is interested and has been trained to lead this type of group. The leadership may be rotated to fit the schedule of the various leaders involved. These meetings are best held late in the day or in the evening to allow working family members to attend.

Education

Conferences and presentations to the medical and nursing staff by the attending liaison psychiatrist about common psychiatric disorders and psychosocial management are useful in helping the staff integrate knowledge as part of their professional skills. Of particular importance are efforts to increase the awareness and sensitivity of physicians to the need for mental health support of the critically ill. The ICU liaison psychiatrist also is in an excellent position to train the psychiatric resident in the principles of consultation-liaison psychiatry on the ICU.

Support Groups

The importance and relevance of nurse support groups has been well-documented. Though early studies were largely anecdotal, recent studies have attempted to be more objective. Support groups can be effective on an ICU only when reasonable efforts are made to make the changes recommended by the groups. Without such efforts, the group members will come to believe that "there's no use talking about matters of concern, because no one tries to do anything to change things."

It is also important that salaried mental health professionals supervise the leaders of the support groups on a regular basis. The time provided by the mental health professional for this purpose should be flexible so that the groups can meet at times that are convenient for all nursing shifts.

Organization and Structure

Physical Space

In general, private rooms with glass walls for ease of observation are recommended to ensure patient privacy. Central monitoring systems help to reduce patient sensory overload and allow the nurses to monitor the patients while charting.

A quiet room away from the immediacy of the ICU is necessary as a place where the nursing staff can relax during breaks. Here, the nurses should be able to be alone without the intrusion of physicians and family members and the need to answer numerous questions.

Separate rooms are needed for teaching, treatment conferences, and family interviews. A comfortable lounge for the families and friends of the patients is also needed.

For the storage of large quantities of supplies a separate room is required. Direct accessibility to supplies reduces the waste of time and the frustration of having to make frequent trips to central supply for needed patient care items. The standardization of supplies, accurate documentation of their use, and contractual bulk ordering promote cost-effectiveness. Additional nursing staff could be hired with the money saved.

Such support services as a blood gas lab and a satellite pharmacy should be located within close proximity to the ICU. A full-time pharmacist is needed for the monitoring of drug incompatibilities and interactions.

Physician Director

A medical director of an ICU can provide the kind of leadership and stability that may not be possible in a system of shared administrative responsibility. In ICUs without a director, interactions between various disciplines are difficult to coordinate. Also, quality assurance can be more easily coordinated and monitored by a physician director, thereby facilitating the treatment of patients' medical and psychiatric problems.

It has been suggested that a physician director could make the ICU a strong income-producing service by ensuring thorough billing for procedures and services and careful documentation of all the equipment and supplies. Centralized decision making makes it easier to coordinate treatment services; it also localizes accountability, simplifies procedures, and eliminates duplication and fragmentation of services. Finally, it makes it easier to institute new methods of evaluation and treatment, and to develop consistency in policies dealing with medical and ethical issues concerning the treatment of chronic and terminal patients.

A medical director can implement organizational changes quickly and improve communication between the various departments that provide services to the ICU. The director is also accountable for seeing that adequate orientation and continuing education programs for the staff are planned and carried out.

The nursing staff can gain support and credibility from a director. The nurses can be trained to be more effective in situations in which a patient's clinical condition deteriorates and a physician is not immediately available on the ICU.

A medical director would be responsible for the coordination of house staff physician teaching and for the continuing education of attendings in critical care. The director would also be responsible for implementing the various psychiatric services in the ICU and for overseeing the process of consultation-liaison.

In order to be truly effective, the medical director should be a full-time physician with advanced training in critical care medicine or in a specialty relevant to the nature of the unit. The director should be easily reached by phone for emergency consultations.

Nursing Staff

The feeling of being part of a special group that prides itself on its teamwork and ability to function well in a crisis helps alleviate much of the anxiety generated among nurses by the ICU environment. Regular group meetings, in which nurses are allowed to express their hostility, guilt, shame, fear, or uncertainty and to share their unique methods of dealing with stressful situations, can also help to decrease anxiety and promote a positive working environment.

The behavioral effects of stress on nurses in the ICU are reflected in a high rate of staff turnover, an increased incidence of absenteeism due to minor illness, exacerbation of emotional problems, and complaints of vague somatic symptoms. A good way to alleviate stress is to reduce role ambiguity and role conflict. Role ambiguity is decreased by ensuring that the nurse has the information needed to carry out the responsibilities of the job. The making of logical and meaningful decisions requires adequate information. Role conflict is reduced when the nurse's relationships with co-workers, other medical disciplines, the unit, and hospital administration are clearly defined. When two or more roles conflict as a result of rigid and conflicting expectations of those in power, little room is left for flexibility or alternatives, and the nurse is set up for failure.

As the largest permanent professional group in the ICU, the nursing staff largely determines the atmosphere of the unit. Helping the nurses cope with stress is the key to creating a positive working atmosphere for the staff and an emotionally healthy environment for the patients. Adequate staffing is also a major factor in the reduction of stress among nurses working in the ICU. Optimal staffing requires a consistent nurse-patient ratio of 1:2, with the option of being able to provide one-to-one care when necessary.

Guidelines for the Care of Critically Ill or Dying Patients

Modern Technology and Aggressive Treatment

Medical technology has made a vast array of life support systems available. These systems can be beneficial, sometimes dramatically so, in treating the critically ill. However, they must be critically assessed, since their use is often intrusive, frequently painful, almost always expensive, and often of little value.

One of the biggest complaints of the nursing staff is that patients are not allowed to die in comfort or with dignity. The nurses are upset by the trauma and consequent suffering when seemingly unnecessary procedures are continued. The nursing staff also feel strongly that it is best to allow patients to die in the ICU rather than be transferred to another ward to die. This allows the patient to stay in an environment that is familiar and in which the nursing staff know the patient and family and can assist during the process of dying.

The use of sophisticated innovative technology that can markedly prolong life is drastically altering the decision-making role of the physician in the ICU. The physician must now deal with issues of informed patient consent, legal issues, societal values, and the costs of long-term medical care. These issues are particularly relevant in the care of the terminally ill patient on life support systems.

Difficulties in making decisions about when to institute or stop aggressive life support measures stem from pressures from those in the public and medical profession who tend to regard such interventions as preferable to an acceptance of the terminal disease process. In fact, the balance between ensuring that patients receive the necessary technical care while, at the same time, adhering to personal, public, or professional values is a delicate one. For their part, the nursing staff appreciate that physicians are under societal and legal pressures to continue aggressive treatments under all circumstances. Yet, by assuming a purely technological approach, physicians abdicate their professional responsibility to be the guardians of the rights of their patients. By taking a passive role and by failing to consider and agonize over the moral consequences of a patient care plan, the physician leaves decision making to the medical technologists. In other words, if the equipment is there, use it.

Consultation and Recognition of Patient Interests

Ideally, treatment should be based on what is in the best interests of the patient. However, the need to make quick decisions in a rapidly changing situation often determines the actual treatment. This often prevents the physician from gaining insight into the patient's personal and cultural values.

A vital element in medical ethics is "the duty to desist from medical care, not only when the patient refuses service but when that service does not, in fact, serve the end of medicine, the correction of disease, and the repair of injury."[9] Frequently, this requires that the focus be changed from supporting life to helping the patient and family adjust to the nearness of death.

The decision of when to institute aggressive treatment is best made in the context of the values and autonomy of the patients and their families. And such considerations are best dealt with by a comprehensive team approach (nursing staff, physician, social worker, and psychiatrist). If this approach is used many, perhaps most, of the ethical and legal issues and the problems of human relationships involved in the situation will be resolved.

In difficult cases, consultation with the hospital ethics committee (if one exists) is recommended. Whenever possible, patient and family participation in such consultation should be obtained, along with that of the nursing staff. The final responsibility for deciding the treatment appropriate for the treatment goals belongs to the primary physician.

Yale Guidelines

Duff has reported on the thoughtful and comprehensive guidelines that the Yale University Department of Pediatrics developed in dealing with the care of its critically ill or dying patients.[10] The guidelines were drawn up by a committee made up of members from several disciplines who held differing opinions on the issues involved. The guidelines have been applied in selected situations and the results presented in various forums. The response by medical professionals, hospital administrators, chaplains, lawyers, theologians, and citizens has been very favorable. Most have agreed that this approach to patient care is in harmony with the finest traditions of caring for people. Following is a summary of Duff's report on the Yale guidelines.

It is of utmost importance that a single physician be responsible for monitoring the care of the patient. The name of the responsible physician, who should be known and approved of by the family and when appropriate by the patient, is noted in the patient's chart. This physician of record must ensure that the decisions for care reflect the patient's and the family's values. Also, the high quality of the psychosocial support and the technical care of the patient must be ensured. The patient's own feelings, thoughts, values and wishes, as well as those of the family, must be considered at all times, regardless of the patient's age.

The responsible physician must exercise judgment in evaluating the patient's problems and must regularly exchange information about the patient's condition with the patient and family. The physician must function as a team member with the patient, family, house officers, nurses, and social workers.

In the event of major disagreements among senior physicians or other health care providers, especially among the nurses and social workers involved in the case, the responsible physician must present the conflicting recommendations to the patient and family members, who may then help to resolve the conflict. The responsible physician may request further consultations from other professionals to help clarify the matter.

If all questions of care are still not resolved, a conference of the differing parties, at times including the patient and family, is convened with the chief of service, or that person's delegate, at the request of the chief resident or responsible physician. This conference is designed to share information. The power to make a decision rests first with the patient and family, and second with the responsible physician.

If the patient or family disagree with the proposed course of treatment, their decision must be reviewed in light of the diagnosis, the expected outcome with or without the treatment (including consideration of the quality of life), the degree of certainty of the outcome, the risks or psychological burdens involved, and the probability of benefit from the treatment. The family may seek legal counsel, and the medical authorities may also obtain legal counsel if the family and patient insist on a choice viewed by the medical professionals as detrimental to the patient. The final decision may then be made by whomever the court designates.

Because of their interpretation of professional norms or because of their own prognostic indicators, values, or conscience, some health professionals may object to a course of treatment that the patient, family, and physician of record have agreed upon. These professionals can make their opposing views known to the physician of record, who will discuss the contested issues with the objecting persons and appropriate others before deciding whether to discuss them with the patient and family.

If the physician of record disagrees with a choice that has been made by the patient and family based on the views of another physician or physicians, the physician of record must make that disagreement known to the patient and family.

The responsible physician classifies the critically ill or dying patient with a very poor prognosis in one of the following three groups:

1. Class A—Maximal therapeutic effort without reservation. Patients in this group are likely to benefit from aggressive treatment to such an extent that those making the decision (patient, family, and health professionals) believe the negative aspects (pain, suffering, reduced quality of life, and cost) associated with such treatment are justified.
2. Class B—Selected limitation of therapeutic measures. Patients in this group will not likely benefit ultimately by the use of maximum therapeutic measures. "The responsible physician must clearly state the reasons for initiating any new major procedure so that all care givers, despite some inevitable disagreement, may be united in their interactions with these patients and families. Patients in this group, along with their families, should be made comfortable, and not abused by inappropriate resuscitative measures."[11]
3. Class C—Discontinuation of life-sustaining therapy. In this group, the patient, family, and medical professionals acknowledge that the illness is irreversible and that the patient is dying. In this terminal phase of life, the primary aims are to comfort and deal with the concerns of the patient and family and to ease the dying process as conscience, prudence, and kindness dictate.[12]

Research

Research at the interface of medicine and psychiatry is important. Depression, anxiety, and delirium are common disorders in medical patients. There is a great need to work out the criteria to differentiate between a depressive disorder associated with a physical illness and a patient's despondent mood in response to such an illness. Also, there is a need for more explicit guidelines on how to distinguish a major depressive disorder from an adjustment disorder with depressive mood. It is often difficult to differentiate between dementia, pseudodementia, and delirium. More knowledge about the clinical features of these disorders would facilitate diagnosis and management. In all of these areas, the liaison psychiatrist should become involved in relevant collaborative research with other medical specialists.

Quality assurance studies and research on the cost-effectiveness of psychiatric liaison programs and aggressive medical treatment are essential. These studies must include the long-term benefits, in terms of morbidity and quality of life, of psychosocial interventions and prolonging life in the terminal chronically ill. The results of such studies may well provide additional support for the payment of liaison services from such sources as insurance reimbursements and agency, hospital, and government funds.

Many research studies have verified that critical care nursing is highly stressful, but there is contradictory evidence as to whether it is more stressful than other types of nursing. This indicates a need for improvements in the types of measurements utilized, for clearly developed and articulated measures of stress and coping, and for research designs that delineate more clearly the important distinctions among various ICUs and medical settings.

Evaluation of the value of different intervention strategies is done only rarely. Many methods have been suggested for reducing patient and staff stress, for example, nurse follow-up of transferred patients, support group intervention, improved in-service education, and periodic rotation of nurses to other services. But there are no studies in which interventions have been tested to determine their effectiveness. Thus, there are wide gaps in our knowledge of the factors that can reduce stress. Clearly, studies and tests of the relevant interventions are needed if nurses are to gain optimal satisfaction from their work, cope effectively, and offer high quality nursing to the critically ill.

REFERENCES

1. James L. Strain, "The Development and Practice of Liaison Psychiatry," in *Consultation-Liaison Psychiatry: Current Trends and New Perspectives*, ed. Jerry B. Finkel (New York: Grune & Stratton, 1983), 11.

2. Gerald Caplan, *Principles of Preventive Psychiatry* (New York: Basic Books, 1964).

3. Strain, "The Development and Practice," 3–24.

4. Ibid., 17.

5. Ibid., 20.

6. Ibid., 21.

7. Ibid., 21.

8. Ibid., 22.

9. A.R. Jonsen, "Dying Right in California, the Natural Death Act," *Clinical Research* 26 (1978): 55.

10. Raymond S. Duff, "Guidelines for Deciding Care of Critically Ill or Dying Patients," *Pediatrics* 64 (July 1978): 17–23.

11. Ibid., 22.

12. Duff, "Guidelines," 17–23.

Chapter 9

Specialized Psychiatric Services to the Cardiac Surgery Service

Jerald Grobman, M.D., and Eugene Wallsh, M.D.

INTRODUCTION

Patients undergoing cardiac surgery have always had an unusually high incidence of psychological difficulties. Most attention in this area has focused on the incidence, etiology, and management of postcardiotomy delirium and/or psychosis.[1-9] Some authors have suggested that this syndrome could be prevented by the use of a preoperative psychiatric interview.[10,11] Others have studied patients' long-term adjustment to cardiac surgery.[12-17] In a effort to predict patients' postoperative psychological responses, Kimball established personality profiles of those who underwent cardiac surgery.[18,19]

Although there are several reports of the use and benefits of a preoperative psychiatric interview for patients scheduled for cardiac surgery,[20,21] there are no reports of a psychiatrist functioning as an integral part of the cardiac surgical team. For the last three years, one of the authors has been working as the consultation-liaison psychiatrist to the cardiac surgical team at Lenox Hill Hospital. In making the psychiatrist an integral part of this team, the authors hoped to:

- extend the benefits of a preoperative psychiatric interview to as many patients as possible
- more thoroughly investigate the psychological problems and needs of patients undergoing cardiac surgery
- more thoroughly investigate the psychological problems and needs of the staff who take care of these critically ill patients

In the period 1981–1984, more than 500 patients have been evaluated in preoperative interviews at Lenox Hill. Of these 500 patients, more than 50 percent have required some form of postoperative psychiatric intervention.

This chapter is a report on certain psychological aspects of these patients, the psychiatric interventions that they required, and aspects of the consultation-liaison work with members of the cardiac-surgical team.

THE SETTING

The Cardiothoracic Surgical Service admits adult patients with primary cardiac and/or major thoracic vascular diseases. The majority of patients for surgery are admitted electively. Some patients for surgery are already in the hospital on the medical service.

Emergency surgical cases, both from within and outside the hospital, are also treated. The patients may also be classified as those who have recent-onset illness, those with chronic illnesses, and a small group of acutely, catastrophically ill patients. Each elective patient is offered an opportunity for a preoperative visit to the surgeon's office. However, few patients actually choose to take advantage of this; most seem to prefer initially seeing the surgeon after entering the hospital.

Most patients admitted for cardiac surgery are admitted directly to a surgical unit, which may also have noncardiac surgical patients on its ward. An intensive care unit of five beds is immediately adjacent to the surgical ward of beds for preoperative and postsurgical convalescent patients. These two areas are separated by the main nursing station. The nursing staff responsible for cardiac surgical patients rotate their coverage between pre- and postoperative patients on the main floor and the open-heart intensive care patients.

The entrance area to the cardiac surgical floor contains a family waiting room. This area is separated by approximately 60 feet from the nearest open-heart cardiac surgical patient bed.

This floor layout, together with the nonhierarchical nursing coverage system, leads to the inevitable mixing of newly admitted patients with those in various stages of convalescence from cardiac surgery. Thus, the patients are exposed to all manner of input from previously admitted patients.

Approximately 250 patients per year are referred to the Cardiothoracic Surgical Service. Most are admitted for either coronary bypass surgery or cardiac valvular replacement surgery. Occasionally, patients are also admitted with congenital cardiac problems or major thoracic vascular catastrophies.

Preoperative Protocol

Cardiothoracic service patients are admitted to the hospital approximately 36 hours prior to surgery. At that time, they establish relationships with the nursing staff and observe and talk to other patients in various stages of recovery. Following the admission, history is taken, physical examination is made by the house staff officer, laboratory bloods are drawn, and x-ray studies are obtained.

Each patient is visited by a floor nurse, who orients the patient to the preoperative protocol. The protocol includes such items as diet, medications, and preoperative surgical preparation. The patient is then seen by a pulmonary therapist and familiarized with the postoperative equipment used to optimize pulmonary function. The patient is also seen preoperatively by a physical therapist who explains the postoperative activity goals and routines. A hospital chaplain from the appropriate religious affiliation is also available, upon request. The patient is then brought to the open-heart recovery room and familiarized briefly with the area. At this time, the patient may or may not encounter a recent postoperative patient. The patient is routinely seen preoperatively by the attending surgeon and anesthesiologist. The members of the staff who see the patient explain their functions on the surgical team and describe their roles in caring for the patient during hospitalization.

When the surgeons feel the patient or family is having difficulty in coping with the scheduled surgery, the patient is referred for a preoperative psychiatric interview. The majority of the patients require this review.

The Preoperative Psychiatric Interview

Each patient referred for psychiatric evaluation is interviewed before surgery. Occasionally, patients scheduled for surgery may be in such emotional distress that several psychotherapy sessions, in addition to the preoperative evaluation, are required. This occurs most commonly when a patient's surgery is postponed one or more days, either because of surgical emergencies or other unforeseen circumstances. The following case illustrates the use of the preoperative interview:

> Mr. B was a 48-year-old man admitted for coronary bypass surgery. In the preoperative interview, he openly discussed how annoyed he was at having been "bumped" from the surgery schedule several times. In addition to the anxiety he felt about his upcoming surgery, he talked about his general problem with anger. In discussing difficulties he had in holding jobs, he responded readily to the psychiatrist's suggestion that he might have problems with authority figures. Without much encouragement, he reviewed how hurt he was by his father's harsh and arbitrary treatment. He was easily able to see how his repeated disagreements with his bosses might be related to his unresolved feelings about his father.

He thanked the psychiatrist, noting that he felt the preoperative interview had been most helpful.

When an unexpected snowstorm prevented the surgeons from coming to the hospital, the patient's surgery once again had to be postponed. He became enraged and threatened to sign out. He agreed to see the psychiatrist. After a highly charged session, in which he was able to ventilate his anger and see that his desire to act out would be counterproductive, he agreed to remain hospitalized and approached surgery with much less anger. His surgery and postoperative course were uneventful.

The preoperative interview lasts from 45 to 60 minutes. When clinically appropriate and logistically possible, the patient's family and/or friends may be included in the last 10 to 15 minutes. The interview has both diagnostic and therapeutic purposes. Under ideal conditions, the interview is conducted in a rather structured manner. The patients are asked to review their present illness and past medical history. Events leading to the need for cardiac catheterization and the recommendation for surgery are reviewed. Throughout the interview, the patients are encouraged to express their feelings about their illness, its effect on them and their families, and their attitudes about the necessity for surgery.

Confused and angry patients need the preoperative and postoperative psychiatric interviews more than other patients. Unfortunately, these patients are the most offended by the recommendation for a preoperative psychiatric interview. However, if the psychiatrist can empathize with the patients' confusion and help them clarify and ventilate their feelings, the psychiatrist can help these patients establish a working alliance with him and the entire surgical team.

Patients are encouraged to ask questions and make specific requests regarding their own management. Patients frequently express different views regarding the management of pain, the need for explanations and information, and fears of being controlled or manipulated by the staff. Nowadays, many patients are well-informed about the technical and emotional aspects of cardiac surgery. For example, several patients have asked about the reported high incidence of postoperative depression. They seem reassured that a psychiatrist is available, should this emotional complication occur.

After the completion of the evaluation interview, the psychiatrist writes an extensive, detailed consultation note in the medical chart. Consultation notes that use anecdotal, that is, specific historical material, are much more effective in the surgical-medical setting than notes that use descriptive (interpretive) and diagnostic psychiatric jargon. The consultation note outlines relevant aspects of the patient's medical and personal history and describes how the patient and family both understand and have been affected by the patient's illness and the need for surgery. It presents any initial conceptualizations of the patient's and family's psychodynamics and includes an assessment of their ego strengths and weaknesses. These formulations alert the other team members to potential pre- and postoperative emotional trouble spots. Specific recommendations regarding the type and extent of preoperative education that is appropriate for the patient are provided. Whenever possible, these findings are conveyed to the staff in person.

The Psychiatrist's Postoperative Role

In the surgical ICU, the psychiatrist manages all cases of postoperative delirium and psychosis. When patients leave the ICU, the psychiatrist follows them for more subtle signs of emotional disturbance. The psychiatrist may be asked to intervene in some cases; in others, the psychiatrist may suggest the intervention. In addition, patients or their families may request psychological help. The psychiatrist may be asked by any member of the surgical team for advice and suggestions to improve their management of certain patients or of their own personal, emotional responses to patients or families. The psychiatrist frequently offers suggestions to the staff for the psychological management of patients—both those the psychiatrist sees and those who refuse the interview.

PSYCHOLOGICAL DYNAMICS

The Patients

Postoperative psychosis and delirium are the most dramatic and closely studied psychological problems encountered by cardiac surgical patients. We agree with the general strategy that has been developed to manage these patients (the use of Haldol and a supportive psychotherapeutic relationship). However, it is our strong impression that the use of a preoperative psychiatric interview reduces the incidence of postoperative psychosis and delirium. In addition to managing the psychotic, delirious patient, the psychiatrist helps family members of these patients. Indeed, without adequate intervention, distraught family members can seriously disrupt the workings of the cardiac service.

Kimball outlined three phases of emotional and physical recovery from cardiac surgery. In addition, he described the use of systematic preoperative psychological interviews to identify the patient's general style of life adjustment, anxiety regarding surgery, and orientation toward the future. From this information, he developed four groups of patients (adjusted, symbiotic, anxious, and depressed) and attempted to correlate specific types of postoperative response.[22,23] We have found this scheme to be a valuable starting point in understanding how to help patients with their psychological responses to cardiac surgery.

In working closely with such patients, we have discovered several other important aspects of their psychological dynamics. Patients clearly bring an individual characterologic style to the experience of surgery, and this colors their emotional responses to it. However, they also come to surgery in a unique emotional context. Many times, they are in the midst of acute, subacute, or chronic unresolved emotional conflicts. These individual emotional conflicts influence their psychological approaches to surgery and postoperative course; in fact, the patients may find these emotional issues more troublesome than the surgery itself. When such issues, as well as those specifically related to surgery, are addressed by the psychiatrist in the preoperative interview, the patient approaches surgery in a calmer, more secure fashion.

Loss is the major unresolved emotional issue that these patients struggle with at the time of surgery. Usually, the loss is that of a spouse, parent, income, or job. Most patients deny the emotional importance of their loss yet show clear manifestations of its unresolved nature. The following case is a dramatic example of this condition.

> A 62-year-old man's wife had died eight years prior to the man's surgery. Shortly after her death, he threw himself into his work with even more intensity than he had before. Within a year, he developed angina symptoms and was managed medically. Seven years later, when his symptoms could no longer be contained medically, he was referred for coronary bypass surgery. In the preoperative interview he was able to review, in an unemotional fashion, all the medical events leading to his need for surgery. When he began to discuss his personal life, he started to weep uncontrollably as he described his wife's death and his subsequent loneliness and guilt. He was more relaxed after the interview but denied that his wife's death still troubled him.

Some patients are able to address their emotional problems at the time of surgery, as in the following case.

> A 28-year-old man seemed to approach mitral valve replacement in a calm and settled way. However, in the preoperative interview he

openly shared with the psychiatrist how much he had hoped to put off the surgery until he was able to come to terms with the emotional impact of the recent death of both his parents. Having been estranged from them for many years, he felt guilty that he had not done more for them before their deaths. In fact, he began to cry when he shared his feeling that he did not deserve to survive his surgery. He felt that at least being able to discuss this conflict with someone enabled him to face surgery in a "better frame of mind."

Frequently, a patient's feelings about unresolved issues will get acted out in inappropriate behavior during the postop course, as in the following case.

A 58-year-old woman approached mitral valve surgery in a state of "complete calm and security," since she had the "most complete sense of confidence and faith in [her] doctors." However, in the preoperative interview, she expressed how guilty she still felt about her mother's death ten years earlier. She felt she still had to cry about it but could not bring herself to do this, as her friends and husband kept telling her she was "ridiculous."

She asked if she were crazy because she still felt a need to cry. She requested further sessions with the psychiatrist after surgery to further explore this. During the early stages of her postoperative course, she was attempting too much activity too soon and refused to ask for help when she needed it. The staff was concerned that she might injure herself. After several psychotherapy sessions in which she continued to cry about her mother's death, her postoperative activity level became more phase-appropriate, and she was more easily able to accept assistance from staff members.

In addition to important unresolved emotional issues, patients bring a particular adaptational style to surgery. This style clearly influences how they psychologically approach and manage their surgery. However, we have found that Kimball's four general adjustment styles (adjusted, symbiotic, anxious, depressed) are not specific enough, either in understanding each patient's individual psychological response to surgery or in designing plans for psychological intervention and management. Rather, we have found that the psychiatrist needs to do a thorough dynamic formulation of each patient's defense mechanisms, coping mechanisms, and object relationships. Once this is accomplished in the preoperative interview, the psychiatrist can more fully understand the nature of the patient's inevitable psychological regression, can more clearly communicate this to staff and family members, and can then design specific ways for intervening to help the patient cope with the trauma of surgery. The following case illustrates this approach.

Mr. B was a 54-year-old man who drove a delivery truck for all of his employed life. He was a reclusive man who enjoyed his solitary job. His greatest pleasure in life was maintaining his modest weekend home. He spoke lovingly in the preoperative interview of chopping wood and sitting by the fire, watching the flames. His wife was a lively, engaging person who was always prodding him to be more social. His overriding memory of childhood was that his parents rarely spoke to him.

Shortly after he was fired from his job, he developed anginal symptoms. These became medically unmanageable, and he was recommended for coronary bypass surgery. Several days after he left the ICU he became mute. He would lie in bed for hours at a time, staring at the ceiling or with his face in the pillow. He refused to eat or participate in the rehabilitation program. His wife and daughters became panic-stricken with the thought that he was going crazy. The medical and nursing staff thought he might have had a stroke. After several psychotherapy sessions in which the psychiatrist conveyed an understanding of the patient's need to withdraw, his becoming upset about his job, and the trauma of surgery, the patient slowly became more communicative, acknowledged the presence of his family, and resumed his rehabilitation activities.

During this period, the psychiatrist needed to have several supportive sessions with the patient's wife and daughter. These sessions helped them understand that withdrawal appeared to be the patient's only way of coping with surgery and that his behavior was most likely temporary. Because their anxiety was contained, they did not distract the nurses or surgeons from attending to much sicker patients.

The Staff

The Cardiothoracic Surgical Service is a busy one. Frequently, all five beds in the ICU are filled. The atmosphere is tense; the nurses are hyper-alert and constantly watching for problems that might arise. This vigilant attitude is especially noticeable in the ICU, where the condition of any of the unit patients may deteriorate at any moment. Knowing this, the nurses in the unit carefully and continuously watch and maintain the many monitoring devices and intravenous lines. It is difficult for them to engage in conversation for prolonged periods of time.

On the floor, the atmosphere is somewhat less tense. But, here too, nurses and rehabilitation personnel busily monitor and treat a large number of patients. Staff members pride themselves on their knowledge, efficiency, and success in working with such high-risk, critically ill patients.

In this setting, how does the psychiatrist establish and maintain a working alliance with medical, nursing, and rehabilitation personnel? Initially, the psychiatrist's main task is to allay the staff's anxiety about the psychiatrist's role. Most staff members have had limited contact with this type of professional and may be quite fearful that the psychiatrist will read their minds, analyze them, or criticize their interactions with each other. The psychiatrist must clearly establish that there is no hidden agenda in this regard.

Most staff members recognize the importance of psychological factors in the development of cardiac disease and of the psychological complications associated with cardiac surgery. However, most staff members have had limited training in psychological assessment and treatment. Despite this, they do their best to understand each patient's psychological needs and to manage their complicated emotional responses to surgery. Still when the psychiatrist arrives, the staff members may become concerned that their work in this area will be scrutinized in a harsh and critical way by "the expert." Their anxieties on this score must be allayed before the psychiatrist can be fully integrated into the team.

Another way the psychiatrist achieves and maintains a working alliance is by establishing a clear and structured role as a member of the team. There are three important aspects to this:

1. taking primary responsibility for the treatment and management of patients' psychological problems
2. teaching staff about patients' psychological responses and needs
3. being available in a supportive role to help the staff as a whole deal with problems of morale

Taking Primary Responsibility for Treatment and Management of Patients' Psychological Problems

Because of tremendous service pressures, staff cannot be expected to learn the complex skills required for the in-depth treatment of patients with psychological problems. By accepting responsibility for patients' psychological treatment, the psychiatrist reduces staff anxiety to the point where staff no longer need to deny or avoid patients' blatant or subtle psychological problems and can appropriately refer them for treatment. When staff anxiety has been reduced to workable levels, staff members can more easily understand and implement management suggestions.

The psychiatrist establishes a direct physician-patient relationship with each patient and intervenes using psychotherapeutic and, when appropriate, psychopharmacologic approaches. Because couples or family sessions are often indicated, the psychiatrist must be flexible. Occasionally, patients and families refuse to be involved with a psychiatrist. In these situations, the psychiatrist must act as supervisor to the staff members who manage the patients and families.

Educating Staff about Patients' Psychological Needs

In dealing with patients' psychological problems medical and nursing staff are more interested in simple, practical management solutions than in theoretical explanations. In this situation acting as a psychological interpreter, the psychiatrist can explain the meaning of each patient's psychological symptoms and how to treat them. In the authors' more than three years of work in this setting, it has become clear that the use of even the most elementary psychiatric terminology can be confusing and therefore anxiety-provoking to staff members. Theoretical concepts regarding a patient's character structure, ego strengths and weaknesses, defensive structure, and regression must be explained in language that can be easily understood. At times, staff members may express interest in learning more about a patient's psychological make-up. By and large, however, the psychiatrist must keep in mind that psychological theory and treatment approaches are not primary areas of interest for most staff members.

After the psychiatrist has established a strong working alliance with staff, the staff members may request help, not only with management issues, but also with their own emotional responses to certain patients. Frequently, these emotional responses are more troublesome than management issues. They should thus be approached in an instructional, educational manner, rather than in an exploratory, questioning one; questions like, "Why do you think you are feeling this way," make staff members much too anxious. In this way the psychiatrist can help staff members understand why certain patients are so provocative.

We have found five types of patients to be the most emotionally provocative for staff. The psychiatrist must be especially alert to patients with these character styles and help staff to anticipate the ways in which these patients regress psychologically and to understand the feelings that such patients invariably stimulate:

1. suspicious, paranoid patients who externalize, blame, and reject staff members
2. obsessional patients who need to be in control and require endless explanations and reassurance

3. manipulative patients who pit one staff member against another, hoping to get "more" for themselves
4. passive dependent patients who need a great deal of support, want to know as little as possible about their surgery, and leave their care up to others
5. self-destructive patients who, after surgery, seemingly flaunt their bad habits in front of the staff

Patients in the last category provoke the most intense emotional responses. In these cases staff members have great difficulty dealing with their own sense of failure, helplessness, inadequacy, anger, and guilt; they feel emotionally so out of control. The following case illustrates well staff difficulties with a self-destructive patient.

Emergency surgery was performed on a 32-year-old lawyer when it was discovered that his progressive heart failure was due to mycotic infections of two heart valves, incurred from "shooting up" cocaine. Postoperatively, he was comatose for one week, then became delirious and agitated. Neurologic evaluation revealed the presence of several brain abscesses. Appropriate antibiotic therapy was started.

During his prolonged stay in the intensive care unit, the patient required a great deal of attention from all support staff. His delirium began to clear, and he made slow but steady progress. It became apparent that he was an articulate, intelligent, highly successful man who was well-regarded in his profession. As his miraculous recovery continued, nursing and medical staff were delighted and gratified. Everyone had become quite fond of him.

When the patient was transferred to the area floor and feeling stronger, he began begging nurses to get cigarettes for him. He started to disregard his dietary and exercise restrictions. He manipulated individual staff members in order to get more than prescribed pain medication. Some staff members attempted to reason with him about the use of cigarettes and the need for a special diet, as well as a gradual increase in physical activity. Others attempted to be firm with him. All efforts that staff made to help him care for himself were rebuffed.

Because of this obvious self-destructive behavior, the patient was referred to the psychiatrist. In psychotherapy sessions, he revealed that all of his family members had a history of violence and self-destructive behavior. Recently his father had attempted suicide. One of his memories from age 12 was of being chased by his grandfather with a power lawnmower. His grandfather subsequently shot his pet rabbit.

Although the patient initially appeared to make appropriate use of psychotherapy sessions, he abruptly refused further treatment. Despite his steady progress, he continued to be self-destructive and even more provocative. He responded only to firm, consistent limit-setting of his manipulative behavior regarding pain medication.

The emotional responses the patient provoked ranged from sorrow and pity to rage, horror, and disgust. He caused tremendous turmoil on the floor. Several staff members appealed to the psychiatrist for help in dealing with their feelings. In several group meetings, nurses shared and expressed their intense frustration and hurt at having their heroic efforts rejected and devalued. In addition to facilitating the group process so that the nurses could ventilate their feelings, the psychiatrist shared examples from his own clinical practice and used selected journal articles to help the nurses understand and manage their own emotional responses.[24,25]

Helping Staff Deal with Problems of Morale

In the care of patients with psychological problems, maintaining morale is an area of ongoing concern and attention. Because the work requires intense vigilance and an involvement with considerable technical machinery, nurses may come to feel dehumanized, to feel they are being forced to treat their patients in a dehumanized way. In such situations, especially when the service is busy, staff feel better when they can share the emotional burden of their workload. They also feel better when they know their patients' emotional needs have not been forgotten in the crush of an exhausting and at times numbing work schedule.

In this setting, the psychiatrist becomes the guardian of the humanitarian interests of patients, staff, and the cardiac service as a whole. The psychiatrist's rounds are especially appreciated by staff members; in these rounds, they are able to take a brief break from their vigilance of patients, pills, and machines and have a moment of human interaction.

Two situations invariably lead to crises in staff morale: (1) deaths that occur in close proximity and (2) patients who have severe complications and become chronic custodial problems. In these cases, the psychiatrist may suggest or may be asked to lead group sessions to help nursing staff deal with their feelings of inadequacy, failure, and anger. The psychiatrist functions best in this setting when acting as an educator and facilitator of group process, rather than as a therapist encouraging deep personal exploration.

SUMMARY

Patients bring a particular character style to the experience of cardiac surgery; they also approach surgery in a very personal emotional context. In the authors' experience, in a great many patients the emotional context appears to involve unresolved issues of one or more types of loss. However if the psychiatrist adequately addresses these issues of loss, as well as those anxieties specifically related to surgery, patients have fewer pre- and post-operative difficulties.

As an integral member of the surgical team, the psychiatrist is in a unique position to understand the overall dynamics of the service and in particular the different needs of the staff. In the busy, tense environment of the cardiac service, the staff's primary interest must be the physical welfare of their patients. Yet, although the staff recognize the serious emotional consequences of cardiac surgery, they rarely have the skill or the time to manage them.

In this critical care setting, the psychiatrist functions best when he takes primary responsibility for the treatment and management of patients' emotional problems precipitated by surgery. The psychiatrist establishes a primary physician-patient relationship with each patient and enlists the staff in implementing a practical, workable management protocol. In working with the staff, the psychiatrist should use a minimum of psychiatric jargon and theory.

Because of the unique nature of the cardiac surgical service, in addition to ongoing problems of staff morale, there are particular problems precipitated by certain situations. Among these are a series of deaths and patients who become chronic. The psychiatrist who is integrated into the team is more likely to be asked for help with these problems. Using a knowledge of group process, the psychiatrist can thereby be helpful to the team as a whole and contribute to its smooth functioning.

REFERENCES

1. P.H. Blachly and A. Starr, "Post Cardiotomy Delirium," *American Journal of Psychiatry* 121 (1964): 371–375.

2. S. Gilman, "Cerebral Disorders After Open Heart Operations," *New England Journal of Medicine* 272 (1965): 489–498.

3. P.H. Blachly and F.E. Kloster, "Relation of Cardiac Output to Post-Cardiotomy Delirium," *Journal of Thoracic and Cardiovascular Surgery* 52 (1966): 422–427.

4. P.H. Blachly and F.E. Kloster, "Treatment of Delirium with Phenothiazine Drugs Following Open Heart Surgery," *Diseases of the Nervous System* 27 (1966): 107–110.

5. R.M. Morse and E.M. Litin, "Post Operative Delirium: A Study of Etiologic Factors," *American Journal of Psychiatry* 126 (1969): 136–143.

6. C.P. Kimball "The Experience of Open Heart Surgery III: Toward a Definition and Understanding of Post-Cardiotomy Delirium," *Archives of General Psychiatry* 27 (1972): 57–63.

7. D.S. Kornfeld et al., "Personality and Psychological Factors in Post-Cardiotomy Delirium," *Archives of General Psychiatry* 31 (1974): 249–253.

8. S.S. Heller et al., "Post Cardiotomy Delirium and Cardiac Output," *American Journal of Psychiatry* 136 (1979): 337–339.

9. W.R. Dubin, H.L. Field, and B.S. Gastfriend, "Post Cardiotomy Delirium: A Critical Review," *Journal of Thoracic and Cardiovascular Surgery* 77 (1979): 586–594.

10. H.R. Lazarus and J.H. Hagens, "Prevention of Psychosis Following Open-Heart Surgery," *American Journal of Psychiatry* 124 (1968): 1190–1195.

11. O.L. Layne and S.C. Yudofsky, "Post Operative Psychosis in Cardiotomy Patients: The Role of Organic and Psychiatric Factors," *New England Journal of Medicine* 284 (1971): 518–520.

12. H.S. Abram, "Adaptation to Open Heart Surgery: A Psychiatric Study of Response to the Threat of Death," *American Journal of Psychiatry* 122 (1965): 659–667.

13. D.S. Kornfeld, S. Zimberg, and J.R. Malm, "Psychiatric Complications of Open-Heart Surgery," *New England Journal of Medicine* 273 (1965): 287–292.

14. S.S. Heller et al., "Psychiatric Complications of Open-Heart Surgery: A Reexamination," *New England Journal of Medicine* 283 (1970): 1015–1020.

15. K.A. Frank et al., "Long-Term Effects of Open-Heart Surgery on Intellectual Functioning," *Journal of Thoracic and Cardiovascular Surgery* 64 (1972): 811–815.

16. K.A. Frank, S.S. Heller, D.S. Kornfeld, "A Survey of Adjustment to Cardiac Surgery," *Archives of Internal Medicine* 130 (1972): 735–738.

17. S.S. Heller et al., "Psychological Outcome Following Open-Heart Surgery," *Archives of Internal Medicine* 134 (1974): 908–914.

18. C.P. Kimball, "A Predictive Study of Adjustment to Cardiac Surgery," *Journal of Thoracic and Cardiovascular Surgery* 58 (1969): 891–896.

19. C.P. Kimball, "Psychological Responses to the Experience of Open-Heart Surgery: I," *American Journal of Psychiatry* 126 (1969): 348–359.

20. Lazarus and Hagens, "Prevention of Psychosis."

21. Layne and Yudofsky, "Post Operative Psychosis."

22. Kimball, "A Predictive Study."

23. Kimball, "Psychological Responses."

24. J.E. Groves, "Taking Care of the Hateful Patient," *New England Journal of Medicine* 298 (1978): 883–887.

25. J.E. Groves, "Management of the Borderline Patient on a Medical or Surgical Ward: The Psychiatric Consultant's Role," *International Journal of Psychiatry in Medicine* 6 (1975): 337–348.

Chapter 10

Psychiatric Services to the Renal Dialysis Unit

Joel Gonchar, M.D.

INTRODUCTION AND BACKGROUND

The treatment of end-stage renal disease (ESRD) through use of an artificial kidney (hemodialysis) became possible in the 1960s. However, it was not until 1973, when Congress amended Title 19 of the Social Security Act to include this modality of medical care, that the treatment became widely available. In the ensuing years, the number of treatment modalities for ESRD has also increased. These modalities include:

- transplantation
- continuous ambulatory peritoneal dialysis (CAPD)
- intermittent peritoneal dialysis (CCPD)
- intermittent peritoneal dialysis (IPD)
- home hemodialysis

Currently, transplantation and CAPD are the most commonly used secondary modalities. However, the majority of patients are still treated by hemodialysis in treatment centers. Most of these treatment centers are located in hospitals, although a number of them are satellite units that either are run by a hospital or are free-standing , privately owned units.

For the most part, this chapter deals with the psychological problems of hemodialysis patients and how they are managed in the dialysis unit of Lenox Hill Hospital.

First, however, some definitions are in order. Patients are diagnosed as having ESRD when their serum creatinine is above ten. This indicates that they have less than 10 percent of their renal function left. Hemodialysis is performed by connecting a patient's vascular system to a machine consisting of a dialyzer or filter and a pump to circulate the blood through the machine. The connection to the patient is made through an access site, which may be one of two types: a fistula or a graft. The fistula, the more commonly used access, is created by joining an artery and a vein surgically. A graft is created by joining a synthetic material, such as gortex, with an artery and a vein. In contrast, in CAPD, a permanent catheter is placed through the abdominal wall into the peritoneal cavity. A specially constituted dialysis fluid is instilled through this catheter and removed after six hours. In this treatment, the peritoneal membrane that covers the internal viscera acts as the filter.

PHYSICAL MILIEU

The hemodialysis unit at Lenox Hill Hospital began as a small section of three beds in the rear of the ICU. About six years ago, the hemodialysis unit moved to its own quarters and expanded to five dialysis chairs and three beds. The unit has a central nursing station, so that the nursing and technical staff can respond quickly to any problems that develop with either the patients or the machines. Each machine has a number of alarms that can be heard going off periodically during the treatments.There is a surrealistic quality to the unit that strikes a visitor who is unfamiliar with this form of treatment. The scene is one of a group of patients scattered around a large room with blood-filled tubing running from their arms to machines by their sides. The beds, by and large, are for the sicker patients who cannot tolerate sitting in the large easy chairs.

Most of the patients are treated as outpatients and leave the unit after their treatment, either on their own or by ambulette. A small proportion of patients are inpatients who have either just started hemodialysis or been admitted for some complication. There is one bed kept in an isolation room and reserved for patients with hepatitis—a not uncommon complication, given hemodialysis patients' frequent need for transfusion.

The rate of turnover of patients is low, with many patients maintained in the unit for years. There may be periods, however, when several patients will die within the same week or two, and this is always distressing for both staff and other patients. ESRD patients are all considered "private;" even if they were begun as "service" cases, in a very short time they are assigned to a private attending nephrologist. The dialysis unit, however, is a "regional" floor; as such, all of its patients are considered teaching cases for medical residents and renal fellows. Currently, there are 47 hemodialysis patients and 12 CAPD patients being treated.

In addition to the large treatment area and nursing station, the dialysis unit contains a patients' lounge with lockers (for street clothing that patients come in with), as well as a patients' bathroom and changing room. Next to these facilities are offices for the head nurse, the chief nephrologist, the renal fellows, and other house staff rotating through the service.

The unit has a chief and an assistant chief nephrologist who receive small stipends from the hospital to administer the unit. They are essentially private practitioners with a strong interest in research and teaching. There are three other attending nephrologists, one of whom has responsibility for the CAPD program. The nursing staff include a head nurse, an assistant head nurse, and a staff of five full-time nurses and one part-time nurse. The technician staff, with a technical coordinator and three technicians, also report to the head nurse. The technicians, who are primarily responsible for the operation of the machines, interact a great deal with patients and are intimately involved in their care. A dietitian is assigned exclusively to the dialysis unit. The full-time social worker spends most of the time on dialysis but also has other responsibilities, such as teaching social work students. The author's position as psychiatrist is a voluntary one, involving three hours a week of service time to the dialysis unit and being available to treat patients privately at other times.

PHYSIOLOGICAL-PSYCHOLOGICAL PROBLEMS OF RENAL DIALYSIS

Dependency

Hemodialysis patients face many of the same problems that other patients with chronic illness have. They must learn to live with the limitations imposed on them by their illness, but with the important further limitation stemming from machine dependency.[1] The need to be continually dependent on a machine, as well as on the staff who run the machine, imposes a special burden on hemodialysis patients. Many of them were previously independent adults. Now, on an average of three days a week for four to six hours at a time, they must put themselves in an abjectly dependent position—and they must do this for the rest of their lives. Frequently, this situation revives conflicts over dependency for which some resolution had previously been achieved. At times, however, the reverse situation may hold true; patients with very strong dependency needs may find hemodialysis an ideal situation in which to have these needs gratified. They may welcome the dependency and become overly passive, in relation to both the treatment and their lives in general.

Compliance

Another limitation faced by hemodialysis patients involves dietary and fluid restrictions.[2] In this crucial area, the success or failure of a patient's overall treatment program is determined. Indeed compliance with dietary and fluid restrictions can be used as a measure of a patient's adaptation to life as a dialysis patient.[3] A number of the issues with which patients struggle can be expressed through noncompliance with these restrictions, for example the need to assert their autonomy or to express anger at their physician or nurse. They may use noncompliance in an effort to deny that they are really sick or to express covert suicidal wishes. In any event it must be recognized that, in having to restrict what they can eat and drink, dialysis patients have to give up an important source of gratification in life.

Losses

Apart from dietary and fluid restrictions, there is a larger general loss for the dialysis patient as a result of the chronicity and specific nature of the disease. As a result of their chronic anemia most hemodialysis patients experience a loss of strength and energy, along with a build-up of toxic metabolic waste products between treatments. Many patients also experience some loss of sexual interest and/or functioning. These problems tend to be greater in men than in women; some studies indicate the extent of impotence may be as high as 50 to 70 percent.[4] Decreased libido and ejaculatory problems also exist. Women patients experience frigidity, decreased libido, and difficulty reaching orgasm.[5]

Other losses may include a loss of position within the family or a loss of power or status at work because of diminished capacities and restrictions imposed by dialysis. The patient and the family may experience a loss of position and power within the community because of the economic strain created. Since patients are still uremic to some degree (which increases between treatments), their cognitive functioning may not return to normal, and they may continue to have some degree of organic brain dysfunction. In such cases, if the patients return to work, there is likely to be some degree of disillusionment and disappointment. Such patients have to learn to pace themselves and adjust their work schedules to dialysis; for example, a lawyer would schedule important meetings only for the day immediately following a dialysis treatment. Finally, some level of depression is an invariable accompaniment of all these losses.

Medical Complications

Once the patients have been able to develop coping mechanisms in the course of their illness, the onset of complications will tax, and often overtax, the mechanisms. Access breakdown, whether it be a fistula or a graft, is a common complication. It is an especially difficult problem for patients in whom it occurs repeatedly; in such cases, it can lead to the possibility of running out of sites. Fluid overload, particularly in a poorly compliant patient, leads to congestive heart failure or pulmonary edema. Hyperparathyroidism with concomitant bone disease occurs because of altered phosphorus excretion; in such cases, the patients often go on to have their parathyroid glands removed.[6] In patients who are poorly compliant with the dietary restrictions, hyperkalemia, with associated dangers of cardiac arrhythmias, can occur.

One coping device is denial; but as this device becomes overused, patients are confronted once again with their vulnerability. At such times, dramatic regressions can occur, with or without accompanying anxiety states. These regressions frequently take the form of extreme dependency and helplessness. In such situations, the staff are asked to take care of patients in ways not previously called for, as illustrated in the following case.

> Mr. T was a 65-year-old diabetic hemodialysis patient who was blind. He had a stroke that involved weakness of the left arm and leg. Although he recovered almost complete function, for a period of about a month he required that someone sit with him and reassure him throughout his treatment or he would become very agitated. Because of the anxiety he was experiencing, he would stand up and start walking around (despite being still connected to the machine), even after the use of tranquilizers.

The regressions may be short-lived, or they may last for weeks until a better way of coping is established. In these periods the staff and families require the attention of the mental health staff, who can explain what is going on and aid in developing strategies to deal with the regression. These strategies may involve such techniques as reassurance or reality testing. The latter technique is illustrated in the following case.

> Mrs. G was a 50-year-old married female hemodialysis patient who developed a heart attack and was hospitalized. After discharge, she became fearful of leaving home and was unable to allow her husband to leave her for fear of becoming ill again with no one there to help. She required brief psychotherapy focusing on the reality of her condition of being fully recovered and her misconception of how fragile she was.

One complication that has not been seen in the Lenox Hill renal dialysis unit is dementia dialytica. This is manifested as a slowly evolving encephalopathy with slurring of speech and gradual loss of intelligibility, progressing over a period of months to death. It is thought to be related to aluminum intoxication stemming from the aluminum in the phosphorus binders patients must take to prevent bone disease.

Effects on Family

The families of dialysis patients also have a great deal of coping to do. Dialysis places great stress on a marriage. For spouses who are accustomed to particular roles, chronic illness in one partner frequently necessitates shifts in roles.[7] An example of this may be seen in a marriage in which a previously strong and dominant husband is now sick and the previously weaker or submissive wife must assume her spouse's role. Neither partner has anticipated the change in roles, and a great deal of friction results. In one case of a couple who were on home hemodialysis, the sick wife, who had formerly been the dominant spouse, could not tolerate being in a dependent and submissive role vis-a-vis her husband. The couple eventually opted for medical center dialysis at the Lenox Hill Hospital dialysis unit until they resolved this conflict; but, ideally, earlier mental health intervention with the couple should have been attempted to try to resolve the role problem. On the other hand, it is important for a dialysis center to be flexible about allowing patients to return to the center if home hemodialysis does not work well.

For unmarried patients with available parents, the illness may mean the return of a formerly independent adult child to the parental home. This situation evokes reactions in both the parents and the adult child. The parents may resent having their later years interfered with when they had expected to be finished with caring for a dependent child. For the adult child, the crisis occurs in terms of having to resume dependency on the parents and giving up some measure of autonomy. The young children of dialysis patients also face problems because of the illness of their parent. They may have unmet needs because of the dependent and regressive position of the parent. Often they are faced with demands to take on new responsibilities. In all of these patient-family problem areas, it is important to remember that one of the most important factors in aiding patients to cope with dialysis is the presence of a stable and supportive family.

Effects on Staff

Along with the problems faced by patients and their families in coping with chronic kidney disease, the stresses imposed on the professional staff require attention by the mental health staff. Since the inception of hemodialysis as a treatment, staff turnover has been an important problem. A major factor in this turnover is the continuing and ongoing nature of the staff contact with ESRD patients, in contrast with the situation in other medical-surgical units where staff involvement with patients is short-lived.[8] Another relevant factor is the fact that chronic renal dialysis patients never get better; their condition either remains the same or deteriorates. Frequently, they are overtly angry, noncompliant, and unappreciative of their doctors and nurses. In such situations of prolonged and frequent staff contact with patients, intense feelings, both positive and negative, are generated. Staff members must bear the brunt of the patients' psychopathology or regressive behavior. Frequently they become the target of feelings the patients have displaced from other areas of their lives. Inevitably, counterreactions are evoked in staff members, who may react angrily or withdraw from patients.[9] When a patient deteriorates or dies, the staff may experience a sense either of loss or of relief accompanied by guilt, depending on what their overall feeling was about the patient. At times when a patient is deteriorating and appears to be suffering, staff members often come to feel that what they are doing for the patient is more harmful than helpful. These are the times when staff morale is particularly poor, and tension is high.

Mental Health Care for Dialysis Outpatients and Staff

Recognizing that these various physiological-psychological problems can have significant effects on the success of treatments for ESRD, Congress has mandated the provision of mental health services to dialysis programs. A variety of mental health professionals has been involved in this care, including social workers, psychologists, psychiatrists, and psychiatric nurse clinicians. The overall goal is to help patients adapt to, and cope with, the limitations inherent in ESRD and thus maximize the quality of their lives.

To date the social worker has been the primary mental health practitioner in dialysis units in this country. Psychiatrists and psychologists have been involved in varying degrees, depending on the type and location of the facility. At university teaching general hospitals or their close affiliates, psychiatric consultation-liaison fellowship programs often assign a psychiatric fellow or a resident to the dialysis unit. In community general hospitals like Lenox Hill with psychiatric consultation-liaison services, a psychiatrist on the private voluntary attending staff is assigned to the dialysis unit as a primary "service" commitment. In general hospitals without such a service, psychiatrists may perform consultations for particular dialysis patients, as requested by the staff, but have no continuing involvement with the unit and its staff.

At Lenox Hill Hospital, in addition to the voluntary attending psychiatrist, a full-time social worker provides mental health services. The two professionals function as members of a team, the other members of which include the nephrologists (attendings and fellows), nurses, technicians, and a dietitian. When a patient is identified as a hemodialysis candidate, the social worker and psychiatrist meet separately with the patient to begin the evaluation of the patient's psychosocial status and to look for areas that may call for intervention. An effort is made to dispel misconceptions and to lessen the anxiety about the dialysis program that inevitably arises before the beginning of treatment. The patient is shown around the unit and is at some point introduced to another patient who has been able to cope successfully with the treatment.

After these initial meetings, the staff members discuss the patient at a team conference. If any serious difficulties are detected at this time, an appropriate intervention is planned. This may consist of short-term or crisis-oriented psychotherapy or it may be an intervention with the family. The latter situation is illustrated in the following case.

> Mr. A is a 29-year-old homosexual male with ESRD related to an immune deficiency syndrome. He refused to consider hemodialysis and was extremely depressed and withdrawn. On interview, he would occasionally answer the questions by shaking his head, but he would not speak. He lived alone and was self-supporting. He was estranged from his family and had not seen his mother in a number of years. Attempts were made to contact the mother and bring her in to help influence the patient. The mother said that their relationship had been stormy and described a rather chaotic childhood that the patient had experienced. Although the mother was dubious about his responding to her, she agreed to come in. The result was a dramatic improvement in the patient's mood and desire to live, and he subsequently agreed to dialysis.

The first six months to a year is often crucial to adaptation and rehabilitation. Consequently, special attention is given to a patient's progress during this period. The social worker meets frequently with the patients and their families to facilitate adjustment and to take care of the practical matters involved in filing for Medicare or disability benefits and, when necessary, arranging for transportation. The following case illustrates one possible problem area during this period.

> Mr. R is a 35-year-old married hemodialysis patient who experienced a depression related to his loss of sexual function, specifically to impotence. By history, he no longer experienced much of

an erection on waking in the morning. Both he and his wife were feeling frustrated, since he refrained from going near her because of his feeling that he would fail sexually. Therapy for this couple involved a process of reorienting their sexual life together, deemphasizing the importance of the "penis-in-vagina" aspect of it, and substituting for it other aspects of sexuality.

The role of the psychiatrist is consultative with patients and educative (liaison) with the staff. In addition to assessing all patients to try to predict problems that might arise, the psychiatrist evaluates patients who manifest evidence of psychopathology or problems with coping. However the major part of the psychiatrist's work consists of liaison with the staff. The psychiatrist routinely visits the dialysis unit twice weekly, meeting on one of the two days with the nursing staff and social worker in order to keep informed of developments on the unit and with the care of particular patients. It is crucial to detect as early as possible any difficulties that seem to be evolving with any of the patients or within the staff, in order to maximize the effectiveness of the related interventions. In these meetings, consultations with individual patients or staff members are scheduled. In 1984, the psychiatrist in the Lenox Hill dialysis unit spent 70 hours seeing patients directly in consultation and for follow-up. The second day of psychiatric attendance is devoted to more formal meetings with the entire staff. The general discussions frequently focus on manifest problems with specific patients. Also didactic meetings on various aspects of dialysis that are of general interest are scheduled during these meetings.

These frequent meetings with the staff are particularly important in that the nursing and technician staff spend most of their time working directly with the patients and thus are likely to detect problems before the physicians do. Some of the topics that come up in meetings with the staff have to do with sensitive and difficult issues, such as overt sexual behavior by patients on the dialysis unit. The following is a case in point.

Mr. B is a 40-year-old male hemodialysis patient who, while on the machine, could be seen clearly to be masturbating himself. This behavior was very disturbing to the nursing staff, who brought it up at one of the meetings with the psychiatrist. After the matter was thoroughly discussed, the psychiatrist met with the patient and was able to ascertain that the patient was insecure about his sexuality. After some continued discussion, the behavior ceased.

Other difficult behaviors that come up for discussion include patients' lack of modesty in undressing while in a public area, in preparation for going on the machine, or while walking around the unit. Also, occasional flirtation or sexual advances to the staff can be very discomfiting. Encouraging discussion by the staff helps alleviate a lot of the distress; placing these behaviors in perspective makes them easier to deal with.

Another difficult problem involves the dying patient on the unit illustrated in the following case.

> Mr. R is a 65-year-old male hemodialysis patient with a severe immune deficiency, which led to a number of complications and frequent hospitalizations. One day, while getting into a new hemodialysis chair that had a plaque attached with the inscription "In Memoriam" on it, the patient joked about his reluctance to sit in a chair that had such a plaque. The staff member who was helping him became very uncomfortable and immediately changed the subject, consciously feeling that closing off this communication from the patient was best for the patient's welfare.

In this situation, discussion with staff about the patient's need for ventilation of fears and exploration of staff feelings concerning the dying patient will enable staff members to gain greater objectivity and reduce anxiety concerning the taboo subject.

As noted, the staff meetings are also a time for presentation of patients who have been management problems for the staff. Efforts are made to work out strategies that the staff can apply to improve management of these patients. The following cases are examples of such efforts.

> Mr. L is a 38-year-old male hemodialysis patient who was very demanding and often demeaning of the staff. He created power struggles with the staff over the control of his treatment. This was particularly manifest in his frequent changes of the negative pressure control settings that determine how much fluid is removed from the body during a treatment. His history revealed medical problems early in life; this had necessitated a number of surgeries that were responsible for his eventual development of ESRD. However, as is frequently true in such a situation, the patient developed a strong sense of entitlement; this underlay his battles with the staff, who were trying to impose limits on him. Making the patient's behavior understandable and suggesting he be encouraged to greater self-care, while at the same time establishing clear and firm limits to his behavior, made the patient considerably more manageable.

> Mrs. D is a 55-year-old hemodialysis patient with a psychiatric diagnosis of "borderline personality disorder." She tended to split

the staff by choosing to hate one staff member, whom she viewed as all bad, while she regarded other staff members as all good. This pattern was very disturbing to the staff member who was being scapegoated and who often, in response, became defensive and hostile to the patient, thereby living out the patient's projection. This pattern also created friction between the hated and loved staff members, thereby impairing their functioning. Exploring this pattern with the staff enabled them to place themselves at a sufficient distance to prevent their reacting personally to the projections, which could justify the patient's original projections.

As noted earlier, family members of the patient also have a great deal of coping to do. Much of the mental health care offered must go to family members, in view of the stresses on them and the important roles they perform in the patient's overall adjustment. This is illustrated in the following case.

Mr. F is a 60-year-old married, childless, male hemodialysis patient who worked as an attorney. Renal failure had come as a great shock to him. At the urging of his wife, he delayed starting hemodialysis and looked for alternative treatments, such as herbs and teas. When he became very ill, the couple could no longer deny his need to be on hemodialysis. Once having begun treatment, he was able to return to work, but his reduced energy level and occasional complications reduced his ability to function. The stance of both the patient and his wife was to blame the staff and the physician for this predicament.

It was important in dealing with this couple to understand and respect their shared paranoid defensive style, while at the same time not let this manner of coping get out of hand and interfere with medical compliance. After a long period of time and the maintenance of a firm but sympathetic stance toward the couple, there was some acceptance of the treatment on their part. However, as the years went by and the patient deteriorated in his cognitive functioning, the wife became symptomatically depressed with suicidal ideation. So great was her fear of his dying and of being left alone that she tried to convince her husband to join her in suicide. Therapy with the wife focused on her grief at the prospect of losing her husband and encouraged her to develop an identity separate from him so that she would be enabled to continue with her life after his expected death.

Another mental health service provided by the Lenox Hill consultative program is "postvention." This involves meeting with family members after a patient dies, in order to minimize the guilt they often feel in connection with this event. Although grief and guilt are universal reactions to the death of loved ones, these emotions may be particularly intense in relatives and close friends of hemodialysis patients because of the ambivalent feelings they may have felt toward the patients as a result of the stresses the patients imposed on their loved ones.

At times, patients cannot adjust to hemodialysis, and fortunately there are other options available, such as continuous ambulatory peritoneal dialysis (CAPD) and kidney transplantation. We have had several patients who were markedly unhappy on hemodialysis and moderately unsuccessful in maintaining the dietary and fluid regimens prescribed and who were consequently recommended for CAPD. For some of them, the new treatment was successful largely because of the greater freedom and independence it afforded.

In other cases, acceptance of the risks involved in a cadaver transplant is the only feasible alternative. Finally, for patients who cannot tolerate hemodialysis and who are not transplant or CAPD candidates because of age, other severe illnesses, or psychopathology, withdrawal from hemodialysis becomes the only option. This usually happens when the patient's quality of life is so poor that the patient's motivation for continuing evaporates. Of course, in such cases one must be careful about reflexively agreeing with the patient's assessment. Care must be taken to determine whether one is really dealing with an underlying depression, which can be treated, thereby improving the patient's quality of life. This situation is illustrated in the following case.

> Mr. P is a 63-year-old diabetic male hemodialysis patient who was hospitalized for skin grafting to a diabetic ulceration of his left foot. He had already undergone amputation of several toes. His kidneys had failed because of diabetes, and he had some visual problems related to diabetes. He felt very despondent and did not wish to go on. After being treated for a week with trazodone, his depression began to remit. Even after he required a below-the-knee amputation, his depression continued to recede until he was back to his usual state.

When the patient's quality of life does in fact warrant withdrawal or the patient cannot be dissuaded from such withdrawal, mental health providers can be helpful in clarifying the decision for the patient, the family, and the staff. If this is done successfully, the patient, the family, and the staff can take leave of each other without being burdened by guilt and recriminations.[10]

PROBLEMS AND RECOMMENDATIONS

The work with renal dialysis patients is stressful for all of the staff involved, including the psychiatrist. Some of the stresses on the psychiatrist stem in part from the underlying physical problems of the patients, from the fact that many of them are deteriorating and will die during the course of the psychiatrist's involvement with them. Another area of stress the psychiatrist often encounters is in the resistance of renal dialysis patients to psychiatric intervention, since they often do not admit to, or feel they have, any emotional problems. Despite this resistance, these patients and their families require a great deal of mental health intervention.

The time that a psychiatrist can devote as an unpaid voluntary attending to meet the multiplicity of needs for involvement in a renal dialysis unit is clearly insufficient. A half-time salaried position (15–20 hours per week) could, however, meet the needs of both patients and health care staff. This position might be concerned mainly with advanced-stage situations, after the initial efforts by the consulting psychiatrist have met with success. In any event in order to integrate the consultant more meaningfully into the unit team, the limited number of hours afforded by the voluntary "service" assignment must be expanded considerably.

REFERENCES

1. Harry S. Abram, Gordon L. Moore, and Frederic B. Westervelt, Jr., "Suicidal Behavior in Chronic Dialysis Patients," *American Journal of Psychiatry* 127 (March 1971): 1199–1204.

2. W.A. Crammond, P.R. Knight, and J.R. Lawrence, "The Psychiatric Contribution to a Renal Unit Undertaking Chronic Hemodialysis and Renal Hemotransplantation," *British Journal of Psychiatry* 113 (November 1967): 1201–1212.

3. J.W. Czaczkes and A. Kaplan-DeNour, *Chronic Hemodialysis As a Way of Life* (New York: Brunner/Mazel, 1978) 99-103, 68-70, 45-48, 137-142.

4. Norman B. Levy, "Sexual Adjustment to Maintenance Hemodialysis and Renal Transplantation," in *Living or Dying*, ed. Norman B. Levy (Springfield, Ill.: C.C Thomas 1974), 127.

5. Frederic O. Finkelstein and Thomas E. Steele, "Sexual Dysfunction and Chronic Renal Failure," *Dialysis and Transplantation* 7 (September 1978): 877.

6. R.G. Wright, P. Sand, and G. Livingston, "Psychological Stress during Hemodialysis for Chronic Renal Failure," *Annals of Internal Medicine* 64 (1966): 611-621.

7. J.H. Steidl, et al., "Medical Condition, Adherence to Treatment and Family Functioning," *Archives of General Psychiatry* 37 (1980): 1025-1027.

8. H.S. Abrams, "Prosthetic Man," *Comprehensive Psychiatry* 11 (1970): 475.

9. A. Kaplan-DeNour and J.W. Czaczkes, "Emotional Problems and Reactions of a Medical Team in a Chronic Hemodialysis Unit," *Lancet* 2 (1968): 937–981.

10. G.M. Rodin, et al., "Stopping Life-Sustaining Medical Treatment: Psychiatric Considerations in Termination of Renal Dialysis," *Canadian Journal of Psychiatry* 26 (1981): 540–544.

Chapter 11

Treatment Aspects of Substance Abuse

Murry J. Cohen, M.D.

DEFINITIONS AND CONCEPTS

The term *addiction* is ambiguous and has been criticized by many writers.[1-4] Ludwig writes that "addiction denotes a behavioral pattern of compulsive drug acquisition and use, combined with a heightened tendency for relapse after a period of abstinence, . . . [and] should not be viewed as equivalent to physical dependence, which can also be produced unwittingly in medically ill persons."[5] Adriani notes that "addiction" and "habituation" are incorrectly used interchangeably by some physicians. He goes on to say that addiction is overused by the general public to indicate any and all forms of drug abuse.[6]

In an attempt to resolve some of the confusion in nomenclature, to provide a method of labeling patients' drug use pattern in an objective, treatment-oriented manner, and to give health care providers a common language with which to speak to one another, the American Psychiatric Association, in 1980, published a new diagnostic nomenclature.[7] The behavioral dysfunction that constitutes and indicates a mental disorder involving improper use of drugs is called a "substance use disorder" (SUD). This disorder has two types: substance abuse and substance dependence.

Three diagnostic criteria are required to establish the presence of substance abuse: (1) pattern of pathological use, (2) impairment in social or occupational functioning due to substance use, (3) a one-month minimum duration of disturbance. The pattern of pathological use is defined by any one of five characteristics:

1. inability to cut down or stop
2. repeated efforts to control use through periods of temporary abstinence or restriction of use to certain times of the day

231

3. intoxication throughout the day
4. frequent use of excessive quantities of the substance
5. two or more overdoses with the substance

The single diagnostic criterion required to establish the presence of substance dependence (for drugs other than alcohol or cannabis) is tolerance or withdrawal.

Often, both conditions—one physiological (substance dependence) and one psychological (substance abuse)—are present in the same patient. Though substance abuse may be present without substance dependence, in most instances a person who abuses a drug is also dependent on it. However, not infrequently, substance dependence is present without substance abuse. This is especially important to remember when treating patients for chronic painful conditions with iatrogenic drug dependence.

The concept of psychological dependence (also called "habituation" or "compulsive drug use," or more recently, "pattern of pathological use") is currently subsumed under the term substance abuse. However, it is insufficient by itself to constitute a diagnosis of substance abuse; such a diagnosis requires in addition a duration factor and an objective demonstration of an area of deterioration in the patient's life. The mere presence of psychological dependence or, for that matter, of physical dependence, is insufficient grounds to label the patient a drug abuser.

Where does the term *addiction* fit in? This term should be used only to indicate the morbid state of a patient whose drug use has become a central issue of life, that is, a priority that dwarfs all other responsibilities and commitments. Such a patient will probably show both substance abuse and substance dependence. However, the term *addiction* has an extremely poor prognosis ability. It should therefore be used only when the patient's life is in such disarray from drug use that the outlook is extremely bleak. When it is used, moral and criminal implications should be avoided; the patient's health and well-being alone should be the normative standard.

OBSTACLES IN THE TREATMENT OF SUBSTANCE USE DISORDERS

Probably in no other branch of medicine does a patient's pathology cause such opposition, anger, and avoidance as in the case of a substance use disorder.[8] Persons with SUDs are often regarded as criminals by physicians or government officials,[9] who sometimes deny that heroin addiction is a disease. At times, physicians' own substance abuse problems interfere with their ability to react appropriately to their patients' problems.[10,11]

Newman, writing on the lack of understanding by the medical community of the problem of SUDs, notes that long-term efforts to treat drug abusers have often been viewed as an "all or nothing proposition: either the treatment is 'successful' and clients remain permanently abstinent, or clients return to drug abuse, and therapy is deemed a failure."[12] He refers to this as a "simplistic dichotomy" that fails to consider the chronic relapsing nature of SUDs and that emphasizes cure at the expense of symptom reduction.[13] Psychiatrists are not exempt from such misapprehensions. Nyswander alludes to the "country-wide wave of moral indignation aroused by narcotic users, [with psychiatry], too, [revealing] a lack of sympathy and empathy by lecturing the patient at length."[14]

The ignorance of the medical community in this area was investigated in 1972 by the Committee on Drug Dependence of the American Medical Association's Council on Mental Health. The committee's report noted that physicians are looked to for leadership in combating drug abuse, are called upon to provide substance abusers with significant amounts of medical care, and prescribe many of the drugs that are abused, yet they have inadequate knowledge and understanding of SUDs.[15] The report recommended that medical school curricula contain SUD educational programs—a recommendation made by others[16-17]—and that studies be made of societal attitudes toward substance abuse and of the patterns of nonabusive substance use, both prescribed and nonprescribed.[18] Chappel advocated that medical societies play a major role in helping physicians reverse their negative feelings toward SUDs, concluding that organized medicine is needed to support the development and evaluation of adequate drug treatment programs.[19]

In 1981, Bluestone, McGahee, and Klein concluded that not as much progress had been made as had been hoped and that the medical community was ambivalent about whether drug abuse was a "disease."[20]

Perhaps the best summary of the situation was made by Wilford, who, in 1981, wrote:

> The psychopathology, behavior and values of drug-dependent persons have provided many physicians with unpleasant experiences. Such patients may leave the hospital against medical advice, refuse to cooperate with treatment recommendations, and . . . fail to get better. . . . The physician is left disappointed, depressed and bitter. He may even conclude that effective treatment is impossible. . . . Physicians often find that their authority is challenged by drug-dependent patients. The medical model is based on a patient voluntarily seeking help and cooperating with the physician in his own treatment. Ideally, such a patient gives accurate information, allows the physician to conduct various tests and procedures, lis-

tens carefully, and follows instructions accurately. The drug abuser, on the other hand, rarely fits this model; he is compliant rather than cooperative and covertly or overtly challenges the physician's authority. To the physician, he is an undesirable patient.[21]

USE OF THE GENERAL HOSPITAL IN THE TREATMENT OF SUBSTANCE USE DISORDERS

Treating patients with SUDs in a general hospital remains a controversial subject. In the past, general hospitals were unwilling to admit SUD patients.[22] Such patients were considered untreatable, as too disruptive and manipulative, and their hospitalizations were regarded as too repetitive. In addition, insurance companies often excluded medical care costs of SUDs as reimbursable medical expenses. As a consequence, physicians-in-training did not have the opportunity to acquire experience and expertise in the management of SUD patients.

However, general hospitals cannot avoid SUD patients. A survey of 150 consecutive, first-visit general medical patients showed that 17 (11.3 percent) used psychoactive drugs or alcohol on a daily basis and considered it an abuse problem.[23] Another survey revealed a high occupancy rate of general hospital beds (20–50 percent) with patients who had alcohol and/or drug-related problems.[24] In addition, as Adriani notes, all categories of physicians—such as surgeons, internists, and anesthesiologists—are faced at some point with the management of drug-abusing or drug-dependent patients whose adverse responses often complicate patient management.[25] Thus, it behooves all physicians who work in the general hospital setting to become knowledgeable about SUDs.

Indeed, several experienced workers in the field including Nyswander[26] believe that a general hospital is especially conducive to the appropriate treatment of SUD patients. Freedman sees four advantages in treating SUD patients in a general hospital: (1) acceptance of the patient as a sick person, (2) the total range of services available (medical, surgical, social), (3) the research possibilities, and (4) the potential for nonpsychiatric physicians becoming interested.[27]

Use of the general hospital for the short-term treatment of the SUD patient occurs in four general locales:

1. inpatient division
2. outpatient clinic division
3. emergency room division
4. consultation-liaison psychiatry division

SUD patients can be successfully treated in any of these divisions. In general, successful treatment depends on physicians who can achieve therapeutic relationships with their patients and who are willing to spend time with them.[28]

Inpatient Division

Inpatient treatment can be subdivided into (1) a scatter-bed psychiatric service, (2) a segregated general psychiatric inpatient unit, (3) a drug detoxification unit, and (4) a detoxification psychiatric unit. In general, SUD patients may be managed on any of these four types of services (although the scatter-bed psychiatric service would be appropriate only for a very selected patient cohort).

A "hard-core" SUD patient would do best on a detoxification unit (if detoxification is a goal of treatment) because such a unit addresses more of these patients' needs. A detoxification unit is staffed by workers who are experienced in dealing with SUD patients, provides for more routine and reliable urine testing, offers group therapy specifically focused on SUD problems, is supported by increased security provisions, and contains locked doors. The hard-core patient is characterized by one or all of the following: (1) a long history of illness, (2) a history of many relapses, (3) a potential for acting out, (4) a severe antisocial character disorder with associated manipulative behavior and lying, (5) the presence of polydrug abuse, (6) a criminal history, (7) a very low frustration tolerance, (8) a major impulse disorder.

If the SUD coexists with another major psychiatric illness (schizophrenia, major depressive disorder, bipolar affective disorder, or other severe character disorder), a detoxification unit that is specially organized for severely disturbed individuals is required. This type of unit is also necessary for those who develop major psychopathology as a result of their SUD (cocaine psychosis, amphetamine-induced violence, psychotogen- or PCP-induced mental disorganization, anticholinergic-induced organic brain syndrome or organic psychosis, or prolonged panic reaction). It should be kept in mind, however, that detoxification units per se often do little more than allow patients to achieve abstinence; they tend to ignore the difficult problem of the patients maintaining abstinence by the development of new coping skills.

A segregated general psychiatric unit is appropriate for SUD patients who do not have hard-core characteristics, are reasonably well-motivated, can form a good therapeutic alliance with their psychiatrist, can tolerate the implicit or explicit negative moral judgments of other patients and staff, and can benefit from the general psychiatric therapeutic approach (individual, group, milieu, activities, occupational, pharmacological). Such individuals, should, however, have sufficient insight to realize that, either as a cause or as a result of their SUD, their psychological dysfunction is severe enough to warrant psychiatric hospitalization. Patients who do not have this insight or whose SUD is relatively short-lived and has not significantly impaired ego function do not do well on a psychiatric unit. They resist therapeutic interventions and tend to sign out prematurely. Such patients should probably be admitted to a unit that is specifically geared to treat different aspects of SUD, that is, a medical, detoxification, acute/subacute rehabilitation, or chronic rehabilitation unit.

Treating SUD patients on a scatter-bed psychiatric service involves similar considerations. Here, however, there is an additional factor. On a scatter-bed service, because of the less formal structure and the (correct) feeling on the part of the staff that they exercise less control over the patient, the staff will have less understanding and be less tolerant of patient acting-out behavior, drug use while in the hospital, manipulativeness, and splitting and thus will tend to neutralize the therapeutic potential for the patient. Also, pathological impulses experienced by the patient are more easily discharged in a scatter-bed environment. For these reasons, only carefully selected cases of SUD should be hospitalized on scatter-bed units.

Outpatient Clinic Division

Outpatient division treatment can occur in the psychiatric clinic, in other clinics, or in a methadone maintenance treatment program (MMTP).

The psychiatric clinic is an appropriate place to treat an SUD patient, provided a few general principles are adhered to:

- If the patient is still abusing or dependent on the substance, the total thrust of the treatment should be to help the patient achieve abstinence, by whatever means necessary.
- Objective techniques should be available to ascertain abstinence (blood or urine toxicology, pentobarbital test, pupillary diameter test, and so on).
- Outpatient detoxification should be undertaken only with great care and deliberation; inpatient detoxification should be insisted upon after repeated failures of the ambulatory attempts.
- Once remission is achieved, appropriate adjunctive techniques to psychotherapy should be strongly encouraged, even insisted upon, to sustain it. Such techniques as methadone maintenance, naltrexone maintenance, acupuncture, or a self-help group like Narcotics Anonymous or Pills Anonymous should be considered.

- The psychotherapy decided upon should suit the needs of the patient; and strong consideration should be given to group therapy, either in addition to or in place of individual psychotherapy.

- A clearly defined therapeutic contract should be established, with the indications to continue or discontinue therapy spelled out.

- Medication should be used only with the utmost care; a categorical approach to pharmacotherapy is ill-advised.

- Meetings with significant others are often necessary, and format flexibility of the therapy is essential.

Other clinics are important in the total treatment of the SUD patient. Often, SUD patients will present with a medical, surgical, or gynecological complication of substance abuse or dependence. Physicians of various specialties must be able to diagnose the complication, initiate the indicated treatment, realize the likelihood of an underlying SUD, know the technique of confronting the patient in a nonthreatening and nonjudgmental manner, and facilitate referral for definitive treatment of the SUD. It is important that physicians maintain their medical stance; without it, their credibility will be undermined and their effectiveness neutralized. Also, if the patient is being treated concurrently in the psychiatric clinic and another clinic, it is vital that the treating professionals in the two clinics maintain a dialogue, sharing information and ideas and constructing a joint treatment plan.

Many opiate-abusing SUD patients refuse hospitalization, ignore their medical and psychiatric needs, avoid therapeutic communities, and visit emergency rooms only when desperate. For many such patients, an MMTP, utilizing a multimodal therapeutic approach that addresses various problem areas (medical, psychiatric, psychosocial, legal, vocational), is the approach of choice. (The basic principles in the operation of such a program are discussed later in the chapter.)

Not infrequently, the emergency room serves as a last resort for many SUD patients. In fact, the emergency room has some unique advantages as an SUD treatment area:

- SUD patients are frequently desperate by the time they visit the emergency room and thus may be receptive to therapeutic interventions they would otherwise reject.

- While being treated for the emergency, the patients are a "captive audience" that may respond better to the psychiatric consultant who is called in.

- With the appropriate liaison between the emergency room and the MMTP, an SUD patient can be seen while in the emergency room by an MMTP staff member, and, if warranted, can be started in treatment immediately. If such treatment is impossible, at least a contact has been established that may provide the crucial difference in outcome.

- The patient may come to the emergency room accompanied by friends or family (or law enforcement officers), thereby making it easier to document a history of SUD.

Since up to 50 percent of patients in general hospital beds have problems related to substance abuse or dependence,[29] it is understandable that psychiatrists on the consultation-liaison service frequently are called to evaluate these problems. Strain and Grossman suggest that, in addition to evaluating the consultation request and the impact the patient has upon the primary care physician, the psychiatrist also evaluates the clinical record, the nurse, the family, the milieu, and the patient.[30]

INPATIENT TREATMENT OF NONIATROGENIC SUBSTANCE USE DISORDERS

Noniatrogenic substance use disorders (NISUDs), commonly called "street drug addiction," present a great challenge with respect to treatment efforts in the general hospital. One of the major purposes of acute hospitalization of the NISUD patient—along with treatment of complications, detoxification, and the initiation of rehabilitation—is to effect referral to a definitive, long-term treatment modality. Wilford notes that the primary care physician has an important role to play in that process. In addition to appropriately diagnosing and referring the patient, he must prepare the patient for treatment, communicate hope, and provide emotional and, at times, chemotherapeutic support.[31]

In spite of these efforts, patient compliance with follow-up care is often poor.[32] This is not surprising, since most NISUD patients enter treatment under duress.[33] Galanter studied this problem and suggested that the closed-system model of treatment—in which medical sequelae or withdrawal problems are treated and regarded as the primary disease process at the expense of long-term rehabilitation—be replaced by a model of medical treatment as a subsystem within which staff-patient communication, coordination of treatment planning, continuity of care, and staff education are also examined and emphasized.[34]

Underlying Psychopathologies

NISUD patients with significant underlying psychopathology present additional problems. The increased incidence of depression in opiate abusers has been widely reported.[35-38] Schizophrenia seems to be less common among methadone maintenance patients than in the general population, although the reasons for this are unclear. There are also widely varying reports concerning the prevalence of schizophrenia among heroin-dependent individuals. In a study of 218 consecutive admissions of drug users to the psychiatric service of a general hospital, schizophrenia was underrepresented and character disorders overrepresented among moderate and heavy drug abusers, and schizophrenics were more likely to relinquish drug use than character disorder patients. Among the 218 patients (118 of whom had a history of drug use), the ratio of character disorders to schizophrenics was 2.5 times greater in heavy drug users than in moderate drug users.[39]

Though the actual prevalence of psychopathology among NISUD patients is unclear, it does appear that there is a direct relationship between the socioeconomic class of the patient and the degree of discernible psychopathology.[40] Kissin calls this the "psychosocial equation—an inverse relationship between the prevalence of drug dependence in a given sex or subculture and the degree of psychopathology in an addicted individual of that same sex or subculture."[41] Thus:

- female alcoholics show greater psychopathology than male alcoholics
- Jewish alcoholics show greater psychopathology than Irish alcoholics
- female heroin addicts show greater psychopathology than male heroin addicts
- white, middle-class heroin addicts show greater psychopathology than black "ghetto" heroin addicts [42]

General Principles

The following fourteen general principles pertaining to the management of hospitalized NISUD patients are derived from published general psychiatric,[43,44] psychoanalytic,[45] and psychopharmacologic sources,[46] as well as the author's own experience:

1. The therapeutic relationship established with the patient must reflect an understanding of the patient's motivation; establish in the mind of the mental health provider strong redeeming features of the patient; regard the patient as a sick person in need of treatment, not as a social deviant;[47] and avoid judging the patient with consequent moralizing and preaching.[48]
2. The treatment should take place in an environment in which the patient feels safe but not engulfed.
3. Every attempt should be made to prevent unnecessary suffering by the patient. The mental health provider should inform the patient of such efforts, but should keep in mind the threat of countertransferen-

tial anger, punitiveness, or sadism. The provider should also be aware of the difficulty of treating physical symptoms in NISUD patients because of the patients' possible secondary-gain-induced motivational deficits, uncontrollable craving for the substance of abuse, and unconscious needs to suffer.[49]

4. Limits must be set and an external structure imposed. Often, these are in the form of a written contract specifying grounds for discharge (for example, using drugs while in the hospital, which has been correlated with postdischarge return to drugs).[50] The provider must maintain some distance, refusing final responsibility for patients' actions. At times, understanding NISUD patients is more important than helping them. The provider must walk the line between expectation and apathy, not pressuring the patients, but at the same time preventing them from feeling abandoned.

5. The provider must be committed over the long term; visit the patient frequently; be active and warm; project interest, concern, personal involvement, and competence; refrain from becoming intrusive; and be able to tolerate long periods of therapeutic stagnation and paralysis.

6. SUD diagnostic considerations should be approached objectively and disinterestedly, utilizing the concepts and principles cited earlier in the chapter. DSM-3 Axis Three medical and surgical diagnoses should be delineated,[51] in addition to other psychiatric diagnoses.

7. A treatment plan that reflects the chronic relapsing nature of SUDs and takes into account the natural course of these disorders should be decided upon, with goals that are realistic and achievable. The plan should be as simple as possible, should address itself to all of the established diagnoses, should employ interpersonal resources as much as possible, and should be presented to the patient and the treatment team clearly and logically. Ideally, patients should take as active a role as possible, contributing to decisions about psychoactive medications (many older patients can guide the physician appropriately in terms of the type and amount of anxiolytic or hypnotic medication),[52] and helping to define the goal of hospitalization (resolution of medical/surgical illness, detoxification, chemotherapeutic maintenance). It should be remembered that drug abstinence is sustained one day at a time and that a return to drug use may constitute a slip, not a relapse or failure of treatment.[53]

8. It may be necessary to meet with the treatment unit staff to discuss and justify the treatment plan and to receive information about the patient that can be used prognostically (for example, socialization with other drug abusers worsens the prognosis).[54] This meeting could

serve as a first step in diluting the individual therapy relationship, if necessary, into family and/or group therapies, conducted by other therapists.

9. Pharmacotherapy should be used if indicated, although new treatments should be utilized judiciously. Chemotherapeutic substitution (methadone, propoxyphene, naltrexone, clonidine, phenobarbital) should be initiated if warranted. If indicated, narcotic analgesics should be used for pain, without excessive worry about narcotic maintenance treatment. However, all drugs with narcotic antagonist properties (pentazocine, buprenorphine, butorphanol, nalbuphine) should be completely avoided in narcotic dependent persons, to prevent precipitation of withdrawal. Psychotropic drugs, especially sedative ones, should be used cautiously. If required, psychotropic drugs with the fewest side effects should be given with night loading and minimal doses, during induction, and with frequent reevaluation of the drug regimen.

10. Detoxification should begin only after resolution of major medical and surgical problems, since a patient with opiate abuse and dependence and in poor physical health from opioid-use complications (hepatitis, endocarditis, AIDS, cellulitis, phlebitis, abscesses, nephropathy, tetanus) often has a complicated withdrawal syndrome.[55] If sedative-hypnotic and opiate dependencies coexist, the patient should be detoxified from one before being detoxified from the other, usually doing the sedative-hypnotic one first.

11. Periodic urine toxicology screens for drugs of abuse should be carried out, the frequency dictated by the particular clinical circumstances.

12. Placebos should be avoided except under the most unusual conditions (for example, in some patients at the very end of methadone detoxifications). Placebos are only temporary in their palliative effects; they prove nothing with regard to differentiating "organic" from other manifestations, and they undermine the patient's confidence in the mental health provider.[56]

13. Self-help groups of the "anonymous" type (Narcotics Anonymous, Pills Anonymous) should be strongly recommended, when appropriate, as integral for the patient's recovery.[57]

14. At times, contingency contracts—a behavioral modification technique—can be established, whereby a patient experiences a preplanned, very unpleasant consequence if found to be using drugs.[58,59] For example, substance-abusing physicians may be confronted with the consequence of losing hospital privileges unless they remain abstinent.[60]

IATROGENIC OPIATE DRUG PROBLEMS IN MEDICAL PATIENTS WITH ORGANICALLY BASED PAIN

Definitions and Misconceptions

Medical patients with organically based pain often develop iatrogenic opiate drug problems. There are questions, however, as to the nature of these problems and how they can best be managed. There has been little written on this most important subject.

First, we must define the population involved. We do not include patients with acute, self-limited pain—either medical or surgical—for whom prescription of narcotics carries practically no SUD liability. Postoperative patients receiving repeated doses of opiates for four to five days not infrequently show a mild abstinence syndrome when the opiate is stopped; the syndrome, consisting of weakness, muscle aches, and a depressed mood, is usually ignored.[61] We also do not include patients with chronic pain who do not show a sufficient organic basis for the pain. In these patients, narcotics should only rarely, if ever, be used.

The population of concern here is one of patients with recurrent, acute pain, exacerbations of acute pain, or persistent chronic pain, due to such illnesses as inflammatory bowel disease or rheumatoid arthritis. These patients have a great exposure to narcotic drugs. What are the risks of using such drugs in these patients in terms of substance abuse or dependence liability? Is it necessary to undertreat their pain to avoid producing iatrogenic opiate drug problems? If opiate dependence does occur, do the patients then slowly become "addicts"?

At this point, our earlier words of caution about the term *addiction* should be kept in mind. "The term[s] 'addiction' and 'habituation' . . . are still used interchangeably (and incorrectly) by some physicians."[62] Addiction should not be viewed as equivalent to physical dependence, which can also be produced unwittingly in medically ill persons.[63] Finally, drug use alone is not the sole factor in the development of addiction, other medical, social and economic conditions play important roles.[64]

Yet, there are still some who believe that patients with chronic organic pain who receive narcotic analgesics are at high risk to become "addicted,"[65,66] despite the overwhelming evidence that points in the other direction.[67]

Physicians generally tend to underuse narcotics to treat medically ill patients with severe pain;[68,69] and they tend to exaggerate the dangers of narcotics. In one study, 73 percent of patients undergoing treatment for pain control still experienced moderate to severe pain.[70] Other authors have concluded that the treatment of severe pain in hospitalized patients is woefully inadequate.[71-74] Morgan, calling the phenomenon "opiophobia," reports that, of 100 patients hospitalized at a major urban teaching hospital, 60 percent were given less than 50 mg meperidine and only 8 percent were given more than 75 mg meperidine intramuscularly; of those patients receiving codeine, 60 percent received less than 30 mg.[75]

Available data show that the dangers and risks of prescribing narcotics for patients with organic pain are minimal. A study of 39,946 hospitalized medical patients, of whom 11,882 received at least one narcotic, showed that only four patients without a previous history of addiction (.03 percent of those receiving the narcotics) showed reasonably well-documented addiction.[76] The fact that the use of a narcotic in the treatment of a chronic painful medical illness is not, in and of itself, addictogenic is confirmed in a study that revealed that, of 225 patients hospitalized because of prescription drug abuse, 60 percent abused more than one drug and 30 percent abused narcotics as part of a polydrug abuse pattern and had a psychiatric history.[77] Stimmel concludes that, although the data are scarce, those available "suggest that the actual incidence of medically induced narcotic dependency, when narcotics are utilized appropriately for severe pain in a hospital setting, is negligible."[78] Others agree that medical use of narcotics is rarely, if ever, associated with the development of addiction.[79,80]

In the case of medically ill patients with pain, even though they often receive enough narcotics to produce dependency—seven to ten continuous days of intramuscular daily use of 40–50 mg morphine, 520–650 mg codeine, 6.0–7.5 mg hydromorphone (Dilaudid), 300–500 mg meperidine (Demerol), 40–50 mg methadone (Dolophine), or 60–75 mg oxycodone (Percodan, Percocet)[81,82]—the situation and the setting are usually not pathogenic. In fact, these patients are quite different from those who go on to develop opiate abuse (or "addiction"). Angell finds that even patients who develop tolerance and physical dependence are unlikely to become addicted. Even among these patients withdrawal can be accomplished easily if the painful stimulus is no longer present.[83]

There are of course patients with chronic, underlying, painful organic illnesses who are, in addition, opioid abusers. These individuals are best managed in conjunction with a methadone maintenance program, to which they should be referred. They are extremely difficult patients to treat, challenging even the most skilled and enlightened practitioner.

General Guidelines

The following guidelines should be followed in the management of opiate dependence in chronic, organically based, pain patients who are on medical or surgical units for their primary illness:

- If the primary physician needs assistance, another physician experienced in this area—a psychiatrist if possible—should be called. The latter physician should be solely responsible for analgesic and psychotropic medications.
- After getting to know the patient, the goals should be mutually decided upon. These goals should be realistic, achievable, and consonant with the patient's problems.
- The unit staff should be informed that the patient is not "an addict." Accordingly, they should not treat the patient as an addict but rather as a sick person who has several medical problems, one of which is drug dependence.
- The consultant should participate in the management of the patient's medical and surgical problems, discuss and explain them with and to the patient, speak with the patient's other physicians, and constantly monitor the clinical record for changes in the conditions.
- The consultant should add psychotropic medications—such as hydroxyzine, amitriptyline, possibly amphetamine, possibly a neuroleptic—that might reduce the need for narcotics by treatment of concurrent psychiatric conditions, potentiation of the narcotic, or both.
- The consultant should visit frequently, be available, write chart notes, speak with family members, and spend a reasonable amount of time with the patient.
- If narcotics are to be continued, the oral route is preferable to injections. This means avoiding narcotics, such as meperidine, that are poorly absorbed. If pills are not absorbed properly—because of malabsorption secondary to Crohn's disease, hypermotility with reduced transit time secondary to inflammatory bowel disease, or short bowel syndrome with jejunostomy—liquid forms of narcotics are desired, such as liquid morphine (one-sixth as potent as parenteral morphine) or liquid methadone (one-half as potent as parenteral methadone, and obtainable only if a special effort is made, since this preparation is used by many methadone programs and is carefully monitored). Hydrocodone (Dilaudid) suppositories may also be used.
- Placebos are to be avoided. Patients should know the details of each dose of medication. A nurse should never mislead a patient regarding dose. The dosage regimen should be discussed and decided upon by patient and consultant. The patient should have a sense of control, but understand, of course, that the physician makes the final decisions.
- As-needed (prn) doses are to be avoided. Standing doses are most desirable, in that the patients do not have to ask for each dose, often experienced as a humiliation; the patients are not subjected to the

disapproval of staff nurses, who often feel that a prn order means that they should try *not* to give the medication; and the patients do not have to wait for a dose with increasing pain. If some flexibility in the dosing schedule is desired, the best approach would be to let patients skip a particular standing dose if they wish to do so.

- The consultant, if a psychiatrist, should begin to engage the patient in supportive psychotherapy, allowing the patient to ventilate, acting as a general health counselor, and trying to understand the patient's psychodynamics. The consultant should act as a liaison between patients and their other physicians, always striving to improve communications between them.

- If detoxification is begun, oral methadone is usually the narcotic of choice because of its potency, oral effectiveness, good absorption, lack of side effects and toxicity, and long-acting property. The patient must understand why methadone—a drug tainted with "street junkie" associations—was selected and must agree to its use. After conversion to equivalent doses of methadone, the rate of detoxification should be individualized for the patient, with flexibility maintained for change on a day-to-day basis if warranted. Clonidine (Catapres) should be considered as a detoxification agent if the patient is on 40 mg of methadone or less.

THE EFFECTS OF OPIATE DEPENDENCY ON PAIN MANAGEMENT IN SURGICAL PATIENTS

The analgesic care of opiate-dependent surgical patients is often fraught with confusion and, too often, results in inadequate pain relief. This results in apprehension and agitation by the patient. The patient often becomes more demanding thereby compounding the problem and causing the staff to withhold appropriate analgesics because they feel that the drug-seeking behavior "obviously" means the patient is an addict. Thus a vicious cycle is established; everyone becomes frustrated and anxious—patient, physician, family, and staff. Staff withholding of adequate analgesics probably also reflects an unconscious staff wish to punish the patient for being opiate-dependent.

Whether or not opiate dependent individuals need larger than normal doses of narcotics to achieve satisfactory analgesia is a matter of some controversy. It is known, however, that, contrary to widespread misconception, such individuals do feel pain in a manner similar to persons who are narcotic free.[84] The same agents used in normal patients are successful in patients on methadone maintenance (except for those narcotic mixed agonist-antagonists, which could precipitate immediate withdrawal);[85] and such patients definitely do not need lower doses to achieve adequate analgesia.[86]

In fact, complete tolerance to the analgesic effects of methadone in the chronically maintained, recovering opiate abuser requires that more opiate be used for analgesia. Yet, frequently the physician undermedicates out of fear or belief that all of the methadone being used by the patient should eliminate the pain, that more narcotic creates the risk of a narcotic overdose, or that more narcotic somehow interferes with patients' rehabilitation by either introducing them to a new drug or by allowing them to reexperience narcotic-induced euphoria. In fact, narcotic tolerance produced by chronic methadone maintenance *protects* patients from narcotic overdose;[87] there have been very few, if any, documented pure narcotic overdoses in patients maintained on methadone. Moreover, investigators have found that the use of additional narcotic agents for pain in no way compromises further rehabilitative progress in the posthospitalization period.[88]

Concerning the dose of narcotic analgesics, the same investigators compared 25 methadone maintenance patients from a major hospital-based methadone program who had been hospitalized for surgical procedures and traumatic episodes with 25 nonhospitalized matched-control methadone maintenance patients from the same facility. They found that the hospitalized patients required only standard doses of narcotic analgesia to control pain.[89] However, other studies have found that a decrease in pain tolerance and threshold in opiate-dependent animals or humans results in the need for larger short-acting opiate doses to achieve satisfactory analgesia.[90-92] It has also been determined that pain threshold, but not pain tolerance, was lower in both drug-free ex-addicts and patients on methadone maintenance, when compared with nonaddicted subjects.[93]

The most satisfactory conclusion to be drawn from all this is that, even though methadone patients may attempt to manipulate their surgical admission to receive unnecessary incremental doses of narcotics,[94] they should receive at least standard doses, and very likely larger than normal doses, of parenteral,[95] short-acting narcotics to achieve analgesia for severe pain, in addition to their usual dose of methadone. Increasing their tolerance level occurs only if the patients receive 10 mg of parenteral morphine (or its equivalent) four or five times a day for seven to ten days.[96] Even if this were to occur, it could be easily managed by temporarily increasing the methadone dose after cessation of narcotics for analgesia and then gradually returning to the preanalgesia maintenance dose.

If the patient is on methadone maintenance and can continue to receive oral medication, the methadone dose should be continued once daily at the prehospitalization level. If the patient is dependent on a different narcotic, that drug could be continued or, preferably, converted to oral methadone. In this regard, 20 mg oral methadone is equivalent to oral doses of 60 mg morphine, 200 mg codeine, 8 mg hydromorphone (Dilaudid), 300 mg meperidine (Demerol), and 30 mg oxycodone (Percodan, Percocet).

If the parenteral route of administration is necessary, the oral methadone dose can be converted to an equivalent amount of parenteral methadone by using one-half to two-thirds of the oral dose and giving one-half of that every 12 hours.[97] If additional parenteral narcotic analgesics are required, they should be used according to the principles outlined in the preceding section. Combining the patient's maintenance and analgesic narcotic requirements into either a single methadone regimen or a single short-acting narcotic regimen are not recommended.[98]

If the admitted surgical patient is noniatrogenically opiate-dependent and not on a methadone maintenance program, attempts should be made to stabilize the patient on oral methadone preoperatively. This is done by titrating the patient initially with 10 mg oral methadone every six hours. It is uncommon for such a patient to require more than 40 mg oral methadone a day; however, if after 12 to 24 hours of titration, it appears that the patient is experiencing signs or symptoms of withdrawal, the methadone dose may be increased (although many hospital pharmacy regulations inappropriately preclude a dose of greater than 40 mg oral methadone per day for patients not registered on a methadone program). Once the total daily amount of methadone is known, it can be given on an 8- or 12-hour basis. This would allow for an oral dose 8 to 12 hours prior to surgery, with conversion to parenteral methadone for the second dose (and third dose, if necessary) postoperatively.[99]

A distinction should be made between patients with medical illness who are iatrogenically opiate-dependent and patients who are either methadone-maintenance patients or active heroin abusers. The relevant principles of management cited earlier should be applied.

THE METHADONE MAINTENANCE TREATMENT PROGRAM IN A GENERAL HOSPITAL

Guidelines

The details and principles of methadone maintenance treatment have been detailed exhaustively in the literature.[100-110] In this section, clinical guidelines for the successful functioning of a methadone maintenance treatment program (MMTP) in a general hospital are presented, based on the author's experiences in two such programs.

It is particularly important that the hospital be committed to the MMTP and that the hospital administration support its operation. Many problems stem from the presence of an MMTP; the hospital administration should help the program to solve these problems, rather than enter into an adversary relationship with the program. For its part, the MMTP should meticulously abide by all hospital regulations and guidelines and not expect special privileges or consideration. On the other hand, those regulations and guidelines should not be prejudicial to MMTP patients, who should be treated like any other patients receiving services at the hospital.

It is helpful if the chief executive officer of the MMTP has a position of some authority in the hospital. To the extent possible, professional staff members (psychiatrists, psychologists, social workers, nurses, administrators, general physicians) of the MMTP should also have appointments in the hospital, in order to integrate the program into the general functioning of the institution.

If possible, a senior member of the hospital pharmacy staff should be given the responsibility of managing the utilization of methadone. This includes ordering the medication, preparing it, providing the nurses with adequate supplies, monitoring the flow of medication, and keeping accurate records. The pharmacist-in-charge should be part of the program's senior staff and attend senior staff meetings.

The medical unit of the MMTP should function as a health maintenance organization, with the ability to refer patients to hospital outpatient specialty clinics, to the emergency room, or to evaluation for hospitalization. In this context, an active liaison should be developed with the emergency room by medical, nursing, and psychiatric staff to facilitate patient care in terms of communication, grievance resolution, and delineation of lines of authority. The emergency room should be responsive to the need of the MMTP for immediate evaluation of a program patient. Conversely, MMTP should support the emergency room in providing care to patients with opiate abuse and dependence. In addition, the MMTP and the emergency room directors must decide on a policy regarding the dispensation of methadone in the emergency room.

When a patient who is being followed psychiatrically at the MMTP is evaluated for hospitalization, an MMTP attending psychiatrist should have input and carry authority regarding the decision to admit, the patient's management, and the discharge planning. The MMTP staff psychiatrist should perform psychiatric evaluations, prescribe psychiatric medications, supervise counselors, participate in case discussions, and, if the budget allows, carry out psychotherapy with selected patients.[111] The MMTP psychiatrist should provide consultations to hospital physicians on patients with drug abuse/dependence problems, facilitate their admission to the MMTP if indicated, and advise regarding other treatment resources.

Staff members of the MMTP should provide didactic and supervisory support to the hospital in the form of lectures, seminars, and resident/ medical, student/social work, intern supervision. The topics should include characteristics and psychological profiles of methadone patients, expected methadone-induced side effects, dosage issues, and such special clinical problems as sexual dysfunction, alcoholism, polydrug abuse, amitriptyline misuse, prenatal care, neonatal characteristics and care of the infant born to a mother on methadone, surgical care, heroin nephropathy, and dialysis. In teaching hospitals, the MMTP should offer an elective clerkship to medical students on the methadone maintenance treatment approach to the problem of opiate abuse and dependence. Ideally, psychiatric residents should rotate through the program as part of their learning experience. At least one staff member should participate in the introduction-to-medicine course for first-year medical students. Members of the hospital staff with expertise in relevant matters (hepatitis, AIDS, dialysis, family therapy, group therapy, psychopharmacology, analgesia) should be invited to give seminars to the MMTP staff.

If an MMTP patient is hospitalized, the methadone orders should be written by the physician in charge of the patient's hospital care *after consultation* with MMTP physicians. Frequent communications between these physicians is crucial, especially just prior to discharge from the hospital. The MMTP staff should inform and educate other hospital staff members regarding methadone detoxification of a patient on maintenance, emphasizing the difficulties involved, establishing the criteria to evaluate the indications to detoxify, and resisting the assumption that all patients should be detoxified.[112-114]

In general, as many services as possible should be provided on-site at the program, since methadone patients are less likely than other patients to follow through with referrals elsewhere. If psychotropic medication seems required, it should be used regularly to treat major psychiatric syndromes, used judiciously to treat symptoms alone, and used very carefully if the medication is either dependency-producing or potentially patient-abused. Methadone patients characteristically tend to misuse diazepam, amitriptyline, and ethchlorvynol; the short-acting barbiturate hypnotics, hydroxyzine, and propoxyphine may also be abused. If psychiatric care is indicated, it will be more successful if the psychiatrist works at the MMTP than if the patient is required to visit the psychiatric clinic.

Federal confidentiality regulations require that MMTP service notes be kept in a special clinical record. However, some mechanism should be developed to enable clinical information from the MMTP record and the general hospital record to be shared, as necessary. The MMTP staff should make periodic presentations at medical, surgical, obstetrical, psychiatric and pediatric grand rounds to inform staff physicians about the services provided, treatment limitations and expectations, and recent findings in the field of substance abuse. Since the Joint Commission on Accreditation of Hospitals holds MMTPs to standards applicable to departments of psychiatry, ongoing input from that department is desirable.

The MMTP should keep its medical orientation, function under the medical model, and retain its position as a key treatment modality within the hospital. It should resist attempts at bureaucratic encroachment and control and maintain its dignity despite irrational community opposition, a hostile press, regulatory agency harassment, or physician misunderstanding. In this regard, the MMTP should act as an advocate throughout the hospital—for MMTP patients in particular and for substance-abusing patients in general.

Side Effects

Most of the side effects of methadone are mild, transitory, and insignificant from the health care point of view; most are gone within six months, as tolerance develops at varying rates and to varying degrees. In general, complete tolerance is achieved for functions mediated by the higher cerebral centers; incomplete tolerance develops for functions mediated primarily by the autonomic nervous system. Tolerance develops most quickly to the analgesic effect; less quickly to euphoria, drowsiness and somnolence; and least quickly to dizziness, nausea, vomiting, urinary hesitancy, and edema. Incomplete tolerance develops only to certain methadone-induced effects: menstrual irregularities, sexual dysfunction, insomnia, constipation, increased sweating, and, possibly, weight gain.

Management of the side effects involves alterations in the maintenance dose and the incremental rate of the induction dose. It is never necessary to use stimulatory, hypertensive, antispasmodic, antiemetic, diuretic, or cholinergic drugs to treat the initial, transient side effects. Increased sweating persists in up to half of the patients, but it is not clinically significant. Constipation persists in a somewhat smaller percentage and often requires a mild stool softener or, at times, a bowel stimulant. Insomnia persists in up to one-third of the patients but usually does not require pharmacotherapy. If sexual and menstrual abnormalities appear, they are probably the result of incomplete tolerance on hypothalamic centers. Up to one-third of patients may have persistent sexual dysfunction—in men, impotence and diminished libido; in women, anorgasmia and irregular menses; in both sexes, occasional dose-related sexual dysfunction. Weight gain is poorly understood, with no specific evidence linking it to methadone; however, increased stimulation of the hypothalamic appetite center is a possibility.

Intolerance to methadone is extremely rare. Anecdotal observations of allergic hypersensitivity have been reported. Other very uncommon occurrences include dysphoric reactions, obstipation with ileus, and spasm of the sphincter of Oddi with increased serum amylase.

Management of the pregnant methadone patient is based on considerable evidence that the vast majority of women who are detoxified after pregnancy is diagnosed revert to heroin use. Since it is safer for the fetus if the mother ingests medically safe amounts of pure methadone rather than injects unknown amounts of contaminated heroin, detoxification should only rarely be recommended. The patient should be maintained on the lowest possible maintenance dose that "blocks" the heroin euphoria (40 mg), and dose changes during the last trimester of pregnancy should be avoided, as they have been correlated with birth complications. Appropriate administration of methadone during pregnancy, when accompanied by good prenatal care, is compatible with an uneventful pregnancy and delivery.

Methadone-maintained mothers often give birth to babies that weigh slightly less than those born to comparable mothers. The specific role of methadone in this regard is unclear. Since methadone crosses the placenta, babies born of methadone-dependent mothers undergo some narcotic withdrawal, usually mild and unnoticed. Some babies, however, do require treatment with paregoric for withdrawal manifestations, which begin two to three days after birth. Since methadone is found in breast milk, it is best not to breast feed those babies. Teratogenicity has not been associated with methadone.

Child abuse occurs with greater frequency among children of methadone-maintained parents than in a comparable population. New York State law requires that suspected cases of child abuse or neglect be reported to the Bureau of Child Welfare (BCW). This law is not superseded by federal laws of confidentiality because of the emergency nature of the circumstances. The hospital should have a committee to deal with this problem; the MMTP can report the case to the committee, which in turn decides whether or not to report it to the BCW.

Patient education should be given priority in MMTPs. It should occur through counseling, orientation sessions, ongoing group sessions, regularly published newspapers, and informal "rap" sessions. Often patients are remarkably ignorant about their methadone treatment, believing various street myths. It is therefore important to provide them with accurate medical information.

REFERENCES

1. A.M. Ludwig, *Principles of Clinical Psychiatry* (New York: Macmillan, 1980).

2. J. Adriani, "Drug Dependence in Hospitalized Patients," in *Acute Drug Abuse Emergencies—A Treatment Manual*, ed. P.G. Bourne (New York: Academic Press, 1976), 231–250.

3. R.J. Cadoret and L.J. King, *Psychiatry in Primary Care* (St. Louis, Mo.: C.V. Mosby, 1983), 177–212.

4. B. Stimmel, *Pain, Analgesia and Addiction* (New York: Raven Press, 1983), 44, 241–302.

5. Ludwig, *Principles,* 268.

6. Adriani, "Drug Dependence."

7. American Psychiatric Association, Task Force on Nomenclature and Statistics, *Diagnostic and Statistical Manual of Mental Disorders,* 3rd ed. (Washington, D.C.: American Psychiatric Association, 1980), 163–179.

8. J.N. Chappel, "Physician Attitudes and the Treatment of Alcohol and Drug-Dependent Patients," *Journal of Psychedelic Drugs* 10 (1978): 27–34.

9. R. Tredgold and H. Wolff, *Psychiatry in Primary Care* (New York: International Universities Press, 1970), 98–104.

10. G.E. Vaillant, J.R. Brighton, and C. McArthur, "Physicians' Use of Mood-Altering Drugs," *New England Journal of Medicine* 282 (1970): 365–370.

11. R.P. Johnson and J.C. Connelly, "Addicted Physicians: A Closer Look," *Journal of the American Medical Association* 245 (1981): 253–258.

12. R.G. Newman, "Planning Drug Abuse Treatment: Critical Decisions," *Bulletin on Narcotics* 30 (1978): 41–48.

13. Ibid.

14. M. Nyswander, *The Drug Addict as a Patient* (New York: Grune & Stratton, 1956), 142.

15. H. Bluestone, C.L. McGahee, and N.R. Klein, "Training and Education," in *Substance Abuse—Clinical Problems and Perspectives,* ed. J.H. Lowinson and P. Ruiz (Baltimore: Williams & Wilkins, 1981), 819–829.

16. J.N. Chappel and S.H. Schnoel, "Physician Attitudes: Effect on the Treatment of Chemically Dependent Patients," *Journal of the American Medical Association,* 237 (1977): 2318, 2319.

17. Tredgold and Wolff, *Psychiatry in Primary Care.*

18. Bluestone, McGahee, and Klein, "Training and Education."

19. Chappel, "Physician Attitudes."

20. Bluestone, McGahee, and Klein, "Training and Education."

21. B.B. Wilford, *Drug Abuse—A Guide for the Primary Care Physician* (Chicago: American Medical Association, 1981), 104–106.

22. M. Nyswander, "The Drug Addict in a General Hospital," in *Frontiers in General Hospital Psychiatry,* ed. L. Linn (New York: International Universities Press, 1961), 263–271.

23. F.S. Tenant, C.M. Day, and J.T. Ungeleider, "Screening for Drugs and Alcohol Abuse in the General Medical Population," *Journal of the American Medical Association* 242 (1979): 533–535.

24. Bluestone, McGahee, and Klein, "Training and Education."

25. Adriani, "Drug Dependence."

26. Nyswander, "The Drug Addict in a General Hospital."

27. A.M. Freedman "Drug Addiction," in *The Psychiatric Unit in a General Hospital,* ed. M.R. Kaufman (New York: International Universities Press, 1965), 216–227.

28. F. Dunbar, *Psychiatry in the Medical Specialties* (New York: McGraw-Hill, 1959), 372–381.

29. Bluestone, McGahee, and Klein, "Training and Education."

30. J.J. Strain and S. Grossman *Psychological Care of the Medically Ill—A Primer in Liaison Psychiatry* (New York: Appleton-Century-Crofts, 1975), 11–22.

31. Wilford, *Drug Abuse.*

32. Freedman, "Drug Addiction."

33. W.R.C. Stewart, Jr., and S.C. Cappannari, "Drug Abuse and Alcoholism," in *Basic Psychiatry for the Primary Care Physician,* ed. H.S. Abram (Boston: Little, Brown, 1976), 117–136.

34. M. Galanter, "Drug and Alcohol Referrals from the General Hospital, II: The Clinical Context," in *Critical Concerns in the Field of Drug Abuse, Proceedings of the Third National Drug Abuse Conference,* ed. A. Schecter, H. Alksne, and E. Kaufman (New York: Marcel Dekker, 1978), 912–916.

35. M.M. Weissman et al., "Clinical Depression among Narcotic Addicts Maintained on Methadone in the Community," *American Journal of Psychiatry* 133 (1976): 1434–1438.

36. P.R. Robbins, "'Depression and Drug Addiction," *Psychiatric Quarterly* 48 (1974): 374–386.

37. S.M. Mirin, R.E. Meyer, and H.G. McNamee, "Psychopathology and Mood during Heroin Use: Acute versus Chronic Effects," *Archives of General Psychiatry* 33 (1976): 1503–1508.

38. B. Prusoff et al., "Psychosocial Stressors and Depression among Former Heroin-Dependent Patients Maintained on Methadone," *Journal of Nervous and Mental Diseases* 165 (1977): 57–83.

39. M. Cohen and D. Klein, "Posthospital Adjustment of Psychiatrically Hospitalized Drug Users," *Archives of General Psychiatry* 31 (1974): 221–227.

40. E. Kaufman, "The Psychodynamics of Opiate Dependence: A New Look," *American Journal of Drug and Alcohol Abuse* 1 (1974): 349–370.

41. B. Kissin, "Alcoholism and Drug Dependence," in *Understanding Human Behavior in Health and Disease,* ed. R.C. Simons and H. Pardes (Baltimore: Williams & Wilkins, 1977), 637–652.

42. Ibid.

43. E.C. Senay, *Substance Abuse Disorders in Clinical Practice* (Boston: John Wright, PSG Inc., 1983), 61–94.

44. M.A. Schuckit, *Drug and Alcohol Abuse: A Clinical Guide to Diagnosis and Treatment* (New York: Plenum Medical Books, 1979), 175–177.

45. L. Wurmser, "Mr. Pecksniff's Horse?" in *Psychodynamics of Drug Dependence,* NIDA Research Monograph No. 12, ed. J. Blaine and D.A. Julius (Rockville, Md.: National Institute of Drug Abuse, 1977), 36–73.

46. B. Salzman, "Substance Abusers with Psychiatric Problems," in *Substance Abuse—Clinical Problems and Perspectives,* ed. J.H. Lowinson and P. Ruiz (Baltimore: Williams & Wilkins, 1981), 758–769.

47. Tredgold and Wolff, *Psychiatry in Primary Care.*

48. R. Wortman, "The Management of the Adolescent Patient," in *Psychiatric Management for Medical Practitioners,* ed. D.S. Kornfield and J.B. Finkel (New York: Grune & Stratton, 1983), 267–287.

49. S. Silverman, *Psychological Aspects of Physical Symptoms* (New York: Appleton-Century-Crofts, 1968), 213–219.

50. Cohen and Klein, "Posthospital Adjustment."

51. American Psychiatric Association, *Diagnostic and Statistical Manual.*

52. Nyswander, "The Drug Addict in a General Hospital."

53. J.I. Walker, *Clinical Psychiatry in Primary Care* (Menlo Park, Calif.: Addison-Wesley, 1981), 180–194.

54. Cohen and Klein, "Posthospital Adjustment."

55. P.A. Berger and J.R. Tinklenberg, "Medical Management of the Drug Abuser," in *Psychiatry for the Primary Care Physician,* ed. A.M. Freeman III, R.L. Sack, and P.A. Berger (Baltimore: Williams & Wilkins, 1979), 359–380.

56. Stimmel, *Pain, Analgesia and Addiction.*

57. Nyswander, "The Drug Addict as a Patient."

58. H. Boudin, "Contingency Contracting as a Therapeutic Tool in the Deceleration of Amphetamine Use," *Behavioral Therapy* 3 (1972): 604–608.

59. R.L. Polakow and R.M. Doctor, "Treatment of Marijuana and Barbiturate Dependency by Contingency Contracting," *Journal of Behavior Therapy and Experimental Psychiatry* 4 (1973): 375–377.

60. N.D. West, *Psychiatry in Primary Care Medicine* (New York: Year Book Medical Publishers, 1979).

61. Adriani, "Drug Dependence."

62. Ibid.

63. Ludwig, *Principles,* 268.

64. R.M. Kanner and K.M. Foley, "Patterns of Narcotic Drug Use in a Cancer Pain Clinic," *Annals of the New York Academy of Sciences* 363 (1981): 161–172.

65. J.D. Parkes, "Diseases of the Nervous System. Relief of Pain: Headache, Facial Neuralgia, Migraine and Phantom Limb," *British Medical Journal* 4 (1975): 90–92.

66. M.A. Kaplan, "Substance Abuse in Inflammatory Bowel Disease," (Unpublished 1984).

67. Kanner and Foley, "Patterns."

68. J.S. Goodwin, J.M. Goodwin, and A.V. Vogel, "Knowledge and Use of Placebos by House Officers and Nurses," *Annals of Internal Medicine* 91 (1979): 106–110.

69. R.M. Marks and E.J. Sacher, "Undertreatment of Medical Inpatients with Narcotic Analgesics," *Annals of Internal Medicine* 78 (1973): 173–181.

70. Ibid.

71. M. Angell, "The Quality of Mercy," *New England Journal of Medicine* 306 (1982): 98–99.

72. J.P. Morgan, personal communication, 1984.

73. Kanner and Foley, "Patterns."

74. Stimmel, *Pain, Analgesia and Addiction.*

75. Morgan, personal communication, 1984.

76. J. Porter and H. Jick, "Addiction Rare in Patients Treated with Narcotics," *New England Journal of Medicine* 302 (1980): 123.

77. D.W. Swanson, R.L. Weddige, and R.M. Morse, "Abuse of Prescription Drugs," *Mayo Clinic Proceedings* 48 (1973): 359–367.

78. Stimmel, *Pain, Analgesia and Addiction.*

79. Porter and Jick, "Addiction Rare."

80. J.P. Morgan, "Watching the Monitors: 'Paid' Prescriptions, Fiscal Intermediaries and Drug-Utilization Review," *New England Journal of Medicine* 296 (1977): 251–256.

81. Adriani, "Drug Dependence."

82. Stimmel, *Pain, Analgesia and Addiction.*

83. Angell, "Quality of Mercy."

84. M. Cohen and B. Stimmel, "The Use of Methadone in Narcotic Dependency," in *Treatment Aspects of Drug Dependence,* ed. A. Schecter and S.J. Mulé (West Palm Beach, Fla.: CRC Press, 1978), 1–31.

85. M.J. Kreek, "Pharmacological Modalities of Therapy: Methadone Maintenance and the Use of Narcotic Antagonists," in *Heroin Dependency,* ed. B. Stimmel. (New York: Stratton Intercontinental, 1975), 232–290.

86. J.A. Renner, Jr., "Drug Addiction," in *Massachusetts General Hospital Handbook of General Hospital Psychiatry,* ed. T.P. Hackett and N.H. Cassem (St. Louis, Mo.: C.V. Mosby, 1978).

87. Stimmel, *Pain, Analgesia and Addiction.*

88. T.G. Kantor, R. Cantor, and E. Tom, "A Study of Hospitalized Surgical Patients on Methadone Maintenance," in *Problems of Drug Dependence 1980, Proceedings of the 42nd Annual Scientific Meeting, The Committee on Problems of Drug Dependence, Inc.,* NIDA Research Monograph No. 34 (Rockville, Md.: National Institute on Drug Abuse, 1981), 243–248.

89. Ibid.

90. Renner, "Drug Addiction."

91. J.E. Martin and J. Inglis, "Pain Tolerance and Narcotic Addiction," *British Journal of the Society of Clinical Psychology* 4 (1965): 224–229.

92. L. Masten, C.H. Hine, and E.L. Way, "Tolerance, Dependence and Lethality in Morphine-Dependent Mice after Repeated Oral Administration of Methadone," *Drug and Alcohol Dependence* 3 (1979): 405–418.

93. A. Ho and V.P. Dole, "Pain Perception in Drug-Free and in Methadone-Maintained Human Ex-Addicts," *Society of Experimental and Biological Medicine* 162 (1979): 392–395.

94. R.B. Rubinstein, I. Spira, and W.I. Wolff, "Management of Surgical Problems in Patients on Methadone Maintenance." *American Journal of Surgery* 131 (1976): 566–569.

95. Stimmel, *Pain, Analgesia and Addiction.*

96. Adriani, "Drug Dependence."

97. Kantor, Cantor, and Tom, "Study of Hospitalized Surgical Patients."

98. Stimmel, *Pain, Analgesia and Addiction.*

99. Rubinstein, Spira, and Wolff, "Management."

100. V.P. Dole and M.E. Nyswander, "A Medical Treatment of Diacetylmorphine (Heroin) Addiction: Clinical Trial with Methadone Hydrochloride," *Journal of the American Medical Association* 193 (1965): 646–650.

101. V.P. Dole, M.E. Nyswander, and M.J. Kreek, "Narcotic Blockade," *Archives of Internal Medicine* 118 (1966): 304–309.

102. V.P. Dole and M.E. Nyswander, "Methadone Maintenance Treatment: A Ten Year Perspective," *Journal of the American Medical Association* 235 (1976): 2117–2119.

103. Kreek, "Pharmacological Modalities."

104. Cohen and Stimmel, "Use of Methadone."

105. J.H. Lowinson, and R.B. Millman, "Clinical Aspects of Methadone Maintenance," in *Handbook on Drug Abuse,* ed. R.I. Dupont, A. Goldstein, and J. O'Donnell (Washington, D.C.: National Institute on Drug Abuse, 1979), 49–56.

106. D.C. Des Jarlais, H. Joseph, and V.P. Dole, "Long Term Outcomes after Termination from Methadone Maintenance Treatment," *Annals of the New York Academy of Sciences* 362 (1981): 231–238.

107. J.H. Lowinson, "Methadone Maintenance in Perspective," in *Substance Abuse—Clinical Problems and Perspectives,* ed. J.H. Lowinson and P. Ruiz (Baltimore: Williams & Wilkins, 1981), 344–354.

108. Senay, *Substance Abuse Disorders.*

109. M.J. Kreek, "Medical Management of Methadone-Maintained Patients," in *Substance Abuse—Clinical Problems and Perspectives,* ed. J.H. Lowinson and P. Ruiz (Baltimore: Williams & Wilkins, 1981), 660–673.

110. J.R. Cooper, F. Altman, B.S. Brown, and D. Czechowicz, eds., *Research on the Treatment of Narcotic Addiction—State of the Art* (Rockville, Md.: National Institute on Drug Abuse, 1983).

111. A. Schiffman, personal communication, 1984.

112. B. Stimmel et al., "Parameters Defining the Ability to Remain Abstinent after Detoxification from Methadone: A Six Year Study," *Journal of the American Medical Association* 237 (1977): 1216–1220.

113. B. Stimmel, J. Goldberg, and M. Cohen, "Detoxification from Methadone Maintenance: Risk Factors Associated with Relapse to Narcotic Use," in *Annals of the New York Academy of Sciences* 311 (1978): 173–180.

114. B. Stimmel, R. Hanbury, and M. Cohen, "Factors Effecting Detoxification from Methadone," *Journal of Psychiatric Treatment and Evaluation* 4 (1982): 377–381.

Chapter 12

The Treatment of Alcoholism

Sheldon Zimberg, M.D.

INTRODUCTION

Alcoholism can be defined as a state in which the repetitive consumption of alcoholic beverages has impaired an individual's physical health, work functioning, social or family relationships, finances, or caused problems with the law. It is a life-long chronic illness with a high potential for relapse, for recovery with treatment, and even for spontaneous remission. Its etiology is unknown; its causes include physiological factors (probably of genetic origin), psychological factors, and sociocultural factors.

There is a high prevalence of this disorder, with an estimated ten million problem drinkers, or four to five percent of the American general population. This includes alcohol abusers and dependent individuals (alcoholics) who are physiologically addicted to alcohol. The lifetime prevalence of alcoholism was the highest DSM III diagnosis in two of three cities, and second highest in the third city, in which a recent survey of psychiatric disorders was conducted.[1]

In any individual, alcoholism varies in severity over time. Moreover, it affects individuals in a variety of ways to produce many behavioral and medical complications. Alcoholism is not necessarily a progressive disease; it can improve with treatment, and in a small percentage of cases (10–15 percent), does so without treatment.

Clearly, alcoholics are not a homogeneous population. The modal group of alcoholics consists of white upper-, middle-, and working-class men. However, other ethnic and socioeconomic groups, less represented in the general population, have higher rates of alcoholism and may require different treatment approaches. Among them are elderly alcoholics, adolescents, women, the socioeconomically deprived, and homeless skid-row types. Thus, all alcoholics cannot be treated alike. This chapter examines the treatment of the modal group of alcoholics cited above. (Information about treatment of various subpopulations of alcoholics can be found in the author's book, *The Clinical Management of Alcoholism.*)[2]

Among the most severe, and most common, manifestations of alcoholism are the medical, surgical, psychiatric, and neurological complications caused by the disease. These complications account for up to 50 percent of the medical inpatients in general hospitals,[3] and for up to a third of emergency room patients with alcoholism.[4] The general hospital setting is thus the obvious place for case finding and treatment services for alcoholic individuals.

DIAGNOSIS OF ALCOHOLISM

A significant number of patients seen in the general hospital are alcoholic, but very few will openly acknowledge a problem with alcohol. It is therefore necessary for the physician to take a thorough history of drinking and sedative drug usage as part of the medical history that is obtained. Also, the physical examination should be done with a high index of suspicion for possible physical effects of alcohol.

In obtaining the drinking history, one should ask how long the patient has been drinking, the frequency of use of alcoholic beverages, what beverages are used, when and where they are used, and for what purpose. Information about the quantity of alcohol consumed is unreliable; most alcoholics will tend to deny or minimize their use of alcohol. If the patient drinks repeatedly to reduce anxiety, to overcome fatigue, or to get through stressful situations, that is evidence of psychological dependence on alcohol.

One should ask about potential problems associated with drinking and what family members say of the patients' drinking. Have there been efforts to cut down or modify drinking by switching to other alcoholic beverages? Have the patients ever been told by a physician to stop drinking, and if so what was their reaction? Do they have tremors in the morning or a history of blackouts or seizures? The use of sedative drugs and minor tranquilizers—for example, chlordiazepoxide (Librium), diazepam (Valium), or meprobamate (Miltown)—often coexists with alcohol abuse; thus, information concerning the use of such drugs should also be sought. Most alcoholics will tend to deny and minimize the use of sedative drugs as well as alcohol.

When information regarding the use of alcohol and its impact on their lives indicates that there is a drinking problem, the patients should be confronted with the information and be told that they have a drinking problem. The diagnosis of alcoholism must be presented to the patients just as the diagnosis of any other chronic disorder (for example, diabetes) is presented, together with the necessary treatment approaches. Most patients will resist and will deny the diagnosis at first. However, it should be pointed out to them that denial is a basic part of the illness and that the patients' very resistance to giving up the use of alcohol is further evidence of their dependence on it.

This straightforward approach can be carried out in the outpatient or inpatient setting when the patient is sober. Most alcoholics who present themselves in the emergency room and are intoxicated may not be able to give a current history. The history should then be obtained from a collateral or when the alcoholic has sobered up to some degree, usually 8 to 12 hours later. (Further details on interviewing the alcoholic and the significant other can be found in *The Clinical Management of Alcoholism*.)[5]

Most physicians are reluctant to proceed in this professional approach because they are unwilling to stigmatize the patient or believe that alcoholism cannot be treated. However, there is currently a growing acceptance of alcoholism as an illness by the health care professions and the general public. Proper diagnosis is the first step in the provision of treatment for alcoholism, an illness that has a high mortality. The author's experience, as well as experience in the management of alcoholism in industry, indicate that up to 80 percent of alcoholics can achieve recovery.[6]

Criteria

The National Council on Alcoholism has established a set of major and minor criteria for the diagnosis of alcoholism.[7] Each set of criteria is divided into two tracks: Track 1 concerns physiological and clinical manifestations of alcoholism; Track II concerns behavioral, psychological, and attitudinal manifestations. Each criterion is assigned a diagnostic level from one to three. Level 1 represents a definitive diagnosis of alcoholism; Level 2 represents probable alcoholism and requires several other criteria for diagnosis; and Level 3 is a possible diagnosis requiring considerably more evidence beyond that of Level 3 criteria. The two sets of objective criteria provide a structured basis for establishing the diagnosis; they also provide the physician with the information needed to substantiate the diagnosis to the many patients who resist accepting alcoholism as a problem. The complete lists of major and minor criteria and their diagnostic levels are presented in Tables 12–1 and 12–2.

Recent reports suggest that the mean corpuscular volume of red blood cells is elevated in alcoholics.[8] This involves a test that is readily available as part of a complete blood count. The macrocytic condition of the red blood cells is due to folic acid deficiency or to the direct toxic effect of

Table 12–1 National Council on Alcoholism: Major Criteria for the Diagnosis of Alcoholism

Criterion	Diagnostic Level
Track I. Physiological and Clinical	
A. Physiological Dependency	
1. Physiological dependence as manifested by evidence of a withdrawal syndrome when the intake of alcohol is interrupted or decreased without substitution of other sedation. It must be remembered that overuse of other sedative drugs can produce a similar withdrawal state, which should be differentiated from withdrawal from alcohol.	
a) Gross tremor (differentiated from other causes of tremor).	1
b) Hallucinosis (differentiated from schizophrenic hallucinations or other psychoses).	1
c) Withdrawal seizures (differentiated from epilepsy and other seizure disorders).	1
d) Delirium tremens. Usually starts between the first and third day after withdrawal and minimally includes tremors, disorientation, and hallucinations	1
2. Evidence of tolerance to the effects of alcohol. (There may be a decrease in previously high levels of tolerance late in the course.) Although the degree of tolerance to alcohol in no way matches the degree of tolerance to other drugs, the behavioral effects of a given amount of alcohol vary greatly between alcoholic and nonalcoholic subjects.	
a) A blood alcohol level of more than 150 mg without gross evidence of intoxication.	1
b) The consumption of one-fifth of a gallon of whiskey or an equivalent amount of wine or beer daily, for more than one day, by a 180-lb individual.	1
3. Alcoholic "blackout" periods. (Differential diagnosis from purely psychological fugue states and psychomotor seizures.)	2
B. Clinical: Major Alcohol-Associated Illnesses. Alcoholism can be assumed to exist if major alcohol-associated illnesses develop in a person who drinks regularly. In such individuals, evidence of physiological and psychological dependence should be searched for:	
Fatty degeneration in absence of other known cause	2
Alcoholic hepatitis	1
Laennec's cirrhosis	2
Pancreatitis in the absence of cholelithiasis	2
Chronic gastritis	3
Hematological disorders:	
Anemia: hypochromic normocytic, macrocytic, hemolytic with stomatocytosis, low folic acid.	3
Clotting disorders: prothrombin elevation, thrombocytopenia.	3
Wernicke-Korsakoff syndrome	2
Alcoholic cerebellar degeneration.	1

Table 12-1 continued

Criterion	Diagnostic Level
Cerebral degeneration in absence of Alzheimer's disease or arterio-sclerosis.	2
Central pontine myelinolysis:	
Diagnosis only possible postmortem.	2
Marchiafava-Bignami's disease:	
Diagnosis only possible postmortem.	2
Peripheral neuropathy (see also beriberi)	2
Toxic amblyopia	3
Alcohol myopathy	2
Alcoholic cardiomyopathy	2
Beriberi	3
Pellagra	3

Track II. Behavioral, Psychological, and Attitudinal

All chronic conditions of psychological dependence occur in dynamic equilibrium with intrapsychic and interpersonal consequences. In alcoholism, similarly, there are varied effects on character and family. Like other chronic relapsing diseases, alcoholism produces vocational, social, and physical impairments. Therefore, the implications of these disruptions must be evaluated and related to the individual and his pattern of alcoholism. The following behavior patterns show psychological dependence on alcohol in alcoholism:

1. Drinking despite strong medical contraindication known to patient	1
2. Drinking despite strong, identified, social contraindication (job loss for intoxication, marriage disruption because of drinking, arrest for intoxication, driving while intoxicated)	1
3. Patient's subjective complaint of loss of control of alcohol consumption.	2

Note: Diagnostic Level 1: Definite diagnosis. Diagnostic Level 2: Probable diagnosis. Diagnostic Level 3: Possible diagnosis.

Source: Reprinted from *The American Journal of Psychiatry,* Vol. 129, pp. 127-135, with permission of the American Psychiatric Association, ©1972.

alcohol on the bone marrow. Liver chemistries are frequently abnormal in alcoholics; this should be looked for as part of the diagnostic process.

Currently, the best approach to the establishment of the diagnosis of alcoholism is to determine that the continued abuse of alcohol has caused problems in the individual's social and family relationships, physical health, employment situation, finances, or legal responsibilities (drunk-driving arrest, for example). These diagnostic problem areas should be understood in the context that alcoholism is not an all-or-nothing phenomenon, that it is rather one of degree, and that the severity of alcoholism can vary in the

Table 12–2 National Council on Alcoholism: Minor Criteria for the Diagnosis of Alcoholism

Criterion	Diagnostic Level
Track I. Physiological and Clinical	
A. Direct Effects (ascertained by examination)	
1. Early:	
Odor of alcohol on breath at time of medical appointment	2
2. Middle:	
Alcoholic facies	2
Vascular engorgement of face	2
Toxic amblyopia	3
Increased incidence of infections	3
Cardiac arrhythmias	3
Peripheral neuropathy (see also Major Criteria, Track I, B)	2
3. Late (see Major Criteria Track I, B)	
B. Indirect Effects	
1. Early:	
Tachycardia	3
Flushed face	3
Nocturnal diaphoresis	3
2. Middle:	
Ecchymoses on lower extremities, arms, or chest	3
Cigarette or other burns on hands or chest	3
Hyperreflexia, or if drinking heavily, hyporeflexia (permanent hyporeflexia may be a residuum of alcoholic polyneuritis)	3
3. Late:	
Decreased tolerance	3
C. Laboratory Tests	
1. Major—Direct	
Blood alcohol level at any time of more than 300 mg/100 ml	1
Level of more than 100 mg/100 ml in routine examination	1
2. Major—Indirect	
Serum osmolality (reflects blood alcohol levels): every 22.4 increase over 200 mOsm/liter reflects 50 mg/100 ml alcohol	2
3. Minor—Indirect	
Results of alcohol ingestion:	
Hypoglycemia	3
Hypochloremic alkalosis	3
Low magnesium level	2
Lactic acid elevation	3
Transient uric acid elevation	3
Potassium depletion	3
Indications of liver abnormality:	
SGPT elevation	2
SGOT elevation	3
BSP elevation	2
Bilirubin elevation	2

Table 12–2 continued

Criterion	Diagnostic Level
Urinary urobilinogen elevation	2
Serum A/G ratio reversal	2
Blood and blood clotting:	
Anemia: hypochromic, normocytic, macrocytic, hemolytic with stomatocytosis, low folic acid	3
Clotting disorders: prothrombin elevation, thrombocytopenia	3
ECG abnormalities:	
Cardiac arrhythmias; tachycardia; T waves dimpled, cloven, or spinous; atrial fibrillation; ventricular premature contractions; abnormal P waves	2
EEG abnormalities:	
Decreased or increased REM sleep, depending on phase	3
Loss of delta sleep	3
Other reported findings	3
Decreased immune response	3
Decreased response to Synacthen test	3
Chromosomal damage from alcoholism	3

Track II. Behavioral, Psychological and Attitudinal

A. Behavioral
  1. Direct effects

Criterion	Diagnostic Level
Early:	
Gulping drinks	3
Surreptitious drinking	2
Morning drinking (assess nature of peer group behavior)	2
Middle:	
Repeated conscious attempts at abstinence	2
Late:	
Blatant indiscriminate use of alcohol	1
Skid Row or equivalent social level	2

  2. Indirect effects

Criterion	Diagnostic Level
Early:	
Medical excuses from work for variety of reasons	2
Shifting from one alcoholic beverage to another	2
Preference for drinking companions, bars, and taverns	2
Late:	
Chooses employment that facilitates drinking	3
Frequent automobile accidents	3
History of family members undergoing psychiatric treatment; school and behavioral problems in children	3
Frequent change of residence for poorly defined reasons	3
Anxiety-relieving mechanisms, such as telephone calls inappropriate in time, distance, person and motive (telephonitis)	2
Outbursts of rage and suicidal gestures while drinking	2

(continued)

Table 12–2 continued

Criterion	Diagnostic Level
B. Psychological and Attitudinal	
1. Direct effects	
Early:	
When talking freely, makes frequent reference to drinking alcohol, people being "bombed," "stoned," etc. or admits drinking more than peer group	2
Middle:	
Drinking to relieve anger, insomnia, fatigue, depression, social discomfort	2
Late:	
Psychological symptoms consistent with permanent organic brain syndrome (see also Major Criteria, Track I, B)	2
2. Indirect effects	
Early:	
Unexplained changes in family, social and business relationships; complaints about wife, job, and friends	3
Spouse makes complaints about drinking behavior, reported by patient or spouse	2
Major family disruptions, separation, divorce, threats of divorce	3
Job loss (due to increasing interpersonal difficulties), frequent job changes, financial difficulties	3
Late:	
Overt expression of more regressive defense mechanisms: denial, projection, etc.	3
Resentment, jealousy, paranoid attitudes	3
Symptoms of depression, isolation, crying, suicidal preoccupation	3
Feelings that he is "losing his mind"	2

Note: Diagnostic Level 1: Definite diagnosis. Diagnostic Level 2: Probable diagnosis. Diagnostic Level 3: Possible diagnosis.

Source: Reprinted from *The American Journal of Psychiatry,* Vol. 129, pp. 127–135, with permission of the American Psychiatric Association, ©1972.

---

individual over time. Alcoholics often try to modify the effects of alcohol on themselves by "cutting down" for periods of time, maintaining short periods of sobriety, restricting drinking to weekends or evenings, or changing from spirits to wine or beer. The efforts of control in the face of evidence of loss of control over the impulse to drink are characteristic of the disorder.

Table 12–3 presents an Alcohol Abuse Scale, developed by the author, that approximates various levels of severity of alcohol abuse, from none to

Table 12–3 Scale of Alcohol Abuse

Level of Severity	Signs and Symptoms
None	Drinks only on occasion, if at all.
Minimal	Drinking is not conspicuous: occasional intoxication (up to four times per year). No social, family, occupational, health, or legal problems related to drinking.
Mild	Intoxication occurs up to once a month, although generally limited to evenings or weekends. Some impairment in social, family relations, or occupational functioning related to drinking. No physical or legal problems related to drinking.
Moderate	Frequent intoxications, up to one to two times per week and/or significant impairment in social, family, or occupational functioning. Some suggestive evidence of physical impairment related to drinking, such as tremors, frequent accidents, epigastric distress, occasional loss of appetite. No history of DTs, cirrhosis, nutritional deficiency, hospitalizations related to drinking, or arrests related to drinking.
Severe	Almost constant drinking, practically every day. History of DTs, cirrhosis, chronic brain syndrome, neuritis, or nutritional deficiency. Severe disruption in social or family relations. Unable to hold a steady job but able to maintain self on public assistance. Two or more arrests related to drinking (drunk or disorderly). Two or more drunk driving citations. One or more hospitalizations related to drinking.
Extreme	All of the characteristics of severe impairment, plus homelessness and/or inability to maintain self on public assistance.

extreme. It is easy to establish the diagnosis of alcoholism at the extreme level (skid-row alcoholics) and the severe level. However, alcoholism is more readily treatable when diagnosed at the mild or moderate levels of severity. The mild stage of severity can be considered a preaddictive stage in which the individual is psychologically dependent on the use of alcohol. The moderate stage is the stage of physiological addiction, as evidenced by the presence of withdrawal signs (tremors) and the beginning of physical consequences and disability and significant social impairment.

The Alcohol Abuse Scale has been found to be extremely useful, practical, and easy to apply by the author in clinical settings and in research programs.[9-11] A high degree of validity and reliability can be obtained when the scale is used with a standardized questionnaire.

TREATMENT OF ALCOHOLISM

Psychodynamic Factors

The major psychodynamic conflict in alcoholics centers around dependency needs. The conflict is based on the childhood deprivations to which many alcoholics have been exposed. Alcoholics have an expectation that they will be rejected. They have a low self-image because of their unmet dependency needs, and they believe that they cannot deal with a crisis. They develop anxiety; and, when faced with a problem or crisis, they habitually turn to alcohol to tranquilize their anxiety. The pharmacological effects of alcohol are such that they cause the alcoholic "to feel no pain."

Alcoholics in crisis will frequently appear in emergency rooms or stressful settings under the influence of alcohol. A common staff response to alcoholics who present themselves in such a state is one of anger and rejection. The rejection the alcoholics experience in their state of heightened dependency confirms their expectations of rejection and feelings of hostility. In order to alter this habitual pattern, the staff must receive alcoholic patients in an accepting fashion and thereby provide a corrective emotional experience.

Chafetz et al. demonstrated that alcoholics who presented to an emergency room and were then treated in an alcoholism unit had a much greater chance of receiving follow-up care if the emergency room staff continued to be available to the patients in the alcoholism clinic than if they were simply referred to other staff.[12] Alcoholics in crisis establish a positive transference to helping staff, since they are looking for support and help because of their unmet dependency needs. Help offered in a nonjudgmental and supportive way can engage alcoholics in treatment. The success of Alcoholics Anonymous is based on an understanding of the psychological needs of alcoholics.

Diagnostic Considerations in the Treatment Process

Psychiatric disorders occur frequently in individuals who abuse alcohol, and their occurrence should always be considered when evaluating alcoholic patients. Among these are schizophrenia, affective disorders, anxiety disorders, neurotic disorders, and personality disorders. Individuals suffering from functional psychoses may use alcohol as self-medication to tranquilize severe anxiety and depression. Alcoholics have a high rate of suicide;

conversely, suicide-prone individuals often resort to combinations of drugs and alcohol in suicidal attempts.

Alcohol produces both acute and chronic toxic effects on the brain that result in organic psychoses. Acute toxic reactions include alcohol intoxication and alcohol idiosyncratic intoxication. Chronic toxic effects on the brain include alcohol amnestic disorder, Korsakoff's psychosis, and dementia associated with alcoholism.

To make a differential diagnosis between primary alcoholism and alcohol secondary to a functional disorder, it is necessary to observe and evaluate the individual in an alcohol-free state. If the history or examination of the patient reveals evidence of psychosis—hallucinations, delusions, suicidal intent, severe depression, severe agitation or excitement—it is best to carry out the evaluation in an inpatient psychiatric setting. Effective psychiatric treatment of the functional disorder can often eliminate alcohol abuse as a problem, and the patients may then be treated in a more extended psychiatric program. Consultation provided by specialists in the field of alcoholism may be helpful in the management of such patients.

In contrast, individuals with coexisting neurotic and personality disorders often can be treated by the primary physician. Psychotherapy for their neurotic or personality disorders can best be provided after sobriety has been well-established. Psychotherapy is clearly not an effective treatment for actively-drinking patients, because the therapeutic process itself produces anxiety that can lead to drinking. Therefore, it is necessary to treat the alcoholism first and to help the patient establish a firm internalized set of controls over the impulse to drink; this can be done through the use of disulfiram (Antabuse), counseling, and/or Alcoholics Anonymous. Once the control over drinking has been established, psychotherapy can be effective in dealing with the neurotic or personality problems.

Alcohol idiosyncratic intoxication is a rare phenomenon. It occurs in individuals who develop a severe change in mental state and behavior after the consumption of a small amount of alcohol. The intoxication is characterized by confusion, transitory delusions, visual hallucinations, and impairment in consciousness. These symptoms may be accompanied by increased activity, rage, aggression, and destructive behavior or by depression and suicidal behavior. Such a state can last from a few hours to a few days. It is best treated with sedation in an in-hospital setting, because the individuals affected can be a serious danger to themselves or others. After a period of sleep, the condition clears and the individual has no memory of the episode.

Other alcohol-related psychoses include alcohol amnestic disorder and dementia associated with alcoholism. Alcohol amnestic disorder is an organic mental syndrome consisting of disorientation, confusion, confabulation, suggestibility, and the inability to recall and retain immediate information. This mental picture is frequently accompanied by polyneuropathy and Wernicke's syndrome. Wernicke's syndrome consists of ataxia, nystagmus, and ocular muscle palsies. It results from necrotic and hemorrhagic lesions of the brain stem; its mental and neurological signs and symptoms result primarily from a thiamine deficiency. The treatment involves immediate admission to a hospital and parenteral administration of 50–100 mg of thiamine daily for four to five days, supplemented by oral B-complex and ascorbic acid.

Dementia associated with alcoholism occurs in individuals with long-standing alcoholism. The clinical picture is one of emotional instability, personality and social disintegration, and subtle signs of dementia. This syndrome was previously thought to be associated with avitaminosis. However, recent evidence of the direct toxic effects of alcohol on the brain indicate that alcohol ingestion alone may be the primary cause. Computerized axial tomographic studies (CAT scans) have found a significant percentage of chronic alcoholics with cerebral atrophy.[13] Such individuals require hospitalization to treat coexisting medical problems, to improve their nutritional status, and to remove them from access to alcohol. Significant improvement can be expected only with treatment of their alcoholism in a long-term residential program.

Treatment of Acute Alcohol Reactions

If the individual is suffering primarily from the effects of alcohol without evidence of psychosis, a determination must be made of the type of reaction—whether it is alcohol intoxication, alcohol stupor or coma, or alcohol withdrawal. Alcohol intoxication of a mild or moderate degree can usually be managed by having the individual sleep it off. This is the usual method of self-detoxification for individuals who become intoxicated, whether or not they are alcoholics. In uncomplicated cases, the patient can be sent home in the company of a responsible person.

Individuals who are stuporous or in coma as a result of alcohol ingestion should be sent to an emergency room where they can be carefully evaluated to rule out other causes. These individuals should be observed and blood alcohol, blood barbiturate, blood urea nitrogen, and blood sugar levels should be measured. Efforts should be directed at maintaining blood pressure and adequate respiration. There should be careful observation for 24–48 hours before a disposition is made. The use of sedatives or tranquilizers should be avoided in such cases because they can potentiate the stupor and lead to respiratory arrest. Stupor should be considered a medical emergency and managed accordingly.

Treatment of Alcohol Withdrawal Syndromes

An alcoholic may appear in a hospital emergency room or outpatient clinic experiencing any of the several manifestations of the syndromes of alcohol withdrawal. Alcohol withdrawal syndromes occur in persons addicted to alcohol who have stopped drinking abruptly or begun reducing alcohol consumption, producing a significant reduction in the blood alcohol level. The severity of the withdrawal cannot be predicted; thus caution should be exercised with anyone manifesting symptoms of alcohol withdrawal. The etiology of withdrawal syndromes is not yet fully understood.

Several levels of alcohol withdrawal have been observed and reported by Victor and Adams.[14] The mildest form is tremulousness, characterized by tremors, vomiting, flushed face, injected conjunctivae, tachycardia, and occasionally agitation. Tremulousness is a common condition among alcoholics, who note that they have the "shakes" upon awakening. This condition will subside with mild sedation, a small amount of alcohol, or eventually with complete abstinence. However, in some cases, the "shakes" if untreated will progress to delirium tremens.

Hallucinosis is a form of alcohol withdrawal syndrome that can occur with or without tremulousness. It is characterized by visual, auditory, or tactile hallucinations. The hallucinations are usually threatening and unpleasant. They are often transitory but can persist for months in some cases. Hallucinations that continue for weeks to months after withdrawal from alcohol and without the resumption of drinking should lead to the suspicion of schizophrenia. Hallucinosis in a chronic alcoholic is most likely an alcohol withdrawal phenomenon and should not be considered a functional psychosis. Alcoholics experiencing acute hallucinosis have often been inappropriately admitted to psychiatric inpatient units. Such individuals risk the danger of developing delirium tremens in an inappropriate setting. It must be remembered that alcohol withdrawal syndromes are primarily medical disorders and require medical treatment.

Seizures, called "rum fits," can be a manifestation of alcohol withdrawal. Individuals who experience seizures related to alcohol withdrawal require primarily medical detoxification from alcohol. The effectiveness of anticonvulsants is somewhat controversial. Some authorities believe they are not of value, except for barbiturates, which have a cross-tolerance with alcohol. However, as a practical matter, most alcohol detoxification units use diphenylhydantoin (Dilantin), 100 mg tid, for alcoholics who experience seizures.

Any of these syndromes of alcohol withdrawal can be self-limiting or lead to delirium tremens. Delirium tremens is clearly a medical emergency, with a mortality rate of from 5 to 30 percent. Delirium tremens consists of tremulousness, hallucinations, disorientation, and a delirious state. Other signs include fever, profuse perspiration, tachycardia, tachypnea, and severe agitation.

Treatment of withdrawal syndromes consists primarily of sedation. Chlordiazepoxide (Librium) and other benzodiazepines have been found to be the most useful drugs in this regard because of the lack of seizure potentiation and the minimum risk of oversedation and adverse effects on the liver. The dosage for the first day consists of Librium 150–200 mg in four doses by mouth, or intramuscularly if the patient is unable to take medication orally. The Librium is gradually reduced over a five-day period. Librium is erratically absorbed intramuscularly; lorazepam (Ativan) is said to be more reliably absorbed intramuscularly, but no clinical trials of its use for alcohol withdrawal have yet been published. In an acute situation with a patient who cannot take medication by mouth, diazepam (Valium) can be used intravenously, giving it very slowly—10 mg over a 60-second period.

In addition to the benzodiazepines, 2 cc of magnesium sulfate, 50 percent, can be given intramuscularly three times a day for the first day and twice daily for the next two days; low serum magnesium may be an etiologic factor in alcohol withdrawal syndromes, and magnesium sulfate's anticonvulsant properties are well-known. Chloral hydrate, 0.5–1.0 gm, can also be given for sleep. Serious sleep disturbances are characteristic of alcohol withdrawal syndromes.

In addition to sedation, thiamine (100 mg IM), B-complex, and multivitamins should be given, because vitamin deficiencies are often found in alcoholics secondary to their poor dietary habits. Intravenous 50-percent glucose and water can be administered if there is a suspicion of hypoglycemia. Because recent evidence indicates that during withdrawal alcoholics are often overhydrated rather than dehydrated, large amounts of intravenous fluids should be avoided unless there is clear evidence of dehydration and the individual is unable to tolerate fluids by mouth.

A number of patients who are experiencing mild to moderate alcohol withdrawal symptoms (mild to moderate tremulousness) can benefit from ambulatory detoxification carried out under close medical supervision in an outpatient clinic or physician's office. Such patients can be treated with oral doses of chlordiazepoxide (Librium), 100–150 mg/day, or diazepam (Valium), 20–30 mg/day, with a decreasing dosage over five to seven days. Diphenylhydantoin (Dilantin) can be administered in doses of 100 mg tid if there is a history of seizures. During ambulatory detoxification, the patient should be seen daily or at least two to three times per week by medical personnel and should be engaged in supportive counseling. The patient should be given no more than a one week supply of medication.

The final stage of alcohol detoxification in an inpatient setting or in an outpatient clinic should be the cessation of all sedative-hypnotic and minor tranquilizing medication. Alcoholics should not, in general, be maintained on sedatives or minor tranquilizers because there is abundant evidence that they frequently come to abuse these drugs.

The treatment of alcohol withdrawal syndromes in moderate to severe states (severe tremulousness, seizures, hallucinations, agitation, delirium) is best carried out in an alcohol detoxification unit or on a medical service in a general hospital. A psychiatric scatter-bed service is also a highly appropriate and effective milieu for this purpose. The duration should be five days of progressive reduction of the benzodiazepine drug and two days of drug-free observation to make sure there are no recurrences of withdrawal signs and symptoms. The detoxification itself is a medical procedure. The equally important procedure of counseling to enhance motivation for treatment after discharge should be carried out by staff who are knowledgeable about alcoholism, some or all of whom are recovered alcoholics. Recovered alcoholic counselors provide a role model of successful treatment for the alcoholic patients as well as for the other staff.

A protracted withdrawal syndrome occurs in some alcoholics after withdrawal from alcohol and can persist for months. The condition includes a fine tremor of the hands, feelings of anxiety and depression, insomnia, irritability, feelings of fatigue, memory impairment, distractibility, and difficulty in concentrating. The syndrome is believed to be due to the prolonged effects of alcohol on the central nervous system. If major clinical depression is present for at least six weeks after detoxification, the patient should be treated with antidepressant medication.

Treatment after Detoxification

Alcoholism is a chronic illness with a high potential for relapse. As in other chronic disorders, continuous care is required, in many cases for life. Alcoholics Anonymous is particularly well-suited to provide this supportive treatment for an indefinite duration. However, professional intervention during the early stages of treatment is necessary to provide detoxification from alcohol, a thorough medical evaluation, and continued support for alcoholics unwilling or unable to make effective use of Alcoholics Anonymous.

Patients with serious depression, psychoses, or severe anxiety states along with alcoholism should be treated for these conditions as well as the alcoholism and should be referred to psychiatrists for the appropriate evaluation and treatment. It has often been found that alcoholism that is secondary to such major psychiatric disorders clears up when the primary disorder is effectively treated. A period of observation in a hospital setting may be required to make a differential diagnosis on such patients.

Directive counseling by the physician during the process of detoxification can enhance an alcoholic's motivation to continue the treatment. Acquainting alcoholics with the physical effects of alcohol on their bodies and the effects on their ability to perform necessary functions should be part of this effort.

Patients should be told that it is necessary to stop drinking. They should be encouraged to go to Alcoholics Anonymous and be started on disulfiram. Directive psychotherapy or counseling should be provided to patients, emphasizing abstinence and helping them to deal with problems and crises without using alcohol. Various modified psychotherapeutic modalities can be applied to alcoholism, including individual therapy, group therapy, couples therapy, family therapy, and psychodrama. (Detailed descriptions of these techniques and their application to alcoholics are provided in *The Clinical Management of Alcoholism*.)[15]

The Use of Disulfiram

The deterrent use of disulfiram (Antabuse) is quite effective. The usual maintenance dose is 250 mg/day, but as little as 125 mg/day may be adequate. The only contraindications for the use of disulfiram are the presence of serious cardiac disorders, decompensating liver disease, psychosis, or brain damage with significant impairment in judgment. Patients should be educated in what to avoid when taking disulfiram and should be given an Antabuse identification card. Few patients on disulfiram will drink. The disulfiram effect lasts about five to seven days after the last dose. Those who do drink and have a disulfiram-alcohol reaction can be treated with oral diphenhydramine (Benadryl), or the patient will remit without treatment. Most serious disulfiram-alcohol reactions require the use of oxygen vasopressors and intravaneous Benadryl.

Disulfiram acts by interfering with the enzymatic breakdown of alcohol at the step of acetaldehyde production. When alcohol is consumed, acetaldehyde is produced in a dose-related amount that produces the toxic reaction, consisting of flushing, nausea, vomiting, anxiety, hyperventilation, and hypotension. This is very rarely a fatal reaction.

Disulfiram can itself occasionally produce a toxic psychosis. Anyone experiencing such a toxic psychosis should be admitted to a hospital and the disulfiram should be discontinued. Minor tranquilizers can be used to control the anxiety. Phenothiazines may be used cautiously if there is severe agitation and overt psychotic symptoms. The reaction usually subsides within a few days.

A history of other medications must be secured from all patients on disulfiram. A number of toxic psychotic reactions have been reported when disulfiram has been used in conjunction with isoniazid; similar reports have been made about the combination of disulfiram and metronidazole (Flagyl). Disulfiram potentiates the effect of diphenylhydantoin (Dilantin), barbiturates, and coumarin anticoagulants. Individuals on amitriptyline (Elavil) and disulfiram may experience an enhanced alcohol-disulfiram reaction if alcohol is ingested.

Referrals to Alcoholism Specialists for Treatment

In general, physicians should refer alcoholics with coexisting major psychiatric disorders to psychiatrists who are knowledgeable about alcoholism. Alcoholics who do not respond to directive counseling, disulfiram, or Alcoholics Anonymous should be referred to specialized alcoholism treatment programs or alcoholism specialists. Local chapters of the National Council of Alcoholism usually have referral and information services and/or directories of such services. These resources should be sought to facilitate the referral of alcoholics who have not responded to initial treatment efforts.

Patients who do not respond easily and quickly should not be a source of discouragement to the physician. In the author's experience, many patients require several efforts at treatment before a therapeutic impact is made. At times, the most reluctant alcoholic will respond when the right approach is applied. Patients desiring insight into their underlying psychological conflicts should be referred to psychotherapists after they have achieved at least a year of sobriety. Psychiatrists who are experienced with alcoholics are probably best equipped to treat such patients, since they can reinstitute disulfiram if a "slip" should occur and can diagnose possible severe underlying psychiatric disorders that might require the use of major tranquilizers or antidepressants. Helping alcoholics recover can be a very satisfying experience, if clinicians recognize their own limitations as well as the tools that are available to assist alcoholics in treatment.

Treatment of Alcoholism in the General Hospital

The results of the Chafetz study,[16] together with an understanding of the psychodynamic conflicts of alcoholics, can aid in clarifying and understanding the nature of hospital emergency services for alcoholics. First, alcoholics who present themselves in a physical or psychosocial crisis will frequently be under the influence of alcohol. Second, although the alcoholics may not remember what transpired in their relationships with care giving persons because of the effects of alcohol, interested and helpful people attending them will have an impact on their motivation to seek treatment for their drinking problems. Third, detoxification is not a treatment for alcoholism; it deals rather with the medical aspects of alcohol withdrawal. Treatment for alcoholism begins after alcohol withdrawal. In light of these observations, careful consideration must be given to the staffing of both medical and psychiatric emergency services.

It is probably not feasible to establish separate 24-hour-a-day emergency services for alcoholics apart from the general hospital emergency service. Neither would it be beneficial to do so, because alcoholism services should be an integrated part of the total health care system. However, emergency services should be staffed by those who are knowledgeable about and receptive to the alcoholic. Most health care professionals cannot be trained quickly, and attitudes toward alcoholism cannot be changed dramatically, to ensure such staffing at all emergency services. However, those professional or paraprofessional staff members who can effectively relate to alcoholics can provide valuable services to such patients, and also provide the rest of the staff with models of effective intervention. Recovered alcoholics can ably perform this function while serving as examples to both patients and staff that alcoholism can be successfully treated.

The emergency room and general medical-surgical inpatient service of the general hospital can serve as focal points for the delivery of emergency acute diagnostic and treatment services for persons suffering from alcoholism. However, these services should be related to an alcoholism detoxification unit, sobering-up station, or alcoholism clinic that provides ambulatory detoxification. After detoxification, comprehensive treatment services for alcoholics that are closely related to the detoxification facilities can be very useful in providing continuity of care. Such service components may include an alcoholism outpatient clinic, a day hospital, a halfway house, a hospital rehabilitation service, a long-term residential care program, a vocational rehabilitation program, and various family-oriented treatment services. The nonavailability of such services undoubtedly results in the loss of treatment to many alcoholics who could otherwise be rehabilitated. In particular, close coordination between general hospital alcoholism services and local Alcoholics Anonymous groups is vital for workable treatment. Alcoholics Anonymous can provide a successful approach for many, if not the great majority, of alcoholics. In the context of a viable working relationship, it can refer and bring alcoholics for emergency hospital treatment and provide follow-up for patients during their hospital stay and after discharge.

DEVELOPING PROGRAMS FOR ALCOHOLICS IN THE GENERAL HOSPITAL

As has been discussed, alcoholism is an extremely prevalent disease and the acute, sub-acute and chronic psychiatric and medical complication makes alcoholics frequent patients in general hospitals. The prevalence of alcoholism requires the development of a systematic approach to the case finding, diagnosis, and treatment of alcoholic patients. The following is a modified version of a ten-part approach advocated by Lewis and Gordon in their development of an alcoholism program at Roger Williams General Hospital in Providence, Rhode Island.[17]

1. *Medical and administrative leadership.* There must be a knowledge-able physician on the staff of the hospital to provide medical leader-ship for the development of an alcoholism program. The physician may be an internist or a psychiatrist. This physician should be able to provide direct care to alcoholic patients, and also provide education to the physicians and physicians-in-training through consultations, lectures, supervision, and conferences on alcoholism. Such a physi-cian can serve as a role model for other physicians in the treatment of alcoholism and provide the administrative leadership to develop pro-gram proposals, grant applications, and program justification to the hospital administration. The hospital administration must be con-vinced of the programmatic value of services to alcoholics and believe that it is fiscally sound policy to provide such services. Only with the support of the hospital administrators can such a program develop.

2. *Availability of special clinics.* In addition to the medical involve-ment, there should be other staff available to provide treatment and consultation services. Such staff should include nurses, social work-ers, and alcoholism counselors. Recovered alcoholics serving as pro-fessionals or alcoholism counselors are particularly effective, since they are experienced and can serve as role models of successful treatment. Alcoholism counselors can provide case finding and treat-ment services under professional supervision. As a highly effective and motivated cadre of staff, they are less costly than more tradi-tional professional groups.

3. *Case finding on inpatient services.* Efforts should be made to find patients admitted to general care beds of the hospital who have alcohol-related (and frequently other) disorders, in order to engage and motivate them for treatment after discharge. The case finding can

be carried out through a consultation-liaison service, which can also provide training in the recognition and diagnosis of alcoholic patients.

4. *Case finding in the emergency room.* Since significant numbers of alcoholics appear in the emergency room, the presence of an alcoholism counselor as an integral member of the emergency room staff can facilitate the diagnosis and referral for treatment of these patients. Without such a specialized staff person, alcoholics are generally not diagnosed as alcoholic, and the treatment rendered is only symptomatic, with discharge affected without referral for treatment.

5. *Establishing an alcoholism program.* A general hospital should provide the following essential services for alcoholics: a small inpatient detoxification unit or detoxification service on a scatter-bed system, an alcoholism clinic, and consultation and case finding services. These basic programs are the ones that a general hospital, among all care givers, is best able to provide. Other programs, such as inpatient treatment programs for alcoholics (rehabilitation), halfway houses, and day hospitals, can be developed based on the size and needs of the alcoholic population served and the availability of such services by other community agencies.

6. *Community liaison.* Referral relationships to other community agencies serving alcoholics should be established so that referrals of patients for diagnosis and acute care treatment at the general hospital can be facilitated. In addition, such community agencies as the department of public assistance and vocational training agencies should be contacted to facilitate the referral for additional services of general hospital patients being treated for alcoholism.

7. *Alcoholics Anonymous and Al-Anon meetings on the premises.* The general hospital should make space available for Alcoholics Anonymous and Al-Anon meetings. This will provide easy access for general hospital patients and their families to these important self-help groups and demonstrate to the hospital community the important role such groups have in the treatment of alcoholism. Staff at the hospital can attend these meetings to learn more about alcoholism.

8. *Employee assistance programs.* An employee assistance program should be established at the hospital, with involvement by the administration, personnel department, and union. Alcoholism is a common problem among employees, and the expertise of the alcoholism program staff can facilitate the development of an effective approach for alcoholic hospital employees. Experience in industry with such employee assistance programs has demonstrated substantial savings to the company in terms of reduced absenteeism, health insurance,

and disability and workers compensation costs and in an increased ability to retain trained effective staff who would otherwise have been fired. Such programs serve not only to indicate a humanitarian approach by the general hospital, they also constitute good business practice.

9. *Staff education.* The alcoholism staff should provide in-service training for physicians, nurses, and social workers to help them diagnose and treat alcoholic patients more effectively. The staff can also provide training for supervisors to help them recognize alcoholic employees and to refer them to available employee assistance programs.

10. *Patient and community education.* The hospital alcoholism staff should provide educational activities through films, lectures, discussion groups, and video cassettes to aid in recognizing problem drinkers. High-risk groups, such as the elderly, children of alcoholics, and adolescents, can be targeted for such educational efforts. There should be outreach efforts aimed at social, business, and community agencies to facilitate case finding and referral of patients for treatment.

This comprehensive ten-step approach will ensure the development of an effective treatment and educational system for alcoholics in the general hospital on a fiscally sound basis and with a high potential for gaining the support of the entire hospital community and the community-at-large.

REFERENCES

1. L.N. Robin et al., "Lifetime Prevalence of Specific Psychiatric Disorders in Three Sites," *Archives of General Psychiatry* 41 (1984): 949–958.

2. S. Zimberg, *The Clinical Management of Alcoholism* (New York: Brunner/Mazel, 1982).

3. J.E. McCusker, C.E. Cherubin, and S. Zimberg, "Prevalence of Alcoholism in General Municipal Hospital Population," *New York State Journal of Medicine* 71 (1971): 751–754.

4. S. Zimberg, "Alcoholism Prevalence in General Hospital Emergency Room and Walk-In Clinic," *New York State Journal of Medicine* 79 (1979): 1533–1536.

5. Zimberg, *Clinical Management.*

6. S.B. Blume, "Is Alcoholism Treatment Worthwhile?" *Bulletin of the New York Academy of Medicine* 59 (1983): 171–180.

7. Criteria Committee, National Council on Alcoholism, "Criteria for the Diagnosis of Alcoholism," *American Journal of Psychiatry* 129 (1972): 127–135.

8. M.H. Eckardt and D.J. Feldman, "Biochemical Correlates of Alcohol Abuse," in *Currents in Alcoholism,* vol. 3, ed. F.A. Seixas (New York: Grune & Stratton, 1978).

9. McCusker, Cherubin, and Zimberg, "Prevalence."

10. Zimberg, "Alcoholism Prevalence."

11. J. Lusins et al.,"Alcoholism and Cerebral Atrophy: A Study of 50 Patients with CT Scan and Psychological Testing," *Alcoholism: Clinical and Experimental Research* 4 (1980): 406–411.

12. M.E. Chafetz et al., "Establishing Treatment Relations with Alcoholics," *Journal of Nervous and Mental Disease* 134 (1962): 395–409.

13. Ibid.

14. M. Victor and R.D. Adams "Alcohol," *Principles of Internal Medicine*, ed. T.R. Harrison, M. M. Wintrobe, and G.W. Thorn (New York: McGraw-Hill, 1974).

15. Zimberg, *Clinical Management*.

16. Chafetz et al., "Establishing Treatment Relations."

17. D.C. Lewis and A.J. Gordon, "Alcoholism and the General Hospital," *Bulletin of the New York Academy of Medicine* 59 (1983): 181–197.

Chapter 13

Child-Adolescent Psychiatric Services in the General Hospital

Leo Kron, M.D.

INTRODUCTION

The general hospital setting has in recent years become increasingly the focal point in the provision of psychiatric services for children and adolescents. At one time, these services were localized primarily in nonmedical, child guidance clinics, which contributed to the development of a distant relationship between the allied areas of general psychiatry and pediatrics. In 1959, child and adolescent psychiatry was formally established as a subspecialty of the American Board of Psychiatry and Neurology. The requirement that training for this subspecialty be hospital-affiliated gave an added impetus to the integration of child psychiatry within the medical community and the general hospital. Heightened awareness of the importance of biological factors in psychiatric illness and recent advances in research into psychiatric disorders in children have further served to remedicalize child and adolescent psychiatry.

St. Luke's/Roosevelt Hospital is a large, 1,300-bed, private, voluntary general hospital serving the upper West Side of Manhattan in New York City. The combined institution was formed in 1979 as a result of the merger of two well-established, but financially troubled, institutions. In 1971, an affiliation agreement had been signed with Columbia University by both St. Luke's and Roosevelt hospitals, providing both institutions with full university hospital status. Although the merged administration of the two departments of psychiatry is now led by one director, in practice each functions largely independently. This chapter is concerned with psychiatric services at the St. Luke's site.

The St. Luke's Hospital Department of Psychiatry, established in 1954, currently comprises the divisions shown in Figure 13-1. The Division of Child and Adolescent Psychiatry was established in 1956 with one child

279

Figure 13–1 Organization of the Department of Psychiatry, St. Luke's/Roosevelt Hospital, St. Luke's Site

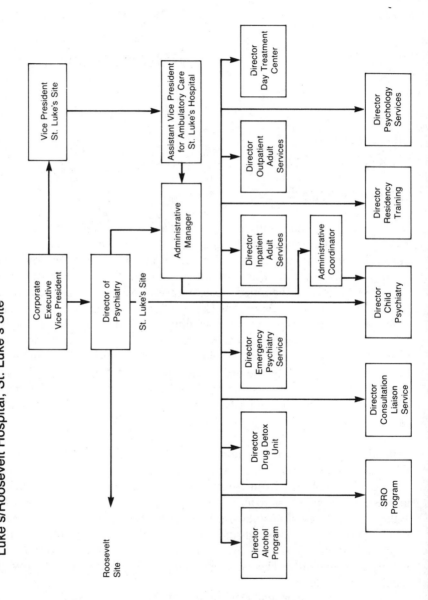

psychiatrist and two psychiatric social workers. It has grown dramatically over the decades, especially in recent years, under the strong and innovative leadership of Dr. Clarice Kestenbaum.

DEFINITIONS AND CONCEPTS

Child and adolescent psychiatry is concerned with the understanding, diagnosis, prevention, and treatment of a wide range of developmental pathologies and psychiatric disorders, as well as with the study and advocacy of normal child development.

According to 1980 census figures, approximately one-third of the American population is composed of persons under the age of 18. Although what constitutes psychiatric or emotional illness in these 62.4 million persons cannot always be precisely defined, prevalence rates for clinical maladjustment in this population have been reported to be between 10 and 15 percent.[1-3] Prevalence of clinical disability within the nation's school systems has been reported to be between 2 and 17 percent,[4] while between 5 and 50 percent of children and adolescents seen by general physicians are found to have psychosocial problems.[5-7] Except for selected disorders, such as anorexia nervosa, prevalence rates for psychiatric disorders are higher in boys, in inner-city communities, among specific ethnic groups, and in the adolescent age group.[8-10] Altogether, it has been estimated that approximately 7.3 million children and adolescents are affected by some form of psychiatric disability.[11] Only a small proportion of these children are receiving the psychiatric care they need.

Children and adolescents are afflicted with the same wide diversity of clinical psychiatric syndromes that is seen in the adult population. In addition, there are those disorders which are specific to childhood. Emotional, behavioral, and developmental disorders include the mild transient adjustment disorders, the affective and anxiety disorders, specific and pervasive developmental lags, and the severe, relentlessly deteriorative psychoses.

Developmental, familial, socioeconomic, and medical factors interact to influence greatly the nature of childhood psychopathology, and these factors require specific consideration in the evaluation and treatment of this population. Comprehensive multiaxial diagnostic and multifaceted therapeutic approaches are often indicated.[12,13]

Certain groups of children have been identified to be at especially high risk for the development of medical and psychiatric disorders.[14,15] Among them are children who live in poverty, those with physical handicaps and chronic illness, foster children, institutionalized retarded children, children of "high-risk" mothers, singly parented children, and the children of racial minorities and migrant workers. Other factors that have been found to increase the risk for psychiatric disturbance in children are parents with psychopathology, abused and abusing parents, adolescent mothers, family discord and violence, prematurity, malnourishment, and environmental toxins.[16-20]

Ideally, psychiatric services for children and adolescents should include prevention and treatment at primary, secondary, and tertiary levels.[21] In the light of our knowledge that developmental deviations and childhood psychopathology leave enduring imprints, it is particularly important that therapeutic interventions be made at the earliest possible opportunity, and especially be provided to at-risk populations. Early case finding is facilitated by liaison and consultation with pediatricians, obstetricians, community schools, the juvenile courts, social agencies, and community representatives. Also, in order that normal, as well as disturbed, children receive optimal care in other settings, it is recommended that child psychiatric services provide support, education, and supervision to other physicians and health care professionals.

Unfortunately, in many clinical settings, it is only when psychiatric illness and psychopathology become well-established and consolidated that interventions are initiated. At play here are deeply ingrained prejudices in both providers and patients against primary and secondary prevention,[22] as well as the priorities forced by insufficient professional and financial resources.

The settings in which child psychiatric services are delivered vary significantly. No one setting is ideally suited to providing all the services children and adolescents require at different levels of disability and chronicity. However, child and adolescent psychiatric services in the general hospital setting are especially well-suited to the provision of optimal care to a large segment of the clinical population. There, the full range of medical services and multidisciplinary professionals necessary to provide the most comprehensive evaluation, diagnosis, and treatment of children is available. This is particularly important for children and families with chronic or recurrent medical and psychiatric problems and for those in an ongoing relationship with the hospital in its role as a frequently used medical resource in the community. In this service context, in-hospital liaison and consultation with other medical services, such as pediatrics and obstetrics, are especially useful in early case finding and programs of primary prevention.

THE TREATMENT PROCESS

Significant variability exists in the kinds of child psychiatric services available in general hospitals. The size of the hospital, its own particular specialty orientation, the availability and orientation of funding, the hospital's proximity and relationship to academic centers, the presence or absence of training programs (in child psychiatry, general psychiatry, and pediatrics), particular research interests, philosophical biases, and the special characteristics of the community in which the hospital is located—all interact to determine the mix of services offered.

In most general hospitals services for children are part of general psychiatric outpatient services. Currently, there are no administratively separate and autonomous departments of child and adolescent psychiatry. However, within the larger hospital centers, there are approximately 100 distinct divisions of child and adolescent psychiatry that often function quite independently of the departments of psychiatry with which they are associated. Few of the general-hospital-based child psychiatry services include a separate inpatient unit for children or adolescents.

Child services therefore range from the most sophisticated to the most rudimentary. The latter comprise only basic diagnostic, consultation, and referral services. Yet, even for these services, minimal staffing requires the expertise of several professionals. These include a child psychiatrist, social worker, child psychologist, and learning disabilities specialist. In larger settings, this core of basic professionals is usually augmented in number by a diversity of diagnostic and therapeutic specialists. Regardless of its size, the child service's basic obligations are to provide evaluation, treatment, and consultation appropriate to the specific needs of the hospital and the community it serves.

The Division of Child Psychiatry at St. Luke's/Roosevelt Hospital serves a socioeconomically and racially heterogeneous population. The hospital has active clinical services in most of the medical-surgical specialties, but of particular relevance to child psychiatry are its active and well-developed Departments of Pediatrics, Obstetrics and Gynecology, and General Psychiatry. All of these departments have long-established training programs. In addition, there is a fellowship training program in child and adolescent psychiatry. Psychiatric care is delivered primarily through outpatient and consultation-liaison settings, although some inpatient psychiatric services are also available.

Inpatient Services

General-hospital-based psychiatric inpatient units for children and adolescents are in short supply. This is primarily due to shortages of professional staff and financial resources. The requirements of such units for highly trained personnel, high staff-to-patient ratios, and educational services makes them expensive to organize and operate. They are most likely to be found in large, urban teaching institutions.

Treatment approaches on inpatient units vary, often according to factors related more to the needs of the providers than to the clinical needs of the patients. Insurance restrictions, which have an adverse impact on middle- and working-class patients within the private general hospital, limit the time available for the implementation of most evaluation, treatment, and disposition strategies to three to four weeks. Medicaid may often provide reimbursement for up to three months. Yet, within these time constraints, a wide variety of inpatient treatment orientations can be found, emphasizing one, or a combination of, the following approaches: developmental, psychodynamic, behavioral, pharmacologic, research-protocol, group, and family.[22-27]

Inpatient treatment of the child or adolescent should be considered as only one aspect of a comprehensive treatment plan, which should include both in-hospital family involvement and thoughtful posthospital outpatient disposition. According to Hersov and Bentovim, hospital admission is considered "the treatment of choice in children:

- "where thought and behavior are so severely irrational and bizarre that outpatient treatment is impossible, or where the child may be a danger to himself or to others,
- "where socially unacceptable behavior arises from a degree of psychiatric disorder which is unaffected by ordinary social measures or outpatient treatment,
- "where a complex psychiatric problem requires skilled observation, assessment and treatment which must be continuous and of an intensity not possible on an outpatient basis, or
- "where the family interaction is so distorted that life at home leads to a continuing or progressive interference with the child's development and progress."[28]

These criteria would include, for example, psychotic, aggressive, suicidal, homicidal, abused, severely impulsive or hyperactive, psychosomatically ill, and diagnostically enigmatic children. (Comprehensive and detailed descriptions of the many issues involved in short- and intermediate-term inpatient psychiatric treatment of children and adolescents can be found in the available literature.)[29-35]

Most general-hospital-based child and adolescent psychiatric services do not have inpatient psychiatric units. Consequently, patients who require admission frequently need to be transferred to other facilities. However, adolescents may often be hospitalized on the hospital's adult psychiatric inpatient unit, if one is available. In addition, scatter beds on the pediatric ward may sometimes be used for appropriately selected child psychiatric patients. Resistance among pediatricians to this utilization tends to be less in units experiencing difficulties in maintaining a high inpatient census.

The St. Luke's Hospital Division of Child and Adolescent Psychiatry, consequent to its location in a large urban setting, has access to several nearby inpatient units for patients requiring admission. Older adolescents who are appropriate for admission to the adult psychiatric unit remain the clinical responsibility of the Division of Child Psychiatry. Child fellows are the primary therapists, while social workers from child psychiatry work with the patients' families. Whenever possible, treatment by the same child fellow is continued on an outpatient basis after discharge.

For several years, pediatric beds at St. Luke's Hospital have been used for the admission of selected child and adolescent psychiatric patients. Comprehensive evaluation, interspecialty consultation, crisis intervention, mobilization of familial resources, protection, and disposition—all are achievable goals during a brief admission to a pediatric scatter-bed ward. Six to eight patients are formally transferred each year to the Psychiatry Service from the pediatric ward and stay for an average of five to six days. Most frequently, these patients have been admitted after a suicidal gesture that initially required medical treatment or observation. Other problems that have occasioned psychiatric admissions include child abuse, depression, noncompliance with medical regimen (for example, as seen in juvenile diabetics), evaluation of physical symptomatology of a possible psychogenic origin, and the monitoring or stabilization of antidepressant treatment with the use of blood levels. Other situations where such admissions might be appropriate include those involving patients with anorexia nervosa; infants with failure to thrive or with a psychogenic growth disturbance; infants with persistent symptoms and no organic documentation, such as is seen occasionally in excessive vomiting, crying, and food refusal; psychosomatic illnesses,[36] and psychosomatic complexes, such as childhood asthma, in which a separation from the family, or a "parentectomy," is sometimes desirable.[37]

After being "medically cleared," these patients become the full clinical responsibility of the Division of Child Psychiatry, although they continue to participate in the usual ward activities. They are seen for daily therapy sessions by either the child psychiatry fellow or the clinical nurse specialist, while their parents are seen by a psychiatric social worker from child psychiatry. Psychological and educational testing are available when indicated. Whenever possible, postdischarge outpatient treatment is conducted by the inpatient therapist.

The main clinical contraindications to such pediatric admission are severely hyperactive or aggressive assaultive symptomatology. Abused children who often show an identification with their abusing parents occasionally may present staff with problems of limit setting. In spite of predictable concerns and staff hesitations regarding the safety of children and adolescents admitted after suicide attempts or gestures, these are rarely substantiated. Constant observation ("CO") has rarely been required for more than one day. No suicidal behavior has occurred on the ward, nor have there been instances of prolonged disruption on the unit. Evaluation, mobilization of resources, and appropriate outpatient disposition can usually be made within a one-week stay on the ward. Only rarely do such patients require transfer to a psychiatric inpatient unit at the time of discharge. Similar experiences have been documented elsewhere.[38,39] In a study of 100 adolescents admitted to an adolescent medicine unit, only 12 of the 100 required further psychiatric inpatient treatment after their brief pediatric stay.[40]

Although not used to its maximum potential, psychiatric admission to pediatric scatter beds presents some substantial difficulties. The disadvantages of using pediatric beds for psychiatric patients become more apparent as the length of the stay increases. Exposure to physically ill children may pose added psychological stress for the disturbed child. The absence of a structured therapeutic milieu too often leaves such patients to their own psychological devices and may encourage regression. The medical and nursing staff, in spite of authentic interest and initial concern, are insufficiently trained in psychological medicine and hence have a limited understanding and tolerance for psychiatric symptomatology. The initial "honeymoon" period for staff seems to last from five to seven days. When beds are in demand, pressures for discharge increase. Heavy caseloads force the attention of the pediatric residents and attendings away from the patient with psychological symptoms, who then may be ignored and become increasingly alienated on the ward.[41]

The substantial presence of a salaried psychiatric attending on the pediatrics ward, along with the clinical nurse specialist and psychiatrically knowledgeable social workers, minimizes these difficulties and extends the scope of possible treatment. The additional expense to the hospital of this kind of adequate psychiatric staffing would be more than made up if otherwise empty pediatric beds could thereby be filled. At a time when the increasing success of outpatient pediatric treatment and evaluation has diminished the need for inpatient care in many general hospitals, the use of pediatric scatter beds for selected psychiatric patients can address both the clinical needs of the patient and the financial concerns of the hospital.

Outpatient Services

Approximately 70 percent of the patients seen in the Division of Child Psychiatry at St. Luke's are black or Hispanic. Approximately 60 percent of clinic visits are reimbursed by Medicaid. The remainder have fees set according to a sliding scale. The entire range of diagnostic entities is seen for evaluation, and only a very small percentage of patients is referred out to more specialized treatment programs (for the retarded, inpatient services, residential treatment settings, and so on). A large proportion of the children seen come from single-parent, multiproblem families. Often, several children (and adults) in the same family repeatedly require psychiatric services during the course of their childhood and adolescent years.

Each child, together with the child's family, receives a comprehensive evaluation by one of several multidisciplinary teams, which then formulates a treatment plan. Each team is composed of (1) an attending child psychiatrist, (2) a fellow in child psychiatry, (3) a social worker, (4) a psychologist, and (5) a learning disabilities specialist. In addition, each child is routinely evaluated in pediatrics and, if indicated, receives a neurological and/or speech and hearing evaluation.

Consultations to the emergency room, provided by the child fellows, are available on a 24-hour basis. During the period of time that a child fellow is responsible for ER coverage, the fellow's team ceases routine evaluations and is available to help the fellow in emergency evaluations, dispositions, and crisis interventions.

The following usual treatment modalities are available within the general Child Psychiatry Outpatient Clinic: individual psychotherapy, pharmacotherapy, behavioral therapy, family therapy, group therapy, language and learning disabilities therapy, paraverbal therapy, occupational therapy, and art therapy. In addition, several programs have been established for children found in the hospital setting or the surrounding community to be at high risk for current and future psychiatric morbidity. Among the goals with these children are primary and secondary prevention and the establishment of ongoing ties with the children and their families as their development proceeds. These special programs include a therapeutic nursery, an adolescent after-school program, a parent-child program, a group therapy program for chronically ill children, and a program for children of psychiatrically disturbed adults.

Therapeutic Nursery

The therapeutic nursery is used for preschool children who manifest significant and often pervasive deviations in ego development. Intensive early intervention with these children and their families maximizes their developmental potential. In addition, efforts are made to mitigate the inevitable pathogenic impact that a severely disturbed young child can have on the entire family.

Referrals to the nursery come from various sources throughout the city, but the nursery serves primarily the hospital catchment area. There is ongoing consultation with pediatricians and several city and community agencies.

Children attend the therapeutic nursery five hours a day, five days a week. Psychotherapy, behavioral therapy, and educational therapy are part of an overall therapeutic milieu. Parents are seen in weekly group sessions, as well as individually, for support and counseling, as indicated. Developmental assessments provide the basis for sound future planning.

Adolescent After-School Program

The adolescents who attend the five-day-a-week, after-school program are primarily from neighboring "ghetto" communities. They are black and Hispanic, largely from broken, fatherless families, raised in poverty and inadequately educated. They are at high risk for psychiatric disorders, school failure, addictions, and sociopathy. Many of these teenagers hear of the after-school program by word of mouth. Others, when younger, have been involved with the clinic and have been "graduated" to the after-school program. Still others are referred from previously mentioned sources in the hospital and from the community.

These adolescents, who otherwise are very difficult to engage in therapy, become involved in various group activities. In addition to "rap" groups, the various groups focus on sports, drama, art, prevocational activities, cooking, video films, and poetry. The program has published three volumes of poetry written by teenagers under the guidance of a state-sponsored "poet-in-residence."[42] The video-film group is taping short, "real-life" stories acted out by the group members. One of the themes acted out is "junkies copping dope."

These activities provide the opportunity for personal discussion, as well as the opportunity to learn skills that might be usable in the future. In addition to the various special group activities, conventional therapeutic modalities are utilized, as indicated. Vocational assessments and counseling are also available.

Parent-Child Program

The parent-child program is aimed at the "high-risk" mother and her child. The mothers are often adolescents who have been abandoned by the fathers of their children, are living in severe poverty, have a psychiatric illness, or have not benefited from adequate prenatal care.

Mothers in the program are referred as a result of liaison activities with the Department of Obstetrics and Gynecology. They are identified prior to, during, or after labor and delivery. Contact is made as early as possible.

Groups have been formed specifically for pregnant women and for adolescent mothers, in addition to the general groups for mothers considered to be at risk because of any of the previously cited factors.

The goals of the parent-child program are to provide assessment, support, treatment, and future planning for the vulnerable mother-child dyad. Mothers and their children attend group sessions together. In addition, the mothers are seen in groups and individually while their children participate in play groups or are evaluated by the developmental psychologist.

Another group participating in the parent-child program is composed of mothers referred by the Bureau of Child Welfare because of suspected child abuse or neglect. The children of these parents tend to be older and, if indicated, are treated in the general Child Psychiatry Clinic.

Group Therapy Programs for Chronically Ill Children

Supportive, self-help, and therapy groups have been established in conjunction with the Department of Pediatrics. Over the years, these groups have involved children with asthma, diabetes mellitus, and sickle-cell anemia. Children requiring more intensive evaluation or treatment are screened and appropriately referred.

Program for the Children of Psychiatrically Disturbed Adults

Environmental and genetic factors place the offspring of psychiatrically ill parents at a higher risk for the development of disturbances. A program, currently in the planning stage, will provide crisis intervention, evaluation, treatment, and follow-up to children whose parents are hospitalized on the general psychiatry inpatient unit. The goals of the program are to provide services for children under significant stress and to identify those children who manifest, or are likely to manifest, psychiatric symptomatology.

Consultation-Liaison Service

As a professional priority, the American Academy of Child Psychiatry has established the goal that "child psychiatrists, through consultation, support, and supervision, provide assistance to other physicians and other providers of care."[43] Schools, courts, child-related agencies, and medical services are areas in which such consultative relationships are useful. With regard to pediatric consultation-liaison, the goals of the interprofessional relationships are:

- to identify and provide treatment to children and adolescents with established psychiatric disorders

- to increase opportunities for primary and secondary prevention of psychiatric disorders in the pediatric population
- to minimize the psychopathogenic impact of hospitalization and illness, acute and chronic[44]

These goals are achieved through direct and indirect consultation,[45] liaison activities, and didactic teaching.

The need for the pediatrician, as primary physician, to be familiar with the principles of normal and aberrant psychological development has long been stressed. Recent studies indicate that approximately 5 percent of all pediatric visits are essentially psychiatric in nature; while up to 50 percent of visits to the pediatrician are related to behavioral, educational, or social concerns.[46] The knowledge and skills that should be imparted to the pediatrician through a closer collaboration between pediatrics and child psychiatry have been articulated extensively.[47-57] Harding, Mattson, and Nathan suggest that, upon completion of a fellowship program in behavioral pediatrics, pediatricians should be able to:

- recognize the normal tasks of various child developmental stages and differentiate healthy responses from developmental deviations
- understand the roles played by acutely ill children in family dynamics
- understand the emotional needs of the hospitalized child
- work with chronically ill and handicapped children, appreciate how the patient and family as a unit cope with the stresses of the problems, and provide anticipatory guidance for the avoidance of further crippling emotional sequelae
- improve communication skills with parents in explaining the mechanisms of common developmental disturbances, such as colic, feeding problems, and enuresis
- understand psychological testing and assessment
- know the needs and crises of adolescence
- recognize and appreciate the emotional and social needs of children in families undergoing divorce and adoption in order to become an advocate for children in such situations
- assess their own capabilities in handling psychological problems in pediatric practice, to improve their ability to determine when referrals should be made for psychiatric consultation and collaboration[58]

These goals are only partially attainable in a consultation-liaison program. Success depends primarily on the availability of resources (time, money, and staff) and the motivation of the child psychiatrists and pediatricians involved. Also, the active support of the directors of pediatrics and medicine is essential for any consultation-liaison service to function smoothly. Without complete cooperation, a negative attitude is quickly absorbed by the house staff, who then can provide many compelling reasons to be distracted from psychosocial issues.

The consultation-liaison activities of St. Luke's Child Psychiatry Service have evolved over many years. Their success has depended largely on the establishment of warm, mutually respectful and beneficial relationships, at both the leadership (director) level and the attending staff level. Given this cooperative and collegial atmosphere, the trainees have absorbed the established role-model relationships and, to some extent, perpetuated them. For example, as an educational exercise for both child psychiatrists and pediatric trainees, visits with pediatric attendings in their private offices were arranged to get a direct awareness of the nature of private pediatric practice and the problems encountered.

Sensitivity to the relevant psychological issues in the treatment of sick children and their families is enhanced by the presence on the pediatric inpatient unit of talented professionals, including social workers and recreational therapists. In addition, the presence of a knowledgeable clinical nurse specialist ensures optimal cooperation and involvement of the nursing staff.

The orientation of the St. Luke's Consultation-Liaison Program is based on a considerable body of literature pertaining to children's reactions to illness and hospitalization,[59-65] and on the principles of consultation and liaison psychiatry.[66-68] The activities of the child psychiatrists include direct clinical case conferences, didactic teaching of normal and aberrant development, and individual supervision of child fellows and the clinical nurse specialist.

Consultation —whether it involves the direct examination of the patient by the child psychiatrist or only the indirect discussion of a patient with the pediatrician—follows the tenets of consultation articulated by Caplan: "The twin goals of consultation are to help the consultee improve his handling or understanding of the current work difficulty and through this to increase his capacity to master future problems of a similar type."[69] Rarely should the child psychiatrist assume the role of the primary physician, even though the pediatrician, who might have become anxious at the prospect of handling psychosocial problems, may wish him to do so.

To be effective, the consultant must be available when most needed. The consultant must be sensitive to the experience of the pediatrician and be able to communicate with that colleague respectfully and in direct practical terms. The consultant must also be available to support ongoing problems, for follow-up, and for disposition planning, as indicated.

The child psychiatrist's participation in multidisciplinary ward rounds facilitates the identification of children and families requiring intervention and the development of appropriate intervention strategies. Participants in the rounds include the attending pediatrician, pediatric residents, the clinical nurse specialist, head nurses, social workers, recreational therapists, the hospital chaplain, child psychiatry fellows, and the attending child psychiatrist. These meetings provide opportunities for the various professionals to exchange data regarding patients from their differing and unique perspectives; they also provide an additional teaching opportunity for the child psychiatrist.

In addition, weekly rounds led by a child psychiatrist are held in the neonatal ICU. In these rounds, psychosocial and developmental issues pertaining to premature and congenitally ill and damaged infants are discussed. These rounds are attended by the ICU nursing staff, pediatric social workers and the unit neonatologist.

The formal teaching activities of the child psychiatrist for the pediatric house staff include a series of 20 lectures. In these lectures, normal development in its various stages is described, and psychiatric disturbances that might be associated with particular stages are identified. Behavioral, observational data are emphasized, and psychological jargon is avoided.

In addition, there are weekly combined conferences for the pediatric residents and child psychiatry fellows. These alternate between clinical case presentations one week, and the discussion of selected topics of interest to both specialties in the following week. Residents, in consultation with a child fellow, present the histories of patients on the ward in which psychosocial issues are prominent. These are discussed from the point of view of the biopsychosocial model of disease.[70] Some of the topics discussed are children's reactions to hospitalization, illness, and medical procedures; the complete psychiatric evaluation of children and adolescents; the dying child and the child's family; and learning disabilities.

The Interfaces of Child and Adolescent Psychiatry and Its Milieu

To achieve common goals, St. Luke's Child and Adolescent Psychiatry Service freely interacts with various hospital departments and community organizations. This collaboration has as its aim the coordination of services, the sharing of relevant information, reciprocal consultation, and mutual education. The interactions may be formal and well-structured, as in regularly scheduled, face-to-face meetings with agendas, or they may be casual, by telephone, and on an as-needed basis.

The Department of Psychiatry

As noted earlier, the Child and Adolescent Psychiatry Service is a division of the combined departments of psychiatry of St. Luke's/Roosevelt Hospital (see Figure 13-1). Although administratively merged under one director, the individual clinical services function independently for the most part, as they did prior to the merger of the two hospitals. Except for the integration of teaching and supervisory activities, this is also true of the child and adolescent psychiatry services. The director of each division is responsible directly to the director of the Department of Psychiatry. The Division of Child and Adolescent Psychiatry maintains strong ties with the Department of Psychiatry in order to coordinate administrative management, clinical services and teaching programs; reach consensus on a variety of operational policies; jointly plan for future programs; and provide resources to each other to deal with problems that arise. The forums for these activities are the weekly departmental steering meetings and the many ad hoc meetings that take place as need dictates.

Contacts with the other divisions in the department may be required in particular clinical situations. Frequently, the parents of children seen in the child psychiatry services are, themselves, patients in the adult outpatient clinic, day hospital, or alcoholism unit, or they may be admitted to the adult inpatient service. Open communications are maintained with psychiatric residents and social workers on the adult inpatient unit for the purpose of identifying and referring to child psychiatry children whose parents are hospitalized. Adolescents admitted to the inpatient unit are primarily the responsibility of the child psychiatry fellows, who must be active in ward rounds and team meetings.

The Division of Child and Adolescent Psychiatry interfaces with the larger Department of Psychiatry on training and educational matters. All general psychiatric residents have an extensive rotation through child psychiatry, during which time they are assigned children and adolescents for evaluation and treatment. They attend diagnostic seminars, as well as the weekly child psychiatry grand rounds. In addition, they participate in lectures on the normal and pathological development of children and on adolescent development.

Each year, one month of the department's grand rounds is devoted to issues germane to child and adolescent psychiatry. This provides an opportunity to bring to a wider audience the clinical concerns of this subspecialty. It also serves to augment each professional's understanding of psychiatric disorders through increased familiarity with developmental perspectives on pathogenesis.

The Hospital Administration

The merger of St. Luke's and Roosevelt hospitals resulted in a complex structure in which two parallel and essentially similar "site" administrative hierarchies are responsible to one encompassing corporate administration. The director of the Department of Psychiatry interacts with a corporate executive vice-president. The psychiatric clinical services at the St. Luke's site, including child psychiatry (through the director and associate director), interact with the department's administrative manager, who is responsible primarily to the director of the Department of Psychiatry but also reports to the assistant vice-president in charge of ambulatory care services at the St. Luke's site. The position of administrative coordinator, reporting to the administrative manager, is currently being established. This office will deal exclusively with the increasing administrative needs of the Child and Adolescent Psychiatry Service (see Figure 13–2).

Interaction with the hospital administration is concerned primarily with financial matters and preparations for reviews or audits by governmental health regulatory agencies. There is steady pressure from the administration to cut costs and increase revenues, while complying with ever-changing and time-consuming governmental regulations. In order to continue the growth of needed services for the patient population, there is also steady clinical pressure for new innovative programs and the professional positions to support them. To this end, it is vital that child psychiatry effectively educate the administration about the complex nature of the clinical problems encountered, the unavoidable expenses incurred in treating these problems, and the obligation not to falter in the pursuit of its undertaking. However, it is also important that child psychiatry, as a responsible part of the hospital, provide services in the most efficient and cost-effective manner possible.

Other Clinical Departments

In addition to the multifaceted manner in which the Division of Child and Adolescent Psychiatry interacts with the Department of Pediatrics, the division maintains communication with the pediatrician of each child initially evaluated in the outpatient clinic and any child in ongoing treatment who requires concurrent medical care. Interactions with the prenatal and maternity services of the Department of Obstetrics and Gynecology involve identification of "high-risk" mothers and facilitation of their referral to the parent-child program.

Nonclinical Hospital Services

To enable the Child Psychiatric Service to function smoothly on a day-to-day basis, ongoing coordination with several nonclinical departments of the

Figure 13–2–Organization of the Division of Child and Adolescent Psychiatry, St. Luke's/Roosevelt Hospital, St. Luke's Site

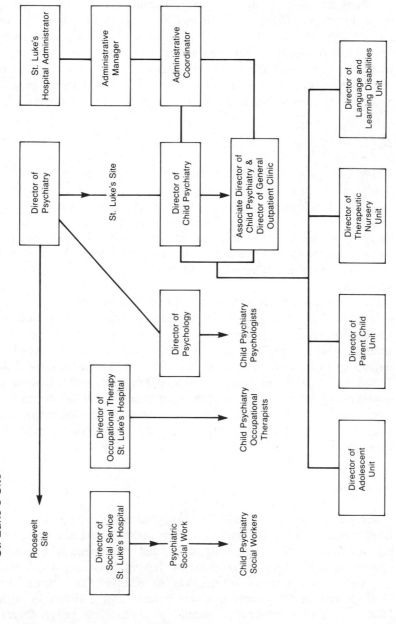

hospital is necessary. The sometimes impulsive, defiant, and provocative behavior of troubled children and adolescents requires that the clinic maintain open communication and good relations with the other services that share the same building, as well as close cooperation with the hospital's security services. Food and refreshments play an important role in the adolescent after-school and parent-child programs, and this necessitates frequent contact with the Food and Dietary Service. The art and occupational therapy groups create special problems for the Housekeeping Service, necessitating open communication to effect ongoing cooperation.

The School System

Ongoing communication with the child's schoolteacher, through written reports and by telephone, is an important part of the child's evaluation and treatment. In addition, discussions with special tutors, the school nurse, or principal, may be necessary. These professionals may serve as valuable observers of the child's intellectual abilities, social interactions, behavior, and symptomatology. In particular, their observations may be necessary to make the appropriate diagnosis or to determine the efficacy of a treatment approach.

The school system provides the child psychiatric services with important access to children and adolescents requiring psychiatric intervention. Referrals are frequently made from the community schools for the evaluation of children who demonstrate abnormal behavior in the classroom or who require assessment to determine the presence and nature of a learning disability. Valuable services can also be provided to the teacher and the school through discussions about difficult children and the strategies to help them adjust in the classroom situation. The principles of consultation discussed with regard to the Pediatric Consultation-Liaison Service are also applicable to school consultation.

Social Service Agencies

Many patients seen in child psychiatry have had previous or concurrent involvement with one or more private or public social agencies, for example, foster agencies, adoption agencies, and the Bureau of Child Welfare. Contact with the latter is required by law in any case where there is a suspicion of child abuse or neglect. In addition, the Bureau of Child Welfare frequently requires that the parents and children in such cases receive psychiatric treatment. Individual assessment, psychotherapy, and group therapy are available for parents suspected of child abuse.

The Courts

Children and adolescents who have come to the attention of the juvenile courts occasionally require psychiatric assessment or treatment as stipulated by the court's decision. Evidence of ongoing treatment may be a condition of parole, in which case communication with the probation officer is required. Child psychiatrists may be called on to act as expert witnesses in proceedings against a child or adolescent; they may also become involved in custody disputes, in which the psychiatrist's assessments may be helpful in the court's determination of what is in a child's best interest.

Community Groups and Organizations

The director and one of the social workers of the Division of Child and Adolescent Psychiatry attend monthly meetings with community groups and agencies in the hospital's catchment area. Other community organizations represented at these meetings include community mental health clinics, the Big Brothers organization, the Children's Aid Society, Direction Services, the Board of Education, school guidance counselors, the city housing authority, day care associations, private social agencies, and parent groups. The goals of these meetings are to exchange information related to the mental health concerns of the community, for example, the current availability of services in the community, the relative length of waiting lists for evaluation and treatment at the various clinics, the effects of local and federal legislation, and funding issues. Opportunities for political lobbying and action are discussed and implemented to further the welfare of young people in the community.

OBSTACLES TO THE DELIVERY OF CHILD-ADOLESCENT PSYCHIATRIC SERVICES

The delivery of optimal psychiatric care to children and adolescents faces many obstacles, which can be broadly categorized as attitudinal, organizational, and economic. These obstacles stem largely from the fact that psychiatric disturbance in children usually reflects a complex interaction of organic, intrapsychic, and intrafamilial pathogenic factors that require comprehensive, coordinated, and protracted treatment by members of several professional disciplines.

Attitudinal Obstacles

An overriding sociocultural impediment to the treatment of emotional problems in children is the tenacious reluctance to acknowledge the existence of the basic aspects of mental life, and hence psychopathology, in children. This phenomenon may reflect a basic human ambivalence toward children.[71] Another expression of the inclination to deny the existence of psychiatric illness in children is the failure to appreciate sufficiently the unexpectedly high prevalence of affective illness in children. Research in this area has in fact documented widespread parental denial of unhappiness and depression in their children.[72] It is as if the child's developmental immaturity confers upon him a lower psychological status.[73] As a consequence of this attitude, the funding priority for mental health care for children remains too low at all levels.

Physician-generated obstacles to the awareness of psychological issues and the emotional concomitants of physical illness are common.[74,75] These obstacles are often found in pediatricians whose residencies have insufficiently prepared them to evaluate adequately and manage effectively the many psychosocial issues they later regularly encounter in hospital and private practice. Exhausted, anxious residents, who rotate through a new service every four to eight weeks and are pressed to learn the critical skills required for each specialty service, do not have the time, appreciation, or continuity of experience with patients to develop the skills that they will later need in practice and that will become an increasingly important source of professional satisfaction to them. Even in private practice, economic pressures, in the form of lower third party reimbursements for psychosocially oriented pediatric interventions, discourage the pediatrician from involvement in these areas.

Attitudinal impediments to successful consultation-liaison are also seen in psychiatrists.[76] These may be manifested in a devaluation of psychosomatic or psychophysiological syndromes, a withdrawal from the medical model, or uncertainty in the psychiatrist's identification as a physician. In the pediatric setting, where action and speedy results are valued, the prolonged, time-consuming endeavors of the child psychiatrist rarely bring immediate improvements, and hence are accorded a relatively low status. This may result in diminished self-esteem, identity conflict, and anxiety in dealing with nonpsychiatric physicians and staff.

Organizational Obstacles

The actual organization and delivery of medical care in general hospital settings often have a direct negative psychological impact on patients, particularly on those with emotional problems. Obvious examples of this are the long waits in crowded, noisy outpatient settings and the confusing myriad of medical personnel confronting the newly admitted inpatient.

Rotations

Continuity of care in all settings is hindered by the frequent rotations of staff. In child psychiatry services, different groups of trainees rotate in and out of the clinic at regular intervals. Though some stay as long as two years (child psychiatry fellows), others stay only a few weeks (medical students). As a result, patient transfers from one therapist to another are unfortunately frequent and exceedingly disruptive.

In pediatric settings, rotations of residents, nurses, and attendings also occur at frequent intervals. Pressures for shorter hospital stays have resulted in a greater number of procedures and tests per unit of time, making the hospital experience even more fragmented for the patient. The formation of a viable physician-patient relationship in this atmosphere is severely obstructed.[77]

Interdisciplinary Frictions

The fact that sick children require the cooperative effort of several professionals for their care can in itself create problems. Interdisciplinary frictions, rivalries, and territorial struggles are evident at the clinical level, both on the ward and in the outpatient clinic. These problems are perpetuated by the hierarchical organization of each profession within the administrative structure of the hospital. On the pediatric inpatient unit, nursing, social work, and pediatric professional loyalties and identifications are very strong. The liaison child psychiatrist is an outsider and must make alliances with each discipline on the basis of mutual concern for good patient care.

In the outpatient clinic, staffing and policy decisions that may significantly determine the quality and quantity of available psychiatric treatment are made within each professional discipline's hospital hierarchy. Too often, these decisions are made with the strategic interests of the discipline in mind, rather than the needs of the patients in the treatment units. Moreover, the ability of the director of a service to develop programs appropriate to patient needs may be quite limited if job descriptions are determined in nonclinical areas. Only ongoing communication and collaboration between the disciplines can eliminate these obstacles. In the clinic, regular team and staff meetings provide the opportunity for the indispensable interdisciplinary interchange.

Government Regulations

The organization of child and adolescent psychiatric services has been greatly affected by the relatively recent explosion of government regulations regarding patient care. Motivated by the need to control medical costs and to monitor the availability, quality, and appropriateness of psychiatric care, the increased regulatory concern is clearly necessary and long overdue. The long-term impact of the new regulatory measures cannot yet be determined, but it is safe to assume that, in the short term at least, some psychiatric services for children have improved as a result of their increased accountability.

However, worrisome obstacles to the delivery of optimal psychiatric care to children have also been created by the new regulations. The need to comply with the differing and continually changing regulations of government agencies that control licensing, reimbursement, and training is a time-consuming task. Each year, a moderately sized clinic is likely to spend hundreds of work hours in preparation for the next comprehensive review audit. Added to this are the hours spent in retraining staff, in completing additional paperwork, and in establishing and implementing procedures for monitoring staff compliance. These are hours that become unavailable for treating patients. Fortunately, recent developments in modern computerized office management procedures can facilitate the monitoring of appointments, statistics, clinical data, and charting procedures and thereby return many of these hours to direct patient-care efforts.

A more difficult obstacle is posed by the fact that many regulations that directly affect patient care and treatment planning are apparently based on therapeutic assumptions appropriate to only a small percentage of clinical problems, that is, those that show a prompt response to behavior therapy or medications. Unfortunately, there is no evidence to support an expectation of such a response in most of the clinical problems encountered in child and adolescent psychiatry. Indeed, one potentially harmful effect of such regulations might be to encourage the inappropriate use of prompt-response treatments at the expense of more suitable ones. The staff time and effort spent in complying with inappropriately conceived treatment guidelines have an overall demoralizing effect on all concerned.

Economic Obstacles

The proper treatment of psychiatrically disturbed children and adolescents is complex and often lengthy. It requires highly trained professionals and comprehensive treatment settings, sometimes specialized residential treatment settings, and, frequently, community support services. According to the 1980 report of the Graduate Medical Education Advisory Committee, to meet the psychiatric needs of children and adolescents by 1990, the number of child psychiatrists would have to treble.[78]

Reduced Funding

Cuts in government grants for training, research, and service have left few general hospital child psychiatry services unaffected. Increased reliance on third party reimbursement has greatly reshaped clinic and hospital practices. Self-pay patients, often the children of lower-middle-income working parents, are ineligible for Medicaid because of their family's income level. They are often denied the psychiatric treatment they need because, at the upper end, self-pay sliding scales may approach private psychiatric fees. The population of children for whom proper psychiatric treatment is not affordable increases in size with each new government restriction or cut in Medicaid.

In efforts to reduce costs, hospital administrators apply constant pressure to increase staff time in revenue-producing activities. Indirect services, such as communication with patients' schools, their physicians, and other agencies involved in their care are clinically necessary but not reimbursable, and are hence discouraged. This phenomenon—as well as the previously described effects of new regulatory guidelines on treatment planning—is an example of "a situation in which the fiscal tail wags the therapeutic dog."[79] It may not in fact be the psychiatrist who makes the treatment decision, based on a clinical assessment; rather, the decision may be influenced primarily by policies determined by people without any clinical background or interest whatsoever.

Because the ability to deliver psychiatric care to children in a general hospital setting is related to the ability of the service to generate revenues, the clinical directors of psychiatric services must be increasingly concerned with basic administrative and managerial issues. Basically, revenues can be increased in two ways: (1) by increasing the number of patients seen, or (2) by ensuring adequate reimbursement for services given. With respect to the first method, the number of patients seen can be increased by enhancing staff productivity and by encouraging the use of treatment modalities, such as group therapies, that are not only clinically efficacious but also increase the number of visits that can be billed.

Missed Appointments

Missed appointments, a frequent problem when working with disturbed and chaotic families, result in significant losses of time and money. Missed appointments by patients in ongoing treatment limit therapeutic gain and can indicate an inappropriate or poorly implemented treatment plan. Appointments for initial evaluation sessions are most frequently missed. Reducing the wait between the referral and the initial appointment may reduce the number of these missed appointments.

Other strategies for reducing the number of missed appointments may include:

- Informing the parents at the time of initial referral that it is important to appear for all appointments as scheduled and that failure to do so can result in the decision to make their time available to the next person on the waiting list. It should be explained that, unlike other hospital clinics they may have attended, child psychiatry has no extended waits because specific times are set aside by staff to see the patients. If they do not appear, the result is lost time, which cannot be used to see anyone else.

- Making contact with patients by telephone on the day prior to their scheduled appointments.

- Using intake-orientation groups, which children and their parents can attend immediately on referral. This eliminates waiting time, allows for orientation, support, preliminary clinical screening, early intervention, and the timely establishment of a relationship between patient and clinic. Attendance in such groups can be scheduled prior to the completion of a comprehensive evaluation. If sufficiently cohesive and homogeneous, they may develop into ongoing therapy groups subsequent to the evaluation period.

- Scheduling more than one patient for each initial referral session. In spite of efforts to stress the importance of keeping these appointments, a substantial number of individuals will miss them. Thus, for cost efficiency, a portion of hours set aside for intake interviews may be "overbooked."

- Establishing initial evaluation sessions on a "walk-in" basis, with staff available during certain blocks of time to see whoever appears.

Unreimbursed Services

Too often, the services that are provided are not reimbursed. For example, consultation services, either inside or outside the hospital, are usually not reimbursable by Medicaid. In some cases, the patients seen may not be correctly registered or may not possess a currently valid Medicaid card. In other cases, reimbursements may be retroactively disallowed if the ongoing documentation and charting procedures are not in compliance with regulations.

Medicaid reimburses only for one visit per patient per day. If another hospital service is required—such as psychological testing, a pediatrics visit, or the services of a learning disabilities specialist—the patient must return on another day in order to be billed for the other service. Unless the hospital is willing to provide services free of charge, the net effect of this stipulation is to deprive many children and their families of the appropriate psychiatric treatments.

Consultation-liaison programs are particularly threatened when funds are short and staffing lines endangered; neither the hospital nor the psychiatrist receives adequate third party reimbursement for many activities provided in these programs. Consultation activities—whether in the hospital, the school, or the social agency—are also hindered by economic constraints on the consultant. The consultant must have adequate resources to free staff and time to discuss and follow a difficult situation; yet such activities are usually not eligible for reimbursement.

Other Funding Problems

Evidence that consultation-liaison activities lead to decreased medical costs has bolstered arguments in favor of continued funding of consultation-liaison programs and positions and prompted a growing interest in cost-effectiveness.[80-82] To date, relevant studies in this area have not been conducted with the pediatric population, where methodological problems are greater than those encountered with adults. Yet, whether in consultation to pediatrics or through direct treatment of children and adolescents, timely and effective interventions can constructively influence the course of a child's psychological development, socialization, behavior, and education. The immeasurable cost to society when such care is not provided is continually reflected in the vast sums spent on maladjusted adults who cannot adequately cope or survive on their own.

Pediatric consultation-liaison functions are considered by the American Academy of Child Psychiatry to be indispensable to the care of hospitalized children. Accordingly, it recommends that the accreditation of facilities treating children be contingent on the availability of consultation-liaison services, in the same way that accreditation is contingent on the availability of other core medical services. It further recommends that insurance reimbursements include consultation-liaison activities.[83]

The cost of psychiatric services for children is often exaggerated because of inappropriate hospital accounting practices. These practices may need to be modified to reflect actual expenses. Because psychiatric services are labor-intensive, with little expenditure on, or use of, expensive capital equipment and ancillary services, their indirect cost allocations should be much lower than those made to other medical services.[84] In view of the fact that ambulatory services are, as a rule, less profitable than inpatient services, the latter should bear a greater proportion of indirect cost allocations to support the maintenance of necessary outpatient services. Ill-conceived plans to reduce hospital expenditures by reducing adequate child psychiatry outpatient services force patients to use the more expensive emergency room to obtain the diagnostic and treatment services they require.

When previous sources of funding can no longer be relied upon, survival requires that new sources be found. Apart from the decreasing number of government grants available for service, training, and research, funds for specialized programs are sometimes available through large corporations. Also, municipal and state governments may have funds earmarked for special projects. And contributions from private foundations and individuals sensitive to the emotional problems of young people can sometimes be found. Finally, pharmacological research and educational and paid consultative activities have served as creative forms of fund generation.[85] Augmenting funds from several of the above sources, the Division of Child and Adolescent Psychiatry at St. Luke's Hospital has raised funds for its parent-child program and adolescent after-school program through a series of educational symposia related to normal and pathological child and adolescent development.

Appropriate funding for child and adolescent psychiatry services requires undaunted efforts to educate administrators, community leaders, and political representatives about the necessity of responding to the emotional needs of children, regardless of short-term and short-sighted concerns about the expense. Although applied originally in the context of supporting general consultation-liaison functions, these words by a well-known hospital administrator should be whispered into the ears of all those in a position to make decisions and initiate special efforts on behalf of the mental health of children: "The ideal will never be approached, unless it is fostered by administrative bias and buttressed by administrative policy and budget lines."[86]

REFERENCES

1. Joint Commission on the Mental Health of Children, *Crisis in Child Mental Health: Challenges for the 1970s* (New York: Harper & Row, 1969).

2. President's Commission on Mental Health, *Report to the President,* vol. 1, No. 040-000-00390-8 (Washington, D.C.: Government Printing Office, 1978).

3. M.S. Gould, R. Wunsch-Hitzig, and B. Dohrenwend, "Estimating the Prevalence of Childhood Psychopathology," *Journal of the American Academy of Child Psychiatry* 20 (1981): 462–476.

4. M.B. Rosen, "Distribution of Child Psychiatric Services," in *Basic Handbook of Child Psychiatry,* vol. 4, ed. J.D. Noshpitz (New York: Basic Books, 1979).

5. A.M. Jacobson et al., "Diagnosed Mental Disorders in Children and Use of Health Services in Four Organized Health Care Settings," *American Journal of Psychiatry* 137 (1980): 559–562.

6. B. Starfield et al., "Psychosocial and Psychosomatic Diagnosis in Primary Care of Children," *Pediatrics* 66 (1980): 159.

7. M.S. Jellinek, "The Present Status of Child Psychiatry in Pediatrics," *New England Journal of Medicine* 306 (1982): 1227–1230.

8. Gould, Wunsch-Hitzig, and Dohrenwend, "Estimating."

9. M. Rutter et al., "Adolescent Turmoil: Fact or Fiction?" *Journal of Child Psychology and Psychiatry* 17 (1976): 35–36.

10. M. Rutter et al., "Attainment and Adjustment in Two Geographical Areas: I. The Prevalence of Psychiatric Disorder," *British Journal of Psychiatry* 126 (1975): 493–509.

11. I. Phillips, R. Cohen, and N. Enzer, *Child Psychiatry: A Plan for the Coming Decades* (Washington, D.C.: American Academy of Child Psychiatry, 1983).

12. M. Rutter, D. Schaffer, and M. Shepherd, *A Multiaxial Classification of Child Psychiatric Disorders* (Geneva, Switzerland: World Health Organization, 1975).

13. American Psychiatric Association, *Diagnostic and Statistical Manual of Mental Disorders, DSM III,* 3rd ed. (Washington, D.C.: American Psychiatric Association, 1980).

14. Rosen, "Distribution."

15. Task Force on Pediatric Education, *The Future of Pediatric Education* (Evanston, Ill.: American Academy of Pediatrics, 1978).

16. Phillips, Cohen, and Enzer, *Child Psychiatry.*

17. C.J. Kestenbaum, "The Child at Risk for Major Psychiatric Illness," in *American Handbook of Psychiatry,* vol. 7, ed. S. Arieti (New York: Basic Books, 1981), 152–171.

18. L. Kron et al., "The Offspring of Bipolar Manic-Depressives: Clinical Features" in *Adolescent Psychiatry,* vol. 10, ed. S.C. Feinstein, J.G. Looney, A.Z. Schwartzberg, and A.D. Sorosky (Chicago: University of Chicago Press, 1982), 273–291.

19. M.M. Weissman et al., "Psychopathology in the Children of Depressed and Normal Parents," *Journal of the American Academy of Child Psychiatry* 23 (1984): 78–84.

20. H.C. Steinhausen, D. Gobel, and V. Nestler, "Psychopathology in the Offspring of Alcoholic Parents," *Journal of the American Academy of Child Psychiatry* 23 (1984): 465–471.

21. I.N. Berlin, "Primary Prevention," in *Basic Handbook of Child Psychiatry,* ed. J.D. Noshpitz (New York: Basic Books, 1979).

22. I.N. Berlin, "Developmental Issues in the Psychiatric Hospitalization of Children," *American Journal of Psychiatry* 135 (1978): 1044–1048.

23. L. Hoffman, *The Evaluation and Care of Severely Disturbed Children and Their Families* (New York: Spectrum Publications, 1982).

24. A.J. Solnit, "Hospitalization: An Aid to Physical and Psychological Health in Childhood," *American Journal of Diseases of Children* 99 (1960): 155–163.

25. F. Nakhla, L. Folkart, and J. Webster, "Treatment of Families as In-Patients," *Family Process* 8 (1969): 79–96.

26. F.T. Main, "Mothers with Children in a Psychiatric Hospital," *Lancet* 2 (1958): 845–847.

27. M. Lynch, M.F. Steinberg, and C. Ounsted, "Family Unit in a Children's Psychiatric Hospital," *British Medical Journal* 2 (1975): 127–129.

28. L. Hersov and A. Bentovim, "Inpatient Units and Day-Hospitals," in *Child Psychiatry: Modern Approaches,* ed. M. Rutter and L. Hersov (Oxford, England: Blackwell Scientific Publications, 1977), 880–900.

29. D. Zinn, "Hospital Treatment of the Adolescent," in *Basic Handbook of Child Psychiatry,* ed. J.D. Noshpitz (New York: Basic Books, 1979), 263–288.

30. Hoffman, *Evaluation and Care.*

31. Hersov and Bentovim, "Inpatient Units."

32. S.A. Szurek and I.N. Berlin, *Inpatient Care for the Psychotic Child* (Palo Alto, Calif.: Science and Behavior Books, 1971).

33. F. Redl, "The Concept of a 'Therapeutic Milieu,' " *American Journal of Orthopsychiatry* 29 (1959): 721–736.

34. D.D. Treffert, "Child-Adolescent Unit in a Psychiatric Hospital," *Archives of General Psychiatry* 21 (1969): 745–752.

35. J.S. Maxmen, G.J. Tucker, and M. Lebow, *Rational Hospital Psychiatry* (New York: Brunner/Mazel, 1974).

36. P.C. Laybourne and H.C. Miller, "Pediatric Hospitalization of Psychiatric Patients: Diagnostic and Therapeutic Implications," *American Journal of Orthopsychiatry* 32 (1962): 566–603.

37. L. Jessner et al., "Emotional Impact of Nearness and Separation for the Asthmatic Child and His Mother," in *Psychoanalytic Study of the Child,* vol. 10 (New York: International Universities Press, 1955).

38. A. Marks, "Management of the Suicidal Adolescent on a Nonpsychiatric Adolescent Unit," *Journal of Pediatrics* 95 (1979): 305–308.

39. R. Radwan and S. Davidson, "Short-Term Treatment in a General Hospital following a Suicide Attempt," *Hospital Community Psychiatry* 28 (1977): 537–542.

40. Marks, "Management."

41. F. Parker, personal communication.

42. *Burning Dreams: Poems by Young Adults* (New York: New York State Poets In The Schools, 1984).

43. Phillips, Cohen, and Enzer, *Child Psychiatry.*

44. M.B. Rothenberg, "Child Psychiatry—Pediatrics Consultation-Liaison Services in the Hospital Setting: A Review," *General Hospital Psychology* (1979): 281–286.

45. M.J. Senn, "The Relationship of Pediatrics and Psychiatry," *American Journal* 71 (1946): 537–549.

46. Jellinek, "Present Status."

47. Ibid.

48. Rothenberg, "Child Psychiatry."

49. Senn, "Relationship."

50. R.S. Louri, "The Teaching of Child Psychiatry in Pediatrics," *Journal of the American Academy of Child Psychiatry* 1 (1962): 477–489.

51. L. Eisenberg, "The Relationship between Psychiatry and Pediatrics: A Disputatious View," *Pediatrics* 39 (1967): 645–647.

52. M.B. Rothenberg, "Child Psychiatry and Pediatrics," *Pediatrics* 60 (1977): 649–650.

53. D.G. Prugh and L.O. Echkhardtt, "Child Psychiatry and Pediatrics," in *Basic Handbook of Child Psychiatry,* vol. 4, ed. J.D. Noshpitz (New York: Basic Books, 1979), 563–576.

54. J.B. Richmond, "Child Development: A Basic Science for Pediatrics," *Pediatrics* 39 (1967): 649–658.

55. R.K. Harding et al., "The Psychiatrist's Role in Behavioral Pediatrics Training Programs," *General Hospital Psychiatry* 1 (1979): 234–239.

56. J.R. Williams, "Teaching How to Counsel in a Pediatric Clinic," *Journal of the American Academy of Child Psychiatry* 22 (1983): 399–403.

57. D.R. Lipsitt, "Some Problems in the Teaching of Psychosomatic Medicine," *International Journal of Psychiatry in Medicine* 6 (1975): 317–329.

58. Harding, et al., "Psychiatrist's Role."

59. A. Freud, "The Role of Bodily Illness in the Mental Life of Children," in *The Psychoanalytic Study of the Child,* vol. 7, ed. R.S. Eissler et al. (New York: International Universities Press, 1952), 69–81.

60. R.H. Thompson and G. Stanford, *Child Life in Hospitals: Theory and Practice* (Springfield, Ill.: Charles C Thomas, 1981).

61. M. Petrillo and S. Sanger, *Emotional Care of Hospitalized Children: An Environmental Approach* (Philadelphia: J.B. Lippincott Co., 1980).

62. D.G. Prugh, "Investigations Dealing with the Reaction of Children and Families to Hospitalization and Illness: Problems and Potentialities," in *Emotional Problems of Early Childhood,* ed. G. Caplan (New York: Basic Books, 1955), 307–321.

63. T. Bergman, *Children in the Hospital* (New York: International Universities Press, 1965).

64. E.N. Plank, *Working with Children in Hospitals* (Cleveland, Ohio: Case-Western Reserve University Press, 1971).

65. A. Mattsson, "Long-Term Physical Illness in Childhood: A Challenge to Psychosocial Adaptation," *Pediatrics* 50 (1972): 810–811.

66. G. Caplan, *The Theory and Practice of Mental Health Consultation* (New York: Basic Books, 1970), 19–30.

67. P.L. Adams, "Techniques for Pediatric Consultation," in *Handbook of Psychiatric Consultation,* ed. J. Schwab (New York: Appleton-Century-Crofts, 1968).

68. J.J. Strain and S. Grossman, "Psychological Care of the Medically Ill: A Primer," in *Liaison Psychiatry* (New York: Appleton-Century-Crofts, 1975).

69. Caplan, *Theory and Practice,* p. 29.

70. G.L. Engel, "The Biopsychosocial Model and the Education of Health Professionals," *Annals of the New York Academy of Sciences* 310 (1978): 169–181.

71. E. Rexford, "Children, Child Psychiatry and Our Brave New World," *Archives of General Psychiatry* 20 (1969): 25–37.

72. Kron et al.

73. W.M. Bolman, "Obstacles to Prevention," in *Basic Handbook of Child Psychiatry,* ed. J.D. Noshpitz (New York: Basic Books, 1979).

74. M.H. Greenhill, "Liaison Psychiatry," in *American Handbook of Psychiatry,* ed. S. Arieti (New York: Basic Books, 1981), 672–702.

75. Z.J. Lipowski, "Consultation-Liaison Psychiatry, Past Failures and New Opportunities," *General Hospital Psychiatry* 1 (1979): 3–10.

76. Ibid.

77. Strain and Grossman, *Psychological Care.*

78. Graduate Medical Education National Advisory Committee, *The Report to the Secretary, Department of Health and Human Services* (Washington D.C.: U.S. Department of Health and Human Services, 1980).

79. Phillips, Cohen, and Enzer, *Child Psychiatry*.

80. F.G. Guggehneim, "Cost Effectiveness and Consultation Psychiatry: Reflecting On, and In, Economic Terms," *General Hospital Psychiatry* 6 (1984): 171–172.

81. H.A. Pincus, "Making the Case for Consultation-Liaison Psychiatry: Issues in Cost-Effectiveness Analysis," *General Hospital Psychiatry* 6 (1984): 173–179.

82. S.J. Levitan and D.S. Kornfeld, "Clinical and Cost Benefits of Liaison Psychiatry, *American Journal of Psychiatry* 138 (1981): 790–793.

83. Phillips, Cohen, and Enzer, *Child Psychiatry*.

84. D.M. Dressler, "Clinical Services within a General Hospital Department of Psychiatry: Conceptual Issues and Operational Guidelines," *General Hospital Psychiatry* 3 (1981): 310–314.

85. Ibid.

86. M. Cherkasky, "Epilogue," in *Psychological Care of the Medically Ill*, ed. J. Strain and S. Grossman (New York: Appleton-Century-Crofts, 1975), 211–214.

Chapter 14

The Multiple Roles of Psychiatric Nurses

Marlene Nadler-Moodie, R.N., M.S.N., C.S.

INTRODUCTION

The psychiatric nurse with expertise in communication skills can be widely used throughout a general hospital to the benefit of many departments and staff members. The specialty of psychiatric nursing has evolved over the last 50 years. Caring for the emotionally disabled in large numbers began with World War II. Before that, only one nursing program offered a psychiatric nursing training course.[1]

Following the progressive use of improved psychiatric therapeutics in patient care, psychiatric nurses, no longer simply custodial keepers-of-keys, moved into a wide variety of settings, including inpatient wards of hospitals, outpatient clinics, long-term facilities, group (boarding) homes, community programs, schools, industries, and health maintenance agencies. Functioning in a multiplicity of roles in these settings, psychiatric nurses have become skilled counselors, supervisors, teachers, program coordinators, and researchers.

The growth of psychiatric nursing accompanied the expansion of the general field of nursing science and the increased recognition of mental health problems and treatments. Closely allied with the resulting rapid growth of community mental health programs, liaison psychiatry also developed. General hospitals were now expected to provide comprehensive service to the community. The large, isolated state hospitals were no longer regarded as the principal means of delivering psychiatric care to those in need. That function was gradually taken over by the acute care community general hospital.

The psychiatrist became an important member of the medical service, consulting with primary care physicians and physically ill patients. Following the psychiatrist's model and stimulated by the growth of the clinical specialist role in nursing, the psychiatric liaison nurse emerged.

AN OVERVIEW OF PSYCHIATRIC NURSING STAFF POSITIONS

Psychiatric nurses first began to function in the psychiatric wards of the older, private, state, and federal (that is, Veterans Administration) hospitals. The nursing services of these institutions were organized generally in the following manner:

Director of Nursing/Supervisor
Head Nurse
Assistant(s) Head Nurse
General Nursing Staff
Nursing Aides

General Staff Nurse

The general staff nurse is a registered nurse (RN). Registered nurses are licensed by the state after they successfully complete a minimum of two years in an approved nursing program and pass a comprehensive examination. Further education in nursing may follow. Thus a registered nurse may have a diploma, an associate's degree, a bachelor's degree, a master's degree, or a doctoral degree. The status of the general staff nurse usually corresponds with the level of clinical practice and experience, as opposed to educational background, although the latter is clearly taken into account.

The general staff nurse has many patient-centered functions, including:

- supervising, coordinating, and assisting psychiatric, medical, and nursing therapists, for example, in amytal interviews, spinal taps, or intravenous infusions
- leading and co-leading therapy and education groups
- administering and monitoring medications and their side effects
- observing and reporting patient behaviors and managing and monitoring aberrant behaviors
- maintaining and ensuring documentation
- maintaining a safe environment
- participating in staff conferences

Most importantly, general staff nurses, constituting the majority of nursing staff members in many hospitals, participate in therapeutic interactions with patients in all areas of unit life.

Assistant Head Nurse

Assistant head nurses are often used as shift coordinators, the nurses-in-charge during evening and night tours of duty. They often work alongside the head nurse, assisting her in the coordination of the unit or ward. Many assistant head nurses are given administrative or nursing staff educational responsibilities. Their presence on the ward fosters direct involvement in the clinical care of patients.

Head Nurse

The head nurse, sometimes called the nursing care coordinator or patient care coordinator, is the general manager of the unit, its patients, and staff on a 24-hour basis. Head nurses are predominantly administrators; they may or may not be involved in direct patient care. In managing the complexities of a psychiatric unit, the head nurse reports to, and receives assistance from, a supervisor. The latter is typically based off the unit and is the link between the unit and the rest of the institution. Both the head nurse and the supervisor have multiple administrative duties, including:

- personnel management
- counseling
- time management
- budget planning
- teaching
- clinical supervision
- future planning
- policy and decision making

Technical Nurses

Many states recognize a category of nonprofessional nurses broadly termed technical nurses. Sometimes they are called practical nurses or vocational nurses. These nurses usually have one year of hospital-based training, and their duties and responsibilities vary from institution to institution. An institution may hire such technical nurses because of a shortage of registered nurses in the area, financial constraints, or concerns with adequate staff-to-patient ratios.

Nursing Aides

Nursing aides—also called nursing assistants, attendants, orderlies or technicians—work under the direction of the nursing staff. While they are unlicensed personnel and are hospital-trained and hospital-monitored, some states offer certification programs that include coursework and practice. California, for example, has both certified nurses aide (CNA) and psychiatric technician categories; each involves brief specialty training and permits expanded duties. In contrast, New York State has no such categories, and its nursing aides are hospital-monitored only.

Generally, nursing aides spend their time in direct patient-care services. These include helping patients carry out such activities of daily living as feeding, grooming, and ambulating. Under the supervision of professional nurses, the aides may also provide one-to-one attendance to patients receiving electroconvulsive therapy (ECT) or to those who pose a potential danger to themselves. Additionally, nurses' aides engage patients in recreational activities and exercises.

Psychiatric Nurse Specialists

The general hospital, with its diagnostically heterogeneous population of patients and its staff, provides a multidimensional opportunity for all levels of psychiatric nurses to utilize their skills. Clinical nurse specialists in psychiatry, if not unit-based in a general hospital, usually function autonomously in less traditional roles (see Chapter 2). These psychiatric nursing specialists are master's degree professionals with clinical and/or teaching expertise. Depending on the specialty, they are variously titled as psychiatric (or mental health) nurse specialists, psychiatric nurse clinicians, psychiatric liaison nurses, psychiatric nurse practitioners, consultation-liaison nurses, or nurse consultants in psychiatry and mental health. The remainder of this chapter focuses on the roles and activities of these nurses. For purposes of clarity and consistency, they will be referred to as psychiatric nurse specialists.

ROLES AND ASSIGNMENTS

Theoretical Framework

The view of human beings functioning in a biopsychosocial framework is one to which psychiatric nurse specialists are naturally inclined. This results from the fact that the majority of today's psychiatric nurse specialists have a common educational foundation in general nursing, which provides a grounding in the biological area, along with advanced specialization in mental health. An exception may be the diploma school graduate from a psychiatric hospital who does not have generalized medical-surgical, clinical-practice training.

Training in Freudian psychoanalysis, Sullivan's interpersonal theory of psychiatry, and Peplau's interpersonal theory of nursing forms a firm foundation for psychiatric nursing practice. Group theory and process are widely applied throughout the general hospital.[2] The crisis intervention model also serves as a valuable conceptual vehicle for nurse clinicians in their daily care of acute- and chronic-care patients. In sum, the tasks of the psychiatric nurse specialist require an eclectic theoretical background that ensures a flexible clinical response based on the needs of the specific situation.

Geography of Assignment

Psychiatric nurse specialists may be found in any of four basic areas in the general hospital:

1. A segregated psychiatric inpatient unit, which, in addition to utilizing psychiatric nurse specialists in caring for its own patients, makes these nurses available to other parts of the hospital on an emergency consulting basis.
2. A psychiatric consultation-liaison service, which utilizes the clinical and educational (liaison) skills of the psychiatric nurse specialist for consultations to staff and patients on medical-surgical wards, outpatient clinics, and in the emergency room.
3. A nursing educational division, from which the psychiatric nurse specialist provides orientation and continuing education programs to all nursing personnel throughout the mental health area, focusing on topics such as interviewing techniques, psychiatric diagnosis and treatment modalities, and psychosocial factors of disease. The psychiatric nurse specialist who functions primarily as an educator may also have some clinical consultation-liaison functions. This is particularly true in those institutions that do not have a formal psychiatric consultation-liaison service.
4. A psychiatric outpatient clinic, in which the psychiatric nurse specialist performs intake, evaluation, and psychotherapy.

Regardless of the area to which the psychiatric nurse specialist is primarily assigned, the educational and clinical needs of the institution frequently require the provision of the specialist's services in other areas as well. All patient care areas need nursing staff members who can provide effective psychosocial care and support. Psychiatric nurse specialists are ideally suited to meet these needs.

In general hospitals that admit patients with primary psychiatric diagnoses to medical-surgical units (scatter-bed systems), the psychiatric nurse specialist is needed to provide support, education, and clinical expertise to the primary care (medical-surgical) nurses. In these cases, the psychiatric nurse specialist also can provide direct specialized nursing care to the patients in a one-to-one therapeutic relationship.

Administrative Accountability and Collaborative Networking

Psychiatric nurse specialists usually report to the department of nursing. However, their placements may vary from hospital to hospital, depending on the institution's historical development. Thus, the specialists may be found in a hospital's education, administration, research, or clinical divisions. In contrast, mental health nurse administrators and staff nurses are almost always placed in nursing administration and clinical services divisions, respectively.

It is important that psychiatric nurse specialists clearly understand to whom they report. An explicit understanding between the specialist and the superiors concerning the priorities of the specialist's role is crucial. If the role is poorly understood, the specialist can be left feeling anxious and isolated. Supervisors who are flexible and colleagues who offer peer support can be enormously helpful in this regard.

When the psychiatric nurse specialist reports directly to the psychiatry department (that is, to the physician chief or director), a collegial, mutually respectful and supportive interdisciplinary relationship is vital to ensure a fruitful ongoing collaboration. In such situations, the patient is the ultimate beneficiary of good clinical teamwork.

Indeed, the psychiatric nurse specialist in a general hospital should foster collaboration with as many members of the health care team as possible. Staff members who may be involved in the total care of a patient could include the dietician who instructs an anorexia nervosa patient, the physical therapist who works with a trauma victim, or the social worker who is involved with a family in determining the type and extent of custodial care for an aged parent.

Consultative Roles

A relatively new role for the psychiatric nurse specialist is that of consultant to other nurses and other health care professionals. Because emergency management situations may arise in which the staff expects the "expert" to work directly with the patient, psychiatric nurse specialists should be equipped with both interpersonal and therapeutic skills. If such is the case, not only will the patient be managed in an appropriately therapeutic manner, the observing and hopefully participating general nursing staff will also learn techniques for dealing with the stressful circumstances. Particularly in the management of violent or assaultive patients on the inpatient wards, psychiatric nursing staff can be utilized in aiding colleagues to intervene more productively and safely.

Educational Roles

Psychiatric nurse specialists have frequent opportunities, through formal and informal didactic presentations, to disseminate to nursing staff knowledge about particular emotional illnesses and psychiatric diagnoses and therapies. Case discussions about clinically challenging patients are excellent vehicles for teaching in the medical-surgical setting. In community outreach programs, psychiatric nurse specialists may serve local citizens by teaching mental health practices. Psychiatric nurse specialists may also directly aid patients and their families by teaching techniques designed to reduce the stresses associated with illness.

Clinical Roles

At all levels, psychiatric nurse specialists, perform a wide range of therapeutic roles. One of the most important is to ensure a safe and therapeutic environment for emotionally disturbed patients. This includes, in the extreme case, careful and constant one-to-one observation of suicidal patients. The administration of medication and assistance with somatic treatments are other important tasks. The psychiatric nurse specialist is expected to have a good knowledge of psychotropic medications and to be prepared to assist with the administration of electroconvulsive therapy (ECT) from the preanesthesia through the recovery phase.

In some hospitals, psychiatric nurse specialists also function as qualified psychotherapists. In this role, brief, supportive, or crisis-oriented therapies may be employed.

Administrative Roles

A general hospital that treats patients with psychiatric disorders on non-segregated (scatter-bed) units may have a specialized therapeutic program for such patients. In such a program, a psychiatric nurse specialist may be responsible for the administrative management of the nursing staff and for coordination of the treatment team. These functions may include patient assignments, performance reviews and evaluation, data management and documentation, and progress reporting.

In general hospitals with separate psychiatric units, the head nurse (patient care coordinator) has traditionally functioned as the manager with administrative responsibility for the nursing staff on the unit. Today, psychiatric nurse specialists have, in some hospitals, replaced head nurses in these positions or, in some cases, even become their supervisors.

CASE STUDIES IN THE PRACTICE OF PSYCHIATRIC NURSING

The case studies in this section focus on the various roles performed by psychiatric nurse specialists in general hospitals. In considering the various "how-to-do-it" aspects of these roles, it is important to keep in mind that, in each case, the personality style of the particular nurse specialist and the character of the institutional setting have considerable influence on the case development and outcome. Each case study is presented in a format that emphasizes the elements of a simple nursing care plan: assessment, plan, intervention, and evaluation (APIE).

The Consultative Role

Case 1: Consultation for a Patient Management Problem

The psychiatric nurse specialist was paged by the assistant head nurse of a medical unit. A 20-year-old female patient, diagnosed as suffering from anorexia nervosa, was being treated for malnutrition by her internist. The patient weighed 74 pounds, was described as "waif-like" in appearance, and was being fed via a nasogastric tube. Although the patient's primary physician was an internist, she was also visited by her private psychiatrist. The assistant head nurse presented her own concerns in these words: "The patient is crazy," "My staff may not know the appropriate thing to say," and "We feel left out of her treatment."

The psychiatric nurse specialist arranged a meeting that included the patient's primary care nurse. In this meeting, more details of the case emerged, and the chart was thoroughly reviewed. Additional concerns were voiced; these included the patient's sabotaging of her regimen by surreptitiously taking her own laxatives, adjusting her feeding tube, and exercising vigorously. Some of the nurses suspected that the patient was hallucinating but did not feel comfortable enough to assess the possibility thoroughly.

The conference group reached agreement that the psychiatric nurse specialist, accompanied by the nurse primarily responsible for the patient's treatment, would make a one-time visit to the patient and perform a psychosocial assessment. The results would be discussed with the staff. The assistant head nurse then obtained the appropriate permissions from the patient and physician. After a discussion between the psychiatric nurse specialist and the physician to clarify the role of nurse consultant, the patient was interviewed.

In the interview, the patient appeared child-like, with a hollow, gaunt face, wide eyes, and a sad expression. Her long, straight brown hair lacked luster. She was wearing a hospital gown which was much too large for her, and she fidgeted anxiously. Occasionally she got up and walked about the room, pulling her intravenous pole with her. She had difficulty maintaining eye contact and spoke in a quiet, high-pitched voice. Her effect and mood were both depressed. She stated that she understood that she had an eating problem but claimed, "I love food; I'll eat more." She wanted to talk mostly about when she could leave the hospital, saying, "I feel just fine now; I'm sure I'm ready to go home now." This denial of the severity of her condition contrasted with her admission to hearing voices, as well as her not following all of the hospital's rules.

The patient's physician was apprised of these observations; and a team meeting, which included the patient's private psychiatrist, was arranged. A patient-focused nursing staff conference was conducted to teach the staff about anorexia nervosa, psychosis, communication techniques, some psychopharmacology, and basic principles in behavior modification. Follow-up conferences were held, as needed, with all members of the health team attending. In this context, the psychiatric nurse specialist functioned as consultant, practitioner, educator, facilitator, and coordinator.

The psychiatric nurse specialist continued to provide support for the nursing staff throughout the patient's treatment. The specialist was especially useful in helping nursing personnel adhere to a care plan, utilizing behavior modification techniques with which they were unfamiliar. The patient gained weight during a prolonged hospitalization and was discharged to outpatient care.

Case 2: Consultation for a Staff Problem

The psychiatric nurse specialist was called by the head nurse of a 37-bed, acute medical unit, a teaching unit for medical interns and residents. The head nurse complained that the staff was "burned out." She reported frequent sick calls by some staff members, necessitating significant amounts of overtime for others; bickering and frank verbal fighting among nurses;

griping among nurses and nursing assistants; and complaints by the nurses about the rotation of house staff. The head nurse admitted that she did not fully understand the role of the psychiatric nurse specialist, aside from the fact that the latter provides specialized patient care, but said that her supervisor had suggested that she consult with the specialist.

The psychiatric nurse specialist arranged a meeting with the head nurse at a mutually convenient time. The head nurse invited her assistant to join them, and the three discussed the issues on a broader basis than originally anticipated. The specialist was interested in patient load, severity of illness of patients currently treated, staff turnover, recent changes on the unit, the manager's perceptions of these problems. The specialist obtained a self-appraisal by both the manager and her assistant of their performances and management styles.

The following week, with the head nurse's permission, the specialist met with the supervisor who had initiated the referral. The specialist shared some concerns about the head nurse's recent performance, although noting that the head nurse seemed well-motivated and bright.

A conference with the staff revealed a shared belief among the over-whelming majority that there was a problem on the unit, but all expressed helpless attitudes about its solution. Despite the press of duties, the staff agreed to continue the ad hoc meetings. Lunch time was recommended, so as not to interfere with what was considered to be a very busy schedule. This demonstrated motivation by the staff was a tremendous asset in getting the group working.

The head nurse and the psychiatric nurse specialist agreed that the specialist should assume a practitioner role for eight weekly meetings and then renegotiate the "contract," as necessary. The specialist, as group leader, managed to maintain neutrality, while attempting to assist the staff in becoming a more cohesive unit. Simultaneously, in leading the group, the specialist became a role model for the head nurse, who planned to assume this function in the future.

The staff meetings proved quite fruitful. The delivery-of-care system was changed from primary nursing to team nursing, and time schedules were adjusted to accommodate staggered hours. The staff seemed to relish the idea of having input to their work environment. For the short term, the staff shared more camaraderie and worked more cohesively toward common goals. After the original contract was completed, the meetings were reduced in frequency to every other week, and the head nurse became group leader. The specialist and the head nurse then arranged a supervisory relationship, which continued on a "prn" basis.

As a byproduct of this endeavor, the psychiatric nurse specialist was sought out by many of the unit's staff members for consultation about their patients. As group participants, some of the nurses were exposed to the psychiatric nurse specialist for the first time, and they now felt comfortable about making these requests. The nurses established more positive relationships on the unit through the group effort. The head nurse reported that verbal communication among her staff had improved and that "the griping has stopped." The problem-solving approaches discussed in the group seemed to be filtering to all areas of the unit. In this case, the psychiatric nurse specialist functioned as consultant, practitioner, and educator.

The Educational Role

Probably the most valuable role of the psychiatric nurse specialist is that of educator. In this capacity, the specialist has the greatest impact. If, through such educative efforts, nursing personnel achieve a better understanding of human emotions, develop more effective techniques for handling psychosocial problems, and improve their communication skills, both patients and staff benefit. Psychiatric nurse specialists who function as nurse educators should be qualified teachers. Thorough preparation from graduate courses and supervised teaching experience are necessary prerequisites.

Two common complaints of in-service educators are poor turnout in the classroom and insufficient time to teach at the bedside. Despite their recognition of the need and desire for continuing education, nursing managers and staff of busy general hospital units often have difficulty setting aside time for in-service education. The psychiatric nurse specialist's sensitivity to this issue, flexible style, perseverance in the face of resistance, and care in scheduling can do much to alleviate these problems.

A variety of program formats offered concurrently throughout the institution at different times is often the best way to address the variety of needs of the broad nursing staff audience. The planning for new psychiatric nursing education programs is best begun within the established patient care system, taking into consideration the 24-hour-a-day, seven-day-a-week, work schedule of the staff. Participation by the psychiatric nurse specialist in the existing orientation program for new nursing staff is a good way to start. This participation might include a short presentation on the operations of available hospital psychiatric services and the roles of the psychiatric nurses who staff them. Didactic presentations could be individually scheduled and advertised, with the more informal case conferences and unit-based staff meetings established on an ongoing basis. Requests should be sent to the individual units regarding their particular educational needs. From the responses, the specialist can identify the areas that are already being overtly addressed. Beyond that, the specialist will need skill and tact to discern the "hidden agendas" and unmentioned problem areas in certain units.

The following education topics, grouped as patient- or staff-centered in focus, are within the realm of the psychiatric nurse specialist who functions as an educator.

Patient-Centered	Staff-Centered
Depression	Interpersonal communications
Suicide	Assertiveness training
Psychosis	Group process
Substance abuse	Stress management
Geriatric psychiatry	Burn-out
Psychopharmacology	Emotional responses to
Management of assaultive patients	patients
Death and dying	
Mysterious illness	
(AIDS)	
Trauma victim	

The mode of presentation may vary. A one-to-one discussion between an educator and a staff nurse is as much an educational intervention as a lecture to 100 nurses about alcoholism. Small classes or large lectures, unit-based or consultation-liaison conferences, multidisciplinary staff meetings—all serve as appropriate forums for different topics. The need for group process and the rapid dissemination of new materials must also be considered. The opportunity to teach on a one-to-one basis should be arranged within the constraints of hectic nursing schedules. Creative time-management skills should be applied in a given situation with the maximum number of involved staff members. The change-of-shift "reporting meeting" offers a wonderful opportunity to make contact for educational purposes with personnel covering two complete shifts (16 hours of the day).

Aside from their services to staff, psychiatric nurse specialists are able to provide teaching directly to patients and their families in many health-care settings. For example, as part of a program in which all postcardiac care unit patients participate, a stress-management group can be conducted by the psychiatric nurse specialist, with teaching, discussion, and relaxation training included. A community affairs program sponsored by a hospital can use psychiatric nursing staff to teach the public about such health topics as alcoholism, depression, anxiety and stress, and interpersonal problems. Finally, intensive care unit nurses can include the psychiatric nurse specialist in a biweekly family group designed to help family members understand the operation of the ICU and their loved ones' illnesses.

The Clinical Role

The role of the psychiatric nurse specialist as clinician is defined to some extent by the department to which the specialist reports, for example, the nursing department or the psychiatry department. Available and permissible sources of referral should be agreed upon between the specialist and that professional's superiors. These sources may be nurses, physicians, social workers, other members of the health care team, or even self-referring patients or their families.

As clinician, the psychiatric nurse specialist begins the nursing process by assessing the referral source and level of urgency. The specialist then reviews the particular patient care situation with the primary nursing staff and physician(s) and carefully reads the medical record. Permission to see the patient is obtained from the primary care provider. A client-centered psychosocial assessment is then made, a plan is formulated, and a client contract is agreed upon, as indicated. Interventions by the psychiatric nurse specialist may include:

- individual psychotherapy
- health maintenance education
- stress management training
- crisis intervention services
- supportive counseling for the dying

The psychiatric nurse specialist is often expected to manage psychiatric emergency situations requiring direct "hands-on" techniques. In such cases, the appropriate medical, legal, and ethical use of the least restrictive restraint should be used for patients who are otherwise uncontrollable and dangerous to themselves or others.

All of the skills that psychiatric nurses employ on a traditional psychiatric unit can be used throughout the general hospital. For instance, the general hospital is well suited for the administration of electroconvulsive therapy (ECT). This procedure usually involves general anesthesia, thus requiring nursing interventions from the "pre-op" through the recovery phase. In addition to having specialty knowledge of the ECT procedure and equipment, psychiatric nurses must be able to monitor vital signs, intravenous therapy, suctioning equipment, and medications. In the medical setting, psychiatric nursing personnel must have a good understanding of general medicine in order to participate in the overall care of patients with concurrent medical problems, which may indeed be the primary reason for the initial hospitalization.

It seems obvious, but it is all too often forgotten, that people with psychiatric illnesses also get "sick." The incidence of alcoholism and depression is at least as high in a hospital as it is in the general population. Patients who survive suicide attempts are most often treated in general hospitals. Paranoid schizophrenics and manic-depressive patients may have cardiac disease or they may accidentally fracture a bone, and thus end up in hospitals. Such patients often require more than the usual level of nursing care. The psychiatric nurse specialist who is able to assist in these difficult patient-management situations can serve as an important adjunct to the primary nurses and enhance the total quality of care.

Case 3: The Clinical Role with a Dying Patient

A 42-year-old woman, admitted for the third time to the same unit with a diagnosis of liver cancer, was referred to the psychiatric nurse specialist because, in the words of the primary care nurse, "she knows she's dying; sometimes she wants to talk about it, and although I try to listen, I don't have the time to share with her that she needs. Maybe, aside from me, you could spend some time with her?" After permissions from physician and patient were obtained, the specialist and the patient agreed upon a contract to spend a half-hour, three times a week, together.

In these meetings, the patient often talked about her past in a reminiscent manner. When new positive or negative changes occurred in her condition, she would review these. The topic of death in general, and specifically her own dying, was discussed. The patient was told about her poor prognosis with liver cancer, and she accepted this news as factual, while sometimes denying its relationship to herself. The patient and specialist developed a warm relationship. Additionally, the patient's family (husband, two sons, and mother) would seek out the specialist to talk about their loved one, as well as about some of their own concerns. When the patient lapsed into a preterminal coma, lasting four days, the specialist continued to visit and included the family more and more in the visits.

Keeping in mind that the initial consultation was requested by the patient's primary nurse, the specialist continued to meet with the nursing staff to discuss the patient's nursing care needs. After the patient's death, it was helpful for both the specialist and the staff to have a last conference about this patient.

Case 4: The Clinical Role in a Complicated Medical-Psychiatric Care
Situation

A 27-year-old man was admitted directly to the operating room after severing his hand, thereby requiring emergency microsurgery. The recovery room nurse called the psychiatric nurse specialist, reporting: "He's awake but not talking yet; he moves around a lot, but his arm must be held in a sling. He has a good chance of saving the hand if he will only cooperate. He has a 'wild' look in his eye and I'm a little afraid of him, I don't know why. Can you come and evaluate him for us?"

Because of the nurse's feeling of urgency, the specialist went directly to the recovery room and interviewed the patient there, with the referring nurse present. A brief psychosocial assessment was done, in consideration of the patient's condition. The patient was psychotic and apparently had a psychiatric history of hospitalizations. In collaboration with the surgical house staff, a psychiatrist was called in as consultant and asked to help manage the patient.

Throughout the patient's stormy surgical and psychiatric course, both the psychiatrist and the psychiatric nurse specialist continued to follow the case. As the patient moved through the system from surgical unit through outpatient department, the support by the psychiatric team proved invaluable to the patient and to those providing his complicated medical care.

Case 5: The Clinical Role in the Case of a Staff Member

A psychiatric nurse specialist was paged by an in-service instructor, who reported, "One of the staff nurses has been acting strange in class. She's been increasingly quiet and even weepy at times. She appears anxious and frequently has called in sick. Most alarmingly, a physician has reported that the nurse was discussing suicide in a philosophical manner." The in-service educator was sufficiently concerned to call and ask what should be done. After further discussion, arrangements were made for the psychiatric nurse specialist to talk to the nurse.

The specialist met with the nurse in an available office on her unit. The nurse was vague and somewhat guarded but did admit to talking about, and currently considering, suicide. After a prolonged interview, in which crisis intervention techniques were used, the nurse agreed to be referred to a psychiatrist. This was facilitated by the specialist. The nurse was subsequently admitted to the hospital on an emergency basis and, after a three-week stay, was discharged. She continued in outpatient treatment and subsequently returned to work.

The Administrative Role

Traditionally, administrative positions for mental health nurses have existed in general hospitals with segregated psychiatric units. But even without such units, the psychiatric nurse specialist may function as an administrator in the hospital setting.

When administration is the only or a major part of the psychiatric nurse specialist's role in a general hospital, the specialist usually must interact with the general nursing management group. This often leads to referrals and consultation requests from members of that group.

Case 6: The Administrative Role on a Scatter-Bed Service

A 700-bed, general hospital without a segregated psychiatric unit established a scatter-bed service for the treatment of a variable number of psychiatric inpatients daily (10–20). The patients were treated for their emotional problems on medical-surgical units, which were selected and designated in advance by the program. An ambulatory psychiatric/mental health staff, in conjunction with the patient's primary physician, provided a wide range of clinical services.

The scatter-bed service staff consisted of a psychiatrist (chief of psychiatric inpatient services), a mental health nurse specialist, a social worker, a staff nurse, an occupational/recreational activities therapist, and two psychiatric nursing aides. The psychiatric nurse specialist was responsible for the support of the staff, administering the program's nursing component, and coordinating the program, in conjunction with the psychiatrist chief. In this nontraditional setting, the psychiatric nurse specialist functioned not only as an administrator but as a consultant, educator, practitioner, and researcher.

ACTIVITIES OF A PSYCHIATRIC NURSE SPECIALIST

The daily routine for psychiatric nurse specialists in a general hospital is quite variable. Psychiatric nurse specialists in a liaison role that is new to the institution may find that they have little "to do" initially. However, over time, and with good promotion and visibility, role-modeling, and demonstration of expertise, they will experience progressively increasing demands for their skills. It is therefore essential that they be in control of their time and utilize it effectively on a priority basis.

Recordkeeping is an important function of a psychiatric nurse specialist. In addition to documentation of activities for periodic and annual reporting and reviews, the specialist must be sure, for both legal and ethical reasons, that the charting of patients' medical records is accurate. These tasks can also be used as teaching tools. For example, accurate and detailed charting can be cited by the psychiatric nurse specialist involved in research as an essential basis for good data collection.

Psychiatric nurse specialists should maintain their own disciplinary styles and personal demeanors, while conducting themselves in an appropriately professional manner. Busy medical nurses look for specialists who are visible, available, and competent. Frequently, consultations occur when the specialist is on general rounds; conversations may be initiated informally in the hallway, cafeteria, or library. However, a nursing staff that operates on a full-time, seven-day/week, 24-hour/day basis appreciates a psychiatric nurse specialist who can be reached whenever necessary. For this purpose, a paging system or an emergency at-home telephone call service can be used. Though, in most instances, nurses are reluctant to call the specialist at home, and usually do not, having the option to do so can decrease staff anxiety.

Psychiatric nurse specialists, probably even more than other health care providers, must maintain confidentiality in order to be effective. They must be particularly sensitive to this issue in a setting where a wide range of people interface and confidentiality may become quickly impaired.

Supervision for the psychiatric nurse specialist can be provided in a variety of ways, as the role function requires. Nursing and psychiatry departments can provide administrative and clinical supervision, as well as educational support. A mentor or peer supervisor can also play valuable roles. Additionally, psychiatric nurse specialists should do their own networking. Reaching out to other professionals to share and broaden one's own scope can be a rewarding experience. Ideally, psychiatric nurse specialists can do this by joining already established peer groups composed of other clinical nurse specialists, educators, consultants, or administrators.

Psychiatric nurse specialists who work in a general hospital have rewarding, albeit taxing, jobs. If they are self-motivated and reflective individuals, they will be able to cope with the many potential role problems. However, overly high expectations and the loneliness that an autonomous role often carries with it, may encourage a feeling of being overwhelmed, which can all too quickly lead to burn-out. Also, in such a situation, a lack of nursing aid or medical staff sophistication about psychiatry can breed an atmosphere of resistance, sometimes to a frustrating degree.

The resulting feeling of powerlessness can pose special problems for psychiatric nurse specialists who find themselves in positions of little or no authority. On the one hand, they may be viewed as experts by the nursing staff, but as with many other nursing staff members, the traditional medical model does not foster concomitant nursing authority. In this context, the lack of feedback, positive or negative, can leave psychiatric nurse specialists without direction.

Yet, even if all these potential problems are taken into account, the valuable multiple roles and services that psychiatric nurse specialists can provide in a general hospital setting can surely be a most satisfying and professionally rewarding experience.

REFERENCES

1. Judy W. Burch and Joan L. Meredith, "Nurses as the Core of a Psychiatric Team," *American Journal of Nursing* 11 (November 1974): 2037–2038.

2. Mary Jo Grace, "The Psychiatric Nurse Specialist and Medical-Surgical Patients," *American Journal of Nursing* 3 (March 1974): 481–483.

Chapter 15

The Psychologist in the General Hospital

Herbert H. Krauss and Lisa A. Aiken

INTRODUCTION AND BACKGROUND

Psychology's Origin

Until the establishment of the first experimental psychology laboratories little more than 100 years ago, psychology was a branch of philosophy.[1] Since then, psychology's emphasis on an empirical foundation and scientific method has ensured that today's psychologists approach epistemology through research in learning and phenomenology through the empirical study of perception. This has been especially true in America, where psychology's establishment was due primarily to the efforts of William James.[2] James infused early American psychology with "pragmatism," the search for meaning and truth in outcomes derived from the application of psychological principles and their verification in correspondence with results derived from experimentation. Required courses in statistics, in the design of experiments, and in principles of measurement have ensured that American psychologists are well-versed in scientific reasoning.

Although the origins of modern psychology are closely linked to the founding of laboratories at academic institutions, psychologists have sought to apply their science to the world outside the academy. James McKeen Cattell, the first professor of psychology at Columbia University in New York City, coined the term *mental test*; in 1894, his laboratory attempted to use such tests to select students for Columbia. In 1896, Lightner Witmer established at the University of Pennsylvania the first psychological clinic in the United States. In his clinic, he attempted to develop treatment regimens for retarded and psychotic children. In 1909, the department of psychology at Clark University in Worcester, Massachusetts, gave Freud and Jung an opportunity to bring reports of their psychodynamic therapies to America.

When the psychiatrist William Healy opened the Juvenile Psychopathic Institute (later the Institute for Juvenile Research) in Chicago in 1909, he included on his staff the psychologist Grace Fernald.[3,4] Yet, in spite of these promising starts and steady progress in a variety of basic and applied areas, psychology remained largely an academic specialty until World War II.

The Growth of Clinical Psychology as a Subspecialty and Creative Discipline

World War II put large numbers of psychologists to work in military psychiatric units. In concert with psychiatrists and social workers, they assessed and treated the mental infirmities of American servicemen. These psychologists left the service determined to make a career for themselves providing health-care services. They were aided and abetted by a government that had committed itself to providing cost-effective care to its physically and emotionally impaired servicemen.

During and after the war, the Veterans Administration (VA) vastly expanded its treatment facilities by including psychologists among its mental health professionals. It also embarked upon a major program to support training in the mental health disciplines. The VA sought to define the professional psychologist as one who held the Ph.D. and was competent in diagnosis, research, and psychotherapy. Soon after, the United States Public Health Service and the newly created National Institute of Mental Health (NIMH) began to contribute training and research funds to the development of psychology as a health treatment profession. NIMH's first research grant was made in 1947 to a psychologist, Winthrop Kelley, who proposed to study the "basic nature of the learning process."[5]

In 1947, responding to increased interest in psychology as a mental health profession, the American Psychological Association (APA) appointed David Shakow to head a select committee to define a philosophy and training model for clinical psychology. The Shakow report provided the paradigm that would dominate clinical psychology for the next 30 years.[6]

In essence, the report argued that the clinical psychologist should possess a doctorate awarded by the graduate school of a university on the recommendation of its department of psychology. Further, an internship in a clinical setting should be mandated. Clinical psychologists were to be scientific psychologists first and clinicians second. They were to be prepared to function fully and autonomously in research, psychological diagnosis, and psychotherapy. To ensure the quality of the candidates' graduate and clinical experience, the American Psychological Association undertook to evaluate and accredit the training sites for academic work and internships.

Though the Shakow committee's scientist-practitioner model continues to dominate training in clinical psychology, recently a number of alternatives have emerged. Among them is the more practice-oriented doctor of psychology degree program. Today clinical psychologists are not only being educated in university graduate departments of psychology but also in professional schools associated with universities (for example, Adelphi, Rutgers) and in such free-standing institutes as the California School of Professional Psychology.[7,8]

The maturation of clinical psychology as a profession has proceeded in step with its development as an identifiable subspecialty within psychology. In 1951, the APA published a tentatively formulated code of ethics for clinical and consulting psychologists. Since then, there have been a number of revisions,[9,10] and the code has been extended to cover all psychologists. The code of ethics articulates standards of appropriate behavior on such issues as client welfare, confidentiality, and test interpretation.

Another sign that psychology was coming of age was its success in achieving legal recognition through licensing and certification laws. Licensing laws restrict certain practices to qualified members of specific professions; certification laws limit the use of a title, in this case "psychologist," to those who meet certain criteria stipulated by statute. As a rule, the APA has favored generic (without regard to subdiscipline) certification over licensing.

Connecticut enacted the first generic certification law in 1945; Virginia followed in 1946.[11] In 1977, Missouri became the 51st legal jurisdiction in the United States to regulate the practice of psychology. Typically, these laws and regulations require, at minimum, the following:

- a doctoral degree in psychology from an approved program or its equivalent
- one or more years of supervised experience in an approved setting
- a demonstration of relevant knowledge on an examination administered by the examining board
- appropriate citizenship, age, and residency
- evidence of good moral character [12]

Because many of the state statutes that certify psychologists are generic (for example, both a qualified clinical psychologist and a qualified social psychologist may be permitted the title "certified psychologist"), the profession has undertaken to identify individual psychologists whose interests, training, and expertise specially prepare them to render health care services. One review body, the National Register of Health Service Providers in

Psychology, publishes a roster ("National Register of Health Service Providers in Psychology") of those psychologists (over 13,000 by 1983) who voluntarily request listing and, at a minimum, meet certain criteria, including licensure or certification, accredited doctoral level education, and two years of supervised in-service training, one year of which must be postdoctoral.[13]

Another review body, the American Board of Professional Psychology, identifies psychologists with exemplary competence in a number of areas of professional psychology, using credential review and examination, one part of which includes an in vivo work sample. Clinical psychology is an area in which this board awards a diplomate.

Clinical Psychology's Relationship to Psychiatry

The institutional relationship between clinical psychology and psychiatry is complex. This is frequently the case when two professions direct their efforts toward providing overlapping services to the same population. In the United States today, this population represents a 17-billion-dollar-a-year market for mental health services.[14] Conflict between the two professions has generally focused on clinical psychology's claim to be an independent health care profession that desires a collegial rather than a worker-supervisor relationship to psychiatry.

Clinical psychology has indeed established itself as an autonomous health care profession, in spite of the opposition of some factions in the medical community. To cite a few examples, the Federal Employees Health Benefit Program and the Civilian Health and Medical Program of the Uniformed Services recognize psychologists as independent providers. By 1983, 38 jurisdictions had enacted legislation that assured consumers with health insurance that mental health services would be reimbursed for treatment provided by qualified psychologists as well as by psychiatrists.[15]

The most recent setting in which clinical psychology's appropriate role in the delivery of health-related services is being defined is the hospital itself. Until recently (July, 1984), the Joint Commission on Accreditation of Hospitals (JCAH) stipulated that hospital medical staffs be limited, unless otherwise permitted by law, to those licensed to practice medicine and dentistry. Arguing that such a state of affairs was not in the interest of individuals in need of treatment and constituted an unfair and monopolistic restraint of free trade, psychologists, acting in coalition with other professional groups, succeeded in having legislation enacted in California, Georgia, and the District of Columbia that forbade their categorical exclusion from the medical staffs of hospitals. These statutes authorized hospitals to grant psychologists privileges regarding admissions, certification of mental illness, treatment and treatment plan authorizations, and discharges.[16,17] Similar legislation is being considered in a number of other jurisdictions. In the meantime, the JCAH has modified its position to some extent. It now allows psychologists to be admitted to medical staffs if permitted by law and by the hospital.[18]

As early as 1932, with considerable prescience, Raymond Cattell described the incipient rivalry between psychiatry and psychology.[19] More recently, in 1983, he suggested a plan to end internecine warfare between the two disciplines. His suggestion was that psychologists, with their expertise in learning theory, psychometrics, and evaluation research, focus upon mental problems, and that doctors of medicine concentrate upon physiological dysfunction—a scenario made more likely by psychiatry's rapprochement with the rest of medicine.[20] Other commentators have taken different tacks. Some have gone so far as to suggest the formation of a new profession, "The Fifth Profession,"[21] combining elements of psychiatry and psychology. However the rivalry is resolved, it is clear that

> when it comes to the actual situation in which psychiatrists and psychologists find themselves working together on clinical problems, mutual contribution is readily reducible to the value which individual colleagues may have for each other in a collaborative effort. To the practicing psychiatrist, clinical psychology is what John Doe, Ph.D. has to offer; for the professional psychologist, psychiatry is represented by the working, teaching, or learning relations established with Richard Roe, M.D.[22]

Clinical Psychology Today

In 1939, the APA had 618 members and 1,909 associates.[23] By 1983, the APA had well over 60,000 members and associates. Stapp and Fulcher estimated that over 57 percent of the members and associates were full-time or part-time providers of health services.[24] Of these health service providers, approximately 10 percent worked in public or private general hospitals.

Though psychologists who are health providers still engage in assessment, treatment, and research, an enormous transformation in their role practices and responsibilities has occurred.[25] While still important, psychometrics is no longer the foremost practice activity of clinical psychologists—psychotherapy is. In turn, psychotherapy, once predominantly psychodynamic, is no longer so. Today psychotherapy as practiced by modern psychologists can only be described as eclectic. Moreover, the number and variety of settings in which clinical psychologists practice have expanded enormously. Beyond their usual academic haunts, clinical psychologists can now be found in private practice, psychiatry departments, autonomous departments of medical psychology and behavioral science in medical schools, general hospitals, community mental health clinics, health maintenance organizations, rehabilitation institutes, consulting firms, and governmental agencies.[26,27]

A CASE STUDY: THE PRACTICE OF PSYCHOLOGY AT LENOX HILL HOSPITAL

Organizational Structure

Lenox Hill Hospital is a moderately-sized, well-established, conservatively administered, medically controlled, private-practice-oriented general medical and surgical hospital without a separate psychiatric ward. It is located on New York's affluent upper East Side, an area in which are located private practice offices of a substantial number of psychiatrists, many of whom are affiliated with the hospital. Historically, clinical psychology has played a minor, peripheral role—indeed a somewhat "traditional" role—at the hospital. Psychologists do have positions of value, but their duties are quite delimited and somewhat removed from central service responsibilities.

The bylaws of the medical staff of Lenox Hill Hospital, following the JCAH mandates in effect at the time (1983), allow psychologists to be appointed to the "affiliate staff" of the hospital.[28] Psychologists are thus barred, de jure, from admitting patients to the hospital; the patient care services they provide must be supervised or directed by a member of the medical staff; and they do not participate directly in the governance of the institution. Within these constitutional parameters, psychologists have some freedom of clinical action, however, and their *de facto* activities are broader than would be indicated by the above restrictions. The organizational structure of psychology at Lenox Hill is depicted in Figure 15–1.

Staffing

The Chief Psychologist

The chief psychologist holds a salaried, 20-hours-per-week position in the Section of Psychiatry, reporting directly to the attending-in-charge. Based in the Psychiatric Outpatient Clinic, the position has a multifaceted charge that extends the chief psychologist's responsibilities widely throughout the hospital. Administratively, the chief psychologist functions as the program

Figure 15-1 The Organization of Psychology at Lenox Hill Hospital

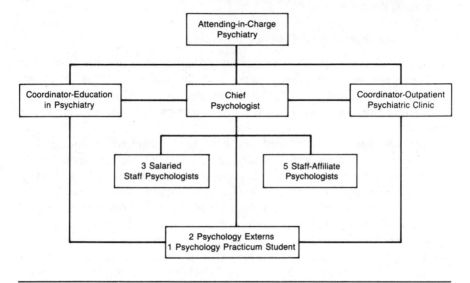

director for psychology within the Section of Psychiatry. The program director's responsibilities are to:

- oversee the performance of all salaried and voluntary clinical psychologists
- coordinate the delivery of psychological services to all inpatients and outpatients inside and outside the Section of Psychiatry
- supervise the development and implementation of psychology's externship and practicum training programs
- foster and advocate the development of psychology's clinical treatment and training roles
- recommend the appointment, reappointment, or nonappointment of all staff-affiliated psychologists
- participate in the deliberations of the executive committee of the Section of Psychiatry

In addition, the chief psychologist provides direct clinical services to psychiatric clinic patients and in-hospital service patients, that is, patients who are admitted to the hospital without having a private physician on the attending medical staff. The chief psychologist also participates in many of the educational activities of the Section of Psychiatry and can offer fee-for-service consultation, psychometric evaluation, and treatment to private patients of the medical staff.

Salaried and Voluntary Staff-Affiliated Psychologists

Presently, three salaried part-time psychologists each provide from 11 to 18 hours per week of clinical service to the patients of the Psychiatry Outpatient Clinic. Most of this time is devoted to individual psychotherapy, with some time devoted to group psychotherapy and the supervision of trainees.

Each voluntary staff-affiliated psychologist is required to donate three hours weekly to the hospital. Usually, the mandated hours are served in the Psychiatric Outpatient Clinic. The particular responsibilities of these psychologists are negotiated on an individual basis, taking into account both the particular expertise of the psychologist and the needs of various hospital programs. Currently, there are five voluntary staff-affiliated psychologists.

Both the salaried and voluntary affiliated psychologists may engage in fee-for-service activities at the hospital. The chance to do so is often an important consideration in psychologists' decisions to seek affiliation. However, it is not the only consideration, nor the one weighed most heavily by all. Also important are the opportunities afforded to participate in the educational programs of the division; to consult about and provide treatment for a variety of patients who may not be encountered in private practice; to supervise and instruct psychology externs, medical students, and psychiatry residents; and to establish professional and personal ties that might prove useful or enjoyable.

In addition to participating in the service and educational functions of the psychology and psychiatry programs, psychologists at Lenox Hill also participate in the governance of the Psychiatry Division. They do so primarily through the formal representation of their views by the chief psychologist on the executive committee. In addition, the chief psychologist's direct collaboration with the attending-in-charge and the coordinator of psychiatric education provides informal vehicles for voicing the concerns of psychologists.

Psychology Externs and Practicum Students

Each year, a few advanced graduate students in clinical psychology are invited to participate in the clinical and educational activities of the Section of Psychiatry. They come from several universities in New York City's metropolitan area. Because these students are involved in course work at their home universities, the time spent at Lenox Hill is limited to the equivalent of two full days per week. When at the hospital, they are supervised by affiliated psychologists. The externs primarily provide psychotherapy to clinic patients; to a lesser degree, they perform psychometric evaluation of clinic and hospital service patients. As indicated in Figure 15-1, there are currently two psychology externs and one practicum student at Lenox Hill.

Psychologist Services

The services of psychologists at Lenox Hill are not distributed equally throughout the hospital's many departments. Concentrated as they are in the Section of Psychiatry, the psychologists participate in the more "traditional" aspects of mental health practice—individual and group psychotherapy with psychiatric outpatients and psychometric assessment of in-hospital patients.[29] The trend toward the traditional is accentuated by a number of factors. One is the contractual obligation of the salaried psychologists to provide potentially reimbursable services to the patients of the Psychiatric Outpatient Clinic. A second is the basic private-practice orientation of the voluntary staff, psychologists and psychiatrists alike. Yet another factor is the emphasis of Lenox Hill Hospital upon tertiary care, that is, the reduction of the consequences of disease processes in patients.[30]

Psychiatric Outpatient Clinic

Not surprisingly, with the greater part of psychology's resources concentrated in the outpatient clinic, the largest part of its service efforts is expended in that setting. Clinic outpatients are referred to psychologists, generally after an intake evaluation by a psychiatrist, on the recommendation of the diagnostic and disposition conference. Assignments are made on the basis of the individual practitioner's expertise and clinical load. On occasion, psychologists perform intake evaluations themselves, especially in cases where patients specifically request behavioral medicine or biofeedback treatments. In large measure, the psychologist, psychiatrist, and social worker provide similar psychotherapeutic services, that is, psychodynamically oriented or occasionally supportive psychotherapy. However, some psychologists are also able to employ behavioral management techniques (such as desensitization and biofeedback), cognitive therapy, and family therapy. Psychological testing falls within the exclusive purview of psychology, whereas pharmacological interventions are exclusively psychiatry's domain.

In any given week, the psychologists of the clinic see an average of 33 patients. This number is somewhat augmented by the work of the two externs and one practicum student. Since the clinic functions as a general, outpatient, community mental health resource, its clientele is quite varied. The one common characteristic of these patients is their lower socioeconomic status; they attend the clinic because they cannot afford private practice fees.

Several basic treatment approaches underlie the therapeutic services provided by psychologists. For the most part, the psychologists at Lenox Hill consider their approach to treatment to be psychodynamic. In contrast, most other psychologists consider their treatment approaches to be eclectic;[31] they attempt to integrate in a coherent fashion elements of each of the major treatment perspectives: psychodynamic, behavioral-cognitive, humanistic existential, sociocultural, and physiological-neuroscience.[32]

The psychodynamic perspective emphasizes the importance of the interaction in the mind of such potent forces as the individual's desires, moral imperatives, and adaptive capacities. The behavioral orientation attempts to alter specific maladaptive behaviors utilizing the laws of learning. The cognitive perspective emphasizes how our beliefs about ourselves and the world influence our moods and actions. The humanistic-existential perspective focuses attention on the way in which individuals experience their world, and on their responsibility to "own" their behavior. The sociocultural orientation conceptualizes the individual as a social being that participates in, and is influenced by, a social field. The neuro-science perspective utilizes the interaction between body and mind to produce, predict, or understand changes in mental and bodily states.

The following cases from the Lenox Hill Psychiatric Outpatient Clinic illustrate the multifaceted nature of the hospital's client population and some uniquely "psychological" strategies in therapeutic intervention.

Case 1. At the time Cindy was seen, she was seven. She had been referred to the Psychiatric Outpatient Clinic by her pediatrician. In the course of the previous year, she had developed a habit that had proved particularly annoying to her parents and, because of their reaction to it, to herself. She would twist tufts of her hair about her fingers ever more tightly until they came loose from her head. Over the course of time, she had created a patchy scalp that embarrassed both her and her parents. Their attempts to end the practice had proved futile. Neither threats, nor punishment, nor ignoring the behavior produced the desired effect, and Cindy seemed unable to resist engaging in it.

As time went on, the tufting increased. Concern mounted that she would grow bald. Her parents feared that Cindy would become an object of derision at school. Family life began to center about Cindy and her hair-pulling. Yet, though her parents found that their concern with her hair-pulling occupied a greater and greater part of the day, they had few other complaints about her. She was performing well at school, and got along normally with peers and her elder sister.

Cindy was interviewed by a clinic psychologist in the presence of her parents. She seemed an adorable, affable child who was slightly immature for her age. She was the baby of the family. Both Cindy and her parents agreed that "hair-pulling" was the problem on which they wished to work. No evidence that there were "deeper" difficulties was uncovered in the interview, in later talks with her parents without Cindy present, or in conversations with Cindy's teacher (parental permission granted). So, the target symptom was to be hair-pulling.

An attempt to describe the typology of the habit proved difficult. No one could pinpoint its inception; no one could describe when it was most likely to occur, aside from an impression that it often occurred when Cindy was doing homework or watching television. Because it had been seen when Cindy slept, she wore a shower cap to bed. As with most such habits, it seemed to be exacerbated by stress. Cindy denied awareness of her hair-twisting until it was too late to stop, until hair had been torn from her scalp. All agreed that every attempt they had made to control the habit had only made things worse.

The treating psychologist decided that a behaviorally oriented, self-management strategy would be likely to produce the most efficacious intervention: Cindy would learn to control her own behavior. The psychologist's reasons for selecting that option were multiple: (1) the problem was specific; (2) Cindy's parents could not watch her all the time and, if they attempted to do so, she might take steps to avoid such intrusive scrutiny; (3) Cindy was interested in possessing and exercising the capacity to control herself.

In general, self-control techniques can be expressed in summary form by the acronym TOTE: T for test; O for operate; T for test; and E for exit.[33] In order to achieve self-regulation, a system must *test* its activities against a standard. If there is a discrepancy between the two, the system must *operate* to reduce it. Then it must *test* to determine whether it has done so successfully. If it has, it may then *exit*.

Cindy knew the standard: no hair-pulling. The rest of the regimen required development. First, she was asked to attempt to note all instances and circumstances in which she engaged in hair-pulling in a given week. When possible, her parents were to verify her tally, independently and separately. At the successful completion of the assignment, Cindy was to have a reward of her own choosing: in this instance, a jigsaw puzzle. At first, her parents rejected this plan as bribery. When it was reinterpreted as a stipend for working on self-regulation, they consented. The next week Cindy returned with a detailed list of hair-pulling incidents. Interestingly, everyone agreed it was largely accurate and that there had been less hair-pulling than usual. The very act of noticing these incidents and writing about them operated to terminate the twisting, a not unusual finding.

Within a month, the hair-pulling was successfully terminated. It did not reappear at follow-up two months later, nor had any symptom been substituted for it.

Case 2. A 35-year-old man, R.T., presented at the psychiatric clinic with complaints of depression and anxiety related to being unable to obtain a satisfactory job. R.T. had a doctorate, but tenured academic appointments in his field were rare and they paid poorly.

R.T. was seen by a psychologist for psychotherapy, who, after several gratifyingly successful months of treating him for his severe depression and anxiety, suggested that he undergo a battery of vocational tests. R.T. willingly agreed, although he probably would not have done so if he had not had a very positive therapeutic experience with the therapist. The vocational tests revealed that R.T. would probably enjoy being a computer programmer, and that he had the skills and personality suited for this field. In addition, it was a field in which he could easily find a well-paying job, with a minimum of time required to retrain himself.

After taking a semester of computer courses, R.T. accepted an excellent job offer to write computer manuals for lay people. In this job he found himself combining his previously acquired academic skills with his computer skills. The patient was glad that he had finally found a well-paying job, with security, that also stimulated him intellectually.

Inpatient Psychiatry Service

As noted earlier, psychologists do not have admitting and discharge privileges at Lenox Hill Hospital. However, if approved by the attending-in-charge, provisions can be made to ensure continuity of care for patients previously under treatment from psychologists during necessary hospitalizations. That is, though such patients are admitted under the primary care of a psychiatrist, psychologists can see them in psychotherapy. With this exception, the psychologists generally do not provide therapy to psychiatric inpatients.

The major task of the psychologist with inpatients is to make psychological assessments on a fee-for-service basis. Psychological tests are integrated into most of these assessments. The tests fall into several broad categories: tests of ability, tests of personality and typical performance, behavioral observations, and self-reports.[34]

In a hospital setting, psychological tests provide reliable and valid information—beyond interviews, case histories, and laboratory tests—that may prove useful in determining a diagnosis, selecting a treatment regimen, or predicting an outcome. The advantages such tests have over more impressionistic methods of gathering and weighing information stem from the extensive research required in their development. In general, the research must show that statistical prediction or classification from quantified results is more accurate and reliable than the clinical decision procedure it replaces. Each test must be accompanied by research that clarifies the legitimate interpretation of results and specifies the probable range of error or accuracy of any given score. Indeed, in some cases, actuarial comparisons may be utilized, relying on statistical data that are unbiased by the clinician's scientific limitations. That is, when thousands of patients with a similar diagnosis have been tested, there may be certain objective similarities in their responses to test questions that will facilitate interpretation. Finally, because objective test results are quantified, changes from baseline can be accurately recorded, and treatments can be modified accordingly.

Psychiatric inpatients have been referred for psychological testing to clarify vocational goals, aid in differential diagnosis, assess treatment progress, and ascertain level of functioning in such areas as memory, learning, and academic skills.

Consultation-Liaison Service

Psychologists also have a consultation-liaison role that, on occasion, takes them throughout the hospital. Medical-surgical patients can be referred in one of two ways. If they are private patients, they are referred directly to the desired psychologist by either the attending physician or the consulting psychiatrist. Service (nonprivate) patients are referred first by the house staff to the chief psychologist. The latter either fulfills the requirements of the referral or assigns it to another psychologist or extern. Since many referral requests are made directly to the voluntary psychologists, it is difficult to estimate the total number of medical-surgical patients seen by the psychology staff; the number is not high, however.

As in the case of inpatient psychiatric referrals, most medical-surgical patients are referred to psychologists for psychological testing. The remainder are sent for specialized treatments, such as biofeedback.

Presently, the consultation-liaison services available from psychologists at Lenox Hill Hospital are underutilized. The full potential of such services could encompass aid to ward staff in dealing with communication or emotional problems arising from care of difficult patients; aid to staff in dealing with patients who are noncompliant with their treatment regimen; application of psychological pain management techniques; aid to patients, staff, and family in dealing with death and dying; and application of life-span developmental psychology to alleviate the reactions of different age groups to hospitalization, illness, and separation.

The following cases illustrate the psychologists' consultation-liaison role at Lenox Hill Hospital.

Case 3. J.M., a twelve-year-old boy with recurrent hydrocephalus, was hospitalized on the inpatient pediatrics unit and referred for school and neuropsychological assessment. J.M. had had repeated hospitalizations and operations since infancy. During his hospital stays he generally received tutoring from family or teachers. The referring social worker wished to know if the child could return to a normal, sixth-grade class after discharge from his latest hospitalization, during which time he was treated for meningitis and hydrocephalus over a four-month period.

Intellectual testing showed that J.M. had a normal IQ. His spelling, reading, writing, and arithmetic skills were all within normal limits for a sixth-grader, although a mild hearing loss was noted. The child was referred back to his regular class upon discharge, with a referral for an audiological work-up.

Case 4. Mr. B., a 45-year-old, white married male, was referred for biofeedback by the physician who was treating him for hypertension. Though medication had significantly reduced his blood pressure, Mr. B. remained a borderline hypertensive (above 140 mm Hg systolic, 95 mm Hg diastolic). He suffered from no other physical or psychiatric dysfunction, was not overweight, and did not smoke.

Subsequent to his acceptance in the program Mr. B. was scheduled for an educational session on the relation of stress to hypertension and the treatment he would be receiving. He was then given an appointment for three-a-week, 45-minute treatment sessions in which he was to be trained in relaxing. He was taught correct breathing techniques, progressive muscle relaxation, and how to use imagery to produce a tension-free state. He was also given a tape containing a relaxation induction that he was to use at home.

After Mr. B. had made sufficient progress in learning the relaxation response, he was introduced to a variety of coping strategies (assertiveness, time management, and other techniques) and to thermal biofeedback.[35] The coping techniques were practiced in the first 20 minutes of each treatment session, and biofeedback was provided in the last 25 minutes. The feedback was auditory. It reflected skin temperature fluctuations measured continuously by electrodes attached to the finger of the nondominant hand. Before and after each session, Mr. B.'s blood pressure was measured. After 31 sessions his blood pressure averaged 120/70 consistently, and he was discharged from the program.

SUMMARY

As noted earlier, Lenox Hill Hospital is a conservatively administered, voluntary, medical-model, care facility without a segregated psychiatric unit. Although there has been substantial expansion of psychiatric services at the hospital in the last decade, and all indicators point to a continuation of that trend, the provision of mental health services has not held the highest priority. Given the private-practice orientation of the institution and its past resistance to psychiatry, it was essential that psychiatry first establish itself in its traditional medical role before it attempted to expand into new territory or to assume its own special responsibilities.

It was inevitable that psychology would follow the same path. There were several initial constraints. First, the psychologists practicing in the outpatient clinic were private practitioners. Second, the clinic's mission was traditional. Third, psychology was organized within the Section of Psychiatry. Finally, psychologists in the hospital did not have primary patient care responsibilities independent of medical sanction.

Thus, when psychiatry expanded its role and services throughout the hospital, it was to be expected that psychology would lag somewhat behind. As the psychiatrists began to earn their own place among the general medical and surgical services, the psychologists, who did not share the bond of medical socialization, continued to have difficulties gaining access to the wards of the hospital. The available psychological services were those that were offered uniquely by psychologists, not those regarded as competitive with psychiatric practitioners. The fact that both the psychologists and the psychiatrists were basically dynamically oriented ensured that the initial services requested from psychologists would be primarily psychometric in nature, not those based on the various therapeutic subroutines of behavioral psychology (desensitization, assertiveness training, and so on).

Today, the role of the psychologist continues to be somewhat restricted at Lenox Hill, compared with other health care settings, for example, other city hospitals, general hospitals affiliated with health maintenance organizations, or community mental health centers.[36-38] Still, psychologists at Lenox Hill enjoy a number of advantages that their professional colleagues elsewhere do not have. Though they are not members of the medical staff of Lenox Hill, they have formal staff privileges; this is relatively rare, especially in New York City.[39] They also have wide latitude to develop close interprofessional relationships throughout the hospital.

Of particular importance is the strong complementary role psychology plays with respect to psychiatry; this ensures that, as psychiatry advances at the hospital, so too will psychology. To some, the price of this symbiotic relationship may seem high, especially if the totally autonomous practice of psychology is taken as the ideal. However, a de jure, strictly autonomous role for psychology at Lenox Hill is not possible at this time. The psychology program thus must depend on the Section of Psychiatry for its representation to the medical staff.

What predictions may be made about psychology's future at Lenox Hill? First, there will be a steady expansion of psychological practice in areas of the hospital not currently covered. In these new areas, the services that are likely to be offered will be those associated with the developing fields of health psychology and behavioral medicine—such health maintenance regimens as cardiological fitness, pain management, and biofeedback programs. Second, psychologists will be asked to assume a greater role throughout the hospital in assessing the efficacy of treatment regimes. As society becomes increasingly concerned with the cost-effectiveness of treatment interventions, psychologists will be asked to bring their research skills to bear on the matter. Third, psychologists will play a larger role in the education of mental health professionals and medical specialists in the hospital. Finally, the psychologists at Lenox Hill will probably eventually gain medical staff privileges.

REFERENCES

1. G. Murphy, "Historical Review," in *Handbook of General Psychology,* 2nd ed., ed. B.B. Wolman (Englewood Cliffs, N.J.: Prentice-Hall, 1973).

2. E. Boring, *A History of Experimental Psychology,* 2nd ed. (New York: Appleton-Century-Crofts, 1957).

3. S.J. Korchin, *Modern Clinical Psychology* (New York: Basic Books, 1976).

4. J.M. Reisman, *A History of Clinical Psychology* (New York: Irvington, 1976).

5. L.B. Silver and J. Segal, "Psychology and Mental Health," *American Psychologist* 39 (1984): 804–809.

6. American Psychological Association, Committee on Training in Clinical Psychology, "Recommended Graduate Training Programs in Clinical Psychology," *American Psychologist* 2 (1947): 539–558.

7. Korchin, *Modern Clinical Psychology.*

8. Reisman, *History.*

9. American Psychological Association, *Ethical Principles of Psychologists* (Washington, D.C.: American Psychological Association, 1981).

10. American Psychological Association, "Psychology as a Profession," *American Psychologist* 23 (1968): 195–200.

11. Reisman, *History.*

12. H.F. Hess, "Entry Requirements for Professional Practice of Psychology," *American Psychologist* 32 (1977): 365–368.

13. Council for the National Register of Health Service Providers in Psychology, *National Register of Health Service Providers in Psychology* (Washington D.C.: Council for the National Register of Health Service Providers in Psychology, 1984).

14. R.B. Cattell, "Let's End the Duel," *American Psychologist* 38 (1983): 769–776.

15. F. Taney, "Hospital Privileges for Psychologists," *American Psychologist* 38 (1983): 1232–1237.

16. Ibid.

17. D.N. Bersoff, "Hospital Privileges and the Antitrust Laws," *American Psychologist* 38 (1983): 1238–1242.

18. Ibid.

19. R.B. Cattell, "Psychologist or Medical Man?" *Schoolmaster* 12 (1932): 330–331.

20. A.M. Calobrisi, "General Psychiatry Update," *Psychiatric Annals* 13 (1983): 598–606.

21. W.E. Henry, J.H. Sims, and S.L. Spray, *The Fifth Profession* (San Francisco: Jossey-Bass, 1971).

22. H.D. Sargent and M. Mayman, "Clinical Psychology," in *American Handbook of Psychiatry,* vol. 2 ed. S. Arieti (New York: Basic Books, 1959), 1711–1732.

23. Reisman, *History.*

24. J. Stapp and R. Fulcher, "The Employment of APA Members: 1982," *American Psychologist* 38 (1983): 1298–1320.

25. L.H. Levy, "The Metamorphosis of Clinical Psychology," *American Psychologist* 39 (1984): 486–494.

26. Stapp and Fulcher, "Employment."

27. Levy, "Metamorphosis."

28. Medical Staff of Lenox Hill Hospital, *Bylaws of the Medical Staff of Lenox Hill Hospital* (New York: Authors, 1983).

29. B.M. Tefft and R.S. Simeonsson, "Psychology and the Creation of Health Care Settings," *Professional Psychology* 10 (1979): 558–570.

30. H. Dorken and J.T. Webb, "The Hospital Practice of Psychology: An Interstate Comparison," *Professional Psychology* 10 (1979): 619–630.

31. Levy, "Metamorphosis."

32. R.R. Bootzin and J.R. Acocella, *Abnormal Psychology: Current Perspectives* (New York: Random House, 1984).

33. J. Iscoe and L.C. Harris, "Social and Community Interventions," *Annual Review of Psychology* 35 (1984): 333–360.

34. L.J. Cronbach, *Essentials of Psychological Testing* (New York: Harper & Row, 1970).

35. M. Acerra et al., "A Preliminary Examination of Thermal Biofeedback Process Data from Essential Hypertension Patients" (Paper presented at the Fifteenth Annual Meeting of the Biofeedback Society of America, 1984).

36. Dorken and Webb, "Hospital Practice."

37. T.H. Budzynski and K.E. Peffer, "Biofeedback Training," in *Handbook on Stress and Anxiety,* ed. I.L. Kutash, L.B. Schlesinger, and Associates (San Francisco: Jossey-Bass, 1980): 413–427.

38. Iscoe and Harris, "Social and Community Interventions."

39. Dorken and Webb, "Hospital Practice."

Chapter 16

The Role of the Social Worker

Natalie Jacobson

INTRODUCTION

One of the questions most frequently asked of general hospital social workers is, "What do you do?" The multiplicity of the social worker's functions and roles has often confused both consumers of health care and professionals in other disciplines. The intent of this chapter is to illustrate and, it is hoped, to clarify the requisite adaptive roles of the social worker in three hospital settings—inpatient psychiatry, outpatient psychiatry, and the emergency room—using the Lenox Hill Hospital as a case example.

The Social Work Department at Lenox Hill consists of a director, two assistant directors and 21 master's-degree social workers, supplemented by a social work assistant, up to four social work graduate students during the academic year, and a secretarial staff of five. Social workers are deployed throughout the hospital; their priority task is to provide relevant services to high-risk patients in need of timely intervention and to aid in posthospital planning. There is no extra charge to hospitalized patients for social work consultation or other social work services (the exception is a fee for service in the Outpatient Psychiatry Clinic).

The philosophy of the Social Work Department is directly related to the Lenox Hill Hospital setting: to enhance patient care by addressing psychosocial factors that affect, and are affected by, medical conditions and treatment. This mission has its roots in the 1918 founding of the department by Abraham Jacobi. Dr. Jacobi was concerned about the welfare of infants and children in the hospital and worked to supplement their care with such services as family counseling, correctional exercises, summer therapeutic camp, recreational outings, nutritional guidance, and the provision of free milk to destitute families.

In 1923, the hospital's trustees voted to have social services available to all patients; by 1931, the social work staff comprised ten full-time medical social work specialists. The mental hygiene clinic (forerunner of the Psychiatry Service) was begun in 1933 under the aegis of a full-time volunteer worker. Since that time, social work services have expanded into all areas of the hospital, offering services and counseling to both medical and psychiatric patients. As the hospital has grown, so has the Social Work Department. Yet, although the field of medicine has become more sophisticated through the years and cost-containment now looms as a major challenge, the Social Work Department remains focused on helping patients to maximize the use of health care services for an optimal and sustained recovery.

At Lenox Hill Hospital, social workers are assigned to the outpatient clinics and to every medical and surgical inpatient unit, including nephrology and pediatrics. They work in conjunction with attending physicians, nurses, house staff, and other health care personnel. The main forum for informational exchange is the weekly discharge planning conference, which is held on every unit. There, patients' medical and psychosocial needs are discussed for the purpose of planning appropriate and timely discharges. On individual cases, the liaison psychiatrist and the social worker may work together as group leaders or staff educators. In contrast to the discharge planning conferences, there is no formal meeting vehicle for the collaboration of the social worker and the liaison psychiatrist, the extent and nature of which varies from unit to unit.

In addition to the direct assignment of social workers to the units, the Social Work Department sponsors group meetings for "relatives and friends of cancer patients," which are led by nurses and social workers, and "middle years" seminars, which are open to the community. Brochures on preparing for hospitalization, returning home and on financing help at home have been made available by the Social Work Department. Augmenting these efforts, volunteers, supervised by a social worker, work as patient advocates in obtaining social welfare entitlements.

All of the social workers offer consultation and counseling to patients and families, consultation to other health care professionals, and linkage to appropriate community resources. At various times, the social worker may function as a counselor, discharge planner, advocate, educator, and psychotherapist.

INPATIENT PSYCHIATRY

Roles and Tasks

On the Psychiatric Inpatient Scatter-Bed Service (see Chapter 2), the social worker is part of a multidisciplinary team consisting of the chief psychiatrist, a mental health nurse specialist, a psychiatric staff nurse, two psychiatric technicians and a coordinator of therapeutic activities. The team's cohesiveness is reinforced through daily rounds and a weekly staff meeting.

The social worker's main functions in the scatter-bed program are to offer counseling to the families of hospitalized patients and assist in discharge planning. Social work treatment plans are reviewed with the admitting psychiatrist, who is the patient's primary therapist. In addition, because the program is a scatter-bed system, the social worker needs to collaborate with nurses on several different nursing units. The patients are frequently elderly, presenting with physical as well as psychiatric problems; thus consultation with physicians is an important part of the social work process. The social worker must also be mindful of utilization review, a process in which the length of a hospital stay is considered within an acute care framework. The Utilization Review Department allots a specific number of days per patient's medical problem and keeps an eye on determining, with the physicians, an appropriate discharge date.

Because of the multiplicity of professional personnel involved with each patient, communication is vital. The unit nurses are a primary source of information, since they have the closest ongoing contact with the patient. In the regular weekly conferences with the nurses on their units, the medical social workers and the nurses exchange information and mutually aid in hospital care and posthospital planning. Because the psychiatric inpatient social worker cannot possibly meet formally with every nurse on each unit, interdisciplinary collaboration is on an ad hoc basis, thus has limited value as an educative or problem-solving tool.

Case Study of Social Worker-Psychiatrist Collaboration in Inpatient Care

E.M., an 82-year-old married man, was admitted for "depression and lethargy," which seemed directly related to a separation of an old hip replacement. He had become increasingly depressed, agitated, and confused after a visit to his orthopedist, who advised him that he was not a candidate for surgery. In addition, Mr. M. had heart disease and osteoarthritis. At admission, he needed help with just about everything—ambulation, eating, hygiene, elimination, and sleeping. The social worker was aware of the patient's admission, and the psychiatrist indicated that the patient needed extensive work-ups, including medical, orthopedic, cardiac, and neurological evaluation, as well as ongoing psychiatric evaluation and treatment.

The patient's wife, 11 years his junior, was coping well and visiting him on a daily basis. According to the psychiatrist, she was not in need of, or requesting, any social work intervention at the time; the nurses on the unit were apparently supportive of her and mindful of her stressful situation. In addition, the psychiatrist was meeting with her frequently. It was clearly a situation, however, about which the social worker needed to be cognizant. An elderly, debilitated, nonambulatory man with an aging wife (there were no children) would probably need help with posthospital planning, even if it were not requested.

Since the social worker was not on the unit on a daily basis, she read the chart notes, noting particularly the findings of the various consulting physicians. She also checked with the district nurse to see how the patient was progressing with activities of daily living. After six days, when it became apparent that Mr. M. was not improving, the social worker discussed with the psychiatrist the advisability of meeting with Mr. M.'s wife. It was agreed that this would be appropriate and timely, and the social worker contacted the wife.

The social worker's interview with the patient's wife had a threefold purpose: (1) to make herself available to the wife to help her cope with the impact of her husband's illness, (2) to assess the couple's psychosocial functioning, and (3) to discuss the potential discharge options. Mrs. M., a dignified European-born woman, who had once been a nurse, was quietly emphatic about being able to care for her husband. She had been doing so for the past 15 years (after the patient had had his hip-replacement surgery) and planned to continue to do so. She would not consider nursing home placement, did not have the funds for employing help at home, and would not apply for public welfare entitlements. In her softly accented voice, she indicated her emotional need for privacy, and pride in her ability to take care of herself and her husband.

Though the patient's condition began gradually to improve, he continued to have fluctuating levels of cognition and poor ambulation. The social worker kept informed about his medical condition, and shared her thinking about possible discharge problems with the psychiatrist, who was meeting with Mrs. M. regularly. The latter was still adamant about not wanting institutional care for her husband but indicated she would consider some help at home if it were available. The social worker contacted a neighborhood agency, which was receptive to the request, could provide minimal service, and would attempt to obtain funds for the couple from a private foundation. When presented with this plan, Mrs. M. was receptive and also noted the need for a wheelchair. The patient was discharged home the following week with home care services and a wheelchair.

While this type of family work is usually considered as a purely social work function, in this instance the social worker and the psychiatrist collaborated in their work with the patient's wife. Because of the psychiatrist's ongoing relationship with Mrs. M., the usual social work role was modified. Mrs. M.'s intact ego strengths and need for privacy and integrity were supported while, at the same time, appropriate discharge planning was pursued.

OUTPATIENT PSYCHIATRY

Roles and Tasks

In the Psychiatry Outpatient Clinic (see Chapter 4), each professional is considered to be a therapist to whom patients can be assigned for treatment. The social worker—like the clinic's two psychiatrists, four psychologists, and psychiatric nurse clinician—carries an individual caseload (the clinic coordinator, who is primarily an administrator, also carries cases).

The outpatient clinic staff has been stable over time and is a cohesive team. Regular staff meetings, case-sharing conferences, and formal and informal staff consultation help to create a mutually respectful working environment. Despite professional differences, the social worker experiences a significant role blending in the clinic; the treating professionals function variously as evaluators, therapists, and as liaison with community agencies. Such overlapping of roles might in some situations be a negative factor;[1] however, at Lenox Hill there is a strong sense of unity among the staff, and professional flexibility is considered the norm.

Case Studies of Social Worker Roles in the Psychiatry Outpatient Clinic

The following two cases illustrate role blurring and role clarity for the social worker in the Psychiatric Outpatient Clinic at Lenox Hill. Both cases were treated in the same clinic and by the same person. On balance, the interdisciplinary collaboration fostered in the clinic has led to less role conflict and more role sharing. The underlying assumptions seem to be (1) that all professionals in the clinic are capable of providing evaluations and psychotherapy, and (2) that each professional can be called upon to perform a discipline-specific task.

Case 1: Role Blurring

The patient, A.P., a 55-year-old, Greek-born woman, was brought to the clinic by a nurse from a medical inpatient floor. The patient's husband had died in the hospital of a heart ailment one month earlier, and the patient had since been a frequent (almost daily) visitor to the nursing unit, coming to look at the room in which her husband had died. The nurse was concerned about the patient's upset condition and persuaded her to come to the psychiatry clinic.

The social worker, on call for intake screening that day, spoke with Mrs. P., who seemed eager to talk, though expressing doubt that this would help, and requesting medication. She agreed to be seen by the psychiatrist for an evaluation, and an appointment was made. It was noted that Mrs. P. had very limited financial assets, but she was too distraught to discuss entitlements.

Mrs. P. was evaluated three days later, and at a team diagnosis and disposition conference was assigned to the social worker for time-limited individual psychotherapy. In addition, the psychiatrist started her on a regimen of antidepressant medication, but she stopped taking this shortly thereafter because of unpleasant side effects. Because the patient was without adequate funds and needed to apply for Medicaid benefits prior to being seen, treatment did not begin until one month later (limited telephone contact took place during this time.)

Mrs. P. and the social worker met for a total of seven visits: the treatment ended with the patient's return to Greece. The focus of treatment was twofold: (1) the patient's feelings about the loss of her husband of 33 years, (2) the patient's return to Greece, at the insistence of her three sons, and her feelings of reluctance and fear about leaving New York. Since the patient was verbal and intelligent, with excellent access to her emotional reactions, she was able to experience a decrease in the overwhelming and confusing anguish with which she initially presented, and she was able to obtain greater mastery over her daily life.

In this case, the therapy could have been conducted by any mental health professional with an understanding of loss and grief (medication ceased to be a treatment factor when the patient discontinued it). A further instance of role-blurring occurred when the psychiatrist discussed financial entitlements with the patient as she was seen for evaluation (she being too upset to discuss this with the social worker at the initial screening interview).

Case 2: Role Clarity

The patient, M.W., a 51-year-old divorced woman, was presented by the evaluating psychiatrist at the diagnosis and disposition conference. Mrs. W., recently discharged from the hospital after having had a stroke, was diagnosed as depressed. She had great difficulty ambulating, had significant speech problems and possibly other brain-function losses. In addition, she had a history of alcoholism and was currently having difficulties with her teenage daughter. The patient lived in a fourth-floor walk-up and had limited insurance coverage.

At the conference, it was suggested that psychological testing might help the staff understand more of Mrs. W.'s deficits. A psychologist was assigned to perform the assessment, and the social worker opted to act as case manager during the evaluation period. When the social worker saw the patient to discuss further evaluation plans, it was evident that Mrs. W. physically could barely make it to the clinic; she walked with a walker and the assistance of a neighbor.

The social worker discussed her observation at the next conference, and it was decided that the psychiatric clinic was not the most appropriate treatment setting for Mrs. W. The patient clearly needed a specialized program that could treat her for both her physical and her emotional problems. A program that included physical therapy, speech therapy, support groups, and individual treatment was a preferable choice. Such a center was located by the social worker. In her two subsequent meetings with the patient, the social worker discussed with her the need for an intensive rehabilitation program. With the patient's consent, an application to the center was initiated, and Mrs. W.'s former employer was contacted about insurance coverage until Medicaid benefits could be obtained. Although Mrs. W. expressed disappointment that she would not be treated at the psychiatry clinic, she did follow through on the referral and reported back that the services were satisfactory.

EMERGENCY ROOM

The psychiatry clinic social worker is responsible for social work services in the emergency room and is on call for such services five days a week, from 9 A.M. to 5 P.M. (the psychiatric inpatient social worker serves as back-up). Unlike an on-site worker who is physically present in the emergency room and who can do active case finding, the on-call social worker is dependent on the ER staff for referrals. The problem categories most frequently referred for social work evaluation are persons in need of emergency lodging; older, fragile persons in need of homemaker services; alcohol and drug abusers; suspected child abusers; and rape victims.

Because the social worker is not physically located in the emergency room, the ideal team approach is somewhat compromised.[2] The social worker must not only make a rapid assessment of the patient's needs, but must, at the same time, "tune-in to" the staff, who both give and receive information about the patient. For an on-site worker, it is much easier to develop rapport; the visibility of the worker, the act of working together over time, and the frequent sharing of common concerns all serve to make the worker a part of the treatment team. Nevertheless, in the ER milieu, the on-call social worker performs valuable functions and can be an effective part of the team.

In the following two cases at the Lenox Hill emergency room, the social worker was called upon to perform rather straightforward tasks—crisis-intervention counseling for a rape victim, and the assessment of a family situation. In the first case, the social worker also provided support and consultation, enabling the nurse to have a better understanding of the rape victim's experience and thus be able to furnish assistance when the social worker was not available. In the second case, the social worker collaborated with another mental health professional to ensure a thorough psychosocial evaluation. In both instances, the social worker accommodated to the needs of the emergency room, recognizing the limitations of the on-call framework and using collaboration as a teaching tool for case finding and referral.

Case 3: Crisis-Intervention Counseling

The social worker was called by the ER nurse to see a 21-year-old woman who had been raped earlier in the day. The woman was shaky, scared, and angry and needed to talk about her experience. She was also amenable to a referral to a specialized, no-fee agency where she could receive ongoing crisis counseling. The nurse, herself young, was concerned about the patient's emotional state and approached the social worker while the latter was writing her report. The nurse, in talking about the patient, voiced her own anger, outrage, and fears. The social worker listened and discussed with the nurse how she might use her own understanding to counsel rape victims at times when the social worker might not be available. The social worker also alerted her to the rape counseling referral list in the ER protocol.

Case 4: Assessment of a Family Situation

The social worker was finishing a chart note when she met the psychiatry resident. He had been called to evaluate the mental status of two girls, aged 11 and 12, who had entered into a suicide pact and together, at school, had taken almost a bottle of aspirin. Found by their teacher in the girls' room and already feeling quite ill, they readily acknowledged their act and were brought to the emergency room. The 11-year-old's parents had come, and plans were made to have her transferred to the hospital where she was already receiving psychiatric treatment.

The other child presented more of a problem. The resident did not think she needed psychiatric admission, although he felt she did need psychotherapy. The patient's mother, however, would not come to the hospital and, in fact, the girlfriend's parents had made some not-too-veiled comments about the mother's fitness. The resident requested the social worker's help in assessing this situation.

After speaking with the mother and the child, the social worker discussed her findings with the resident. The patient's mother was confined to her home with severe back problems and also was being treated for depression; she was separated from her husband, the child's stepfather. Although sounding emotionally stressed, the mother voiced concern about her daughter and frustration at not being able to come to the hospital. She thought, also, that the patient might benefit from psychiatric treatment. The social worker then talked with the child, who was now better able to express her fears about her mother's physical condition and depression; she consented to give psychotherapy a try. It was agreed and arranged that the patient's stepfather would pick her up from the hospital and that the family would make an appointment in the psychiatry clinic. The social worker subsequently informed the charge nurse about the treatment plan, and the patient was discharged from the emergency room.

SUMMARY

It is clear that there is a great variety of social work roles in the hospital setting. Even within the same service, social workers are constantly required to reassess their values and boundaries. Compounding the complexity, social work priorities are often affected by hospital budgetary considerations and productivity expectations. Thus, discharge planning (with its potential fiscal penalties for the hospital if not done in a timely fashion) continues to increase in priority, while counseling (which does not involve discharge planning) becomes more and more of a luxury. Nevertheless, interdisciplinary collaboration remains the backbone of all social work services.

In each of the services discussed in this chapter, collaboration served as the underpinning for delivery of social work services. Generally, the requisite collaboration consists of:

- assessing the psychosocial needs of the patient and the patient's family
- determining the ethos of the service
- exchanging information, diagnostic impressions, and treatment considerations with other professionals
- maximizing the consultative role of the social worker

Given the increasing pressures for cost containment and the growing emphasis on a more efficient provision of services, adaptation to a multifaceted social work role is both a reasonable and appropriate goal.

REFERENCES

1. Phillips and Dawson, "Problems of Institutional Change," *Canadian Psychiatric Association Journal* 17 (December 1972): 443–448.

2. John Farber, "Emergency Department Social Work: A Program Description," *Social Work in Health Care* 4 (Fall 1978): 7–18.

Chapter 17

Approaches to Mental Health and the Law in the General Hospital Setting*

Richard Rosner, M.D.

INTRODUCTION

There are two major areas in which psychiatric administrators and clinicians must have a general understanding of the relationship of mental health to American law. The first devolves from the legal regulation of psychiatric practice. The second entails the field of forensic psychiatry. Both of these areas of concern are changing as the law itself changes; thus it is more important to understand how to think about problems related to mental health and the law than to memorize specific statutes, cases, and administrative codes (although such information may be relevant to the resolution of specific problems that may arise). This chapter emphasizes approaches to thinking about legal problems in mental health and presents several case situations illustrating relevant general principles in the general hospital setting.

LEGAL REGULATION OF PSYCHIATRY

Applicable Laws and Regulations

Because of the multiplicity of constitutions, legislated statutes, and case law interpretations in the legal and regulatory structure of the United States, it is not possible to set forth a single set of legal guidelines for psychiatrists. In each instance, the laws of the state in which the psychiatrist is located address the general practice of medicine and, often, the specific practice of psychiatry and allied mental health professions. In the state of New York,

*Adapted from *Critical Issues in American Psychiatry & the Law*, Vol. 2, by Richard Rosner with permission of Plenum Publishing Corporation, ©1985.

for example, a large proportion of the relevant laws are included in the mental hygiene law of the state. Other bodies of law—for example, the criminal procedure law—may also contain regulations that are relevant to the area of psychiatry. However, even within a single state, it is difficult to find in one volume all the laws that are relevant to the regulation of psychiatry. Thus, it is essential the psychiatrist work cooperatively with a lawyer to find and understand the laws that are applicable to psychiatric practice in a particular locale.

In acting on behalf of their patients, the authority that physicians possess is ultimately derived from the lawful and delimited power of established federal and state governments. For example, the license to practice medicine is delegated by the government, not by the National Board of Medical Examiners. Thus, a surgeon who invades a patient's body is not liable to charges of assault and battery because the act is allowed under laws that govern physician-patient relationships. In short, how one may practice, upon whom one may practice, when one may practice, where one may practice and what one may practice—all are defined and delegated by law.

In general, the legal regulation of psychiatry not only defines psychiatrists' legal obligations to their patients, it also specifically delineates the conditions under which:

- a psychiatrist-patient relationship may be said to exist
- a psychiatrist may treat a patient
- a psychiatrist may not treat a patient
- a psychiatrist may be held liable for injuries sustained by a patient in the course of medical treatment
- a patient may be treated against the patient's will
- a child, an unconscious person, or an adjudicated incompetent person may be treated
- a psychiatrist may reveal secrets confided by a patient

All of these conditions involve issues that relate, not to the science and art of medical diagnosis/therapy and technology, but to the ways and means by which medical science and art may be lawfully practiced in the area of psychiatry.

Involuntary Hospitalization and Competency

Thus, the legal regulation of psychiatric practice is, in principle, no different from the legal regulation of any other profession, skilled trade, or business. This is particularly evident when the psychiatrist is obligated to act against the wishes of a patient, for example, in an involuntary hospitalization procedure. By what right does the psychiatrist deprive patients of their liberty and confine them to a mental hospital? Again, the power to do so is not derived from the profession of medicine but is rather granted by law and, as such, must be implemented by procedures specified by the law. In the case of an involuntary psychiatric hospitalization, one legal criterion is whether the person is judged to be a clear and present danger to others and, if so, whether mental illness is causing the danger. If a deinstitutionalized psychiatric patient is merely unsightly, odoriferous, or a nuisance, community complaints about the patient are not in themselves legal criteria for involuntary hospitalization. Only if the criterion of a clear and present danger is met may such a person be involuntarily hospitalized.

A second legal criterion justifying the restriction of personal liberty, one that is well-founded in the *parens patriae* power of government, derives from the right of the government to care for those who are legally not entitled to care for themselves, for example, orphaned children, persons adjudicated to be incompetent by the courts, and mentally ill persons who meet legal criteria for intervention into their privacy. Thus, in the latter case, another legal justification for involuntary hospitalization in a mental institution may be that the person is gravely disabled by mental illness and cannot function safely outside a hospital setting. However, though many psychiatrists may readily accept and apply this criterion, it is not highly regarded by civil rights lawyers. For example, many deinstitutionalized psychiatric patients are able to function safely outside a hospital, even though they live in a manner that the average citizen disparages; by their own atypical standards, they may not be gravely disabled.

The Role of the Courts

Legal regulation of psychiatry is designed to ensure that psychiatrists exercise their lawfully delegated power in ways that are consistent with constitutional guarantees that no person may be deprived of life, liberty, or property without due process of law. Thus, a psychiatrist may believe that a patient has become incompetent to consent to treatment, but the person remains legally competent until adjudicated to be incompetent by a court. The relevant analogy here is that of a person who may have ceased to live but who is not legally dead until declared so in accordance with law. In both cases, the physician expresses a judgment regarding the patient's condition, but the legal decision is made by a judge.

Why should a judge decide? As a representative of the judicial branch, the judge is vested with constitutional authority to make decisions in legal disputes. In the case of a patient judged to be incompetent to consent to treatment, the dispute is between the patient who feels personally competent and the medical staff member who believes that the patient is not competent. The judge hears both sides and renders a legally binding decision as to which of the two parties is right. Many psychiatrists are not accustomed to being in this type of adversary relationship with their patients; they tend to adhere to the adage, "Doctor knows best." An important responsibility of a psychiatric administrator in the general hospital setting is to assist the clinical medical staff in developing a realistic understanding of the legal limits of psychiatrists' authority.

In New York State, a government agency, the Mental Health Information Service, must be advised of the involuntary hospitalization of psychiatric patients. This agency is charged with the legal representation of the patient's interests, often in opposition to the recommendations of the psychiatric staff of a hospital or other institution. In other states, a special division under the public defender or public advocate may represent the rights of involuntary mental patients. Such a case might develop from a situation where a patient wants to leave the hospital against medical advice, but the psychiatric staff believe that the patient should be involuntarily hospitalized for further treatment; or it might arise in a situation where a patient does not want to take medications, but the psychiatric staff believe that the medications are essential for the treatment of the patient's psychosis and urge that the patient be involuntarily medicated.

At times, a conflict of values may lead to disagreements between the psychiatrist and the lawyer. Generally, in the medical profession, health is a principal value; in the legal profession, liberty is a principal value. For the physician, persons who insist on the freedom to remain sick (for example, mentally ill patients who refuse treatment because they enjoy being manic and who hire a lawyer to sue for their release from a hospital) are problems in medical management. For the lawyer, when the price of health is involuntary hospitalization and the patients prefer to be free and ill, they are problems involving civil liberties. There are no villains in this context; health and liberty are both major values. Thus, in the case of disagreements between psychiatrists and lawyers, it is important to evaluate the facts in the context of both health-centered and liberty-centered principles.

FORENSIC PSYCHIATRY

Definitions and Roles

One definition of forensic psychiatry is that it is the application of psychiatric expertise to legal ends (as compared with the application of psychiatric expertise for therapeutic ends, which is clinical psychiatry). In forensic psychiatry, the psychiatrist frequently evaluates someone who is not a patient. In such cases, it is extremely important that the psychiatrist advise the person of the absence of a physician-patient relationship. In such a relationship, the person being evaluated may reasonably expect that what is discussed will be kept confidential and that the information will be used for the patient's benefit. In contrast, in the relationship between the forensic psychiatrist and the person being evaluated, the information will not automatically be held confidential; in fact, it may be used against the interests of the person being examined.

One of the best examples of this type of relationship between the forensic psychiatrist and the person being evaluated can be seen in the military. The psychiatrist in the armed forces may be called upon to help someone get well enough to go back into a war zone and risk death. The military psychiatrist's primary duty is not to help the soldier escape active duty, on the grounds that it would be better for the soldier's health to stay far away from the bullets and shrapnel. Moreover, in such a setting, confidentiality does not necessarily apply. While the role of the military psychiatrist is admittedly a special one, it is an example of ways forensic psychiatrists must apply their skills on behalf of interests beyond the well-being of the person being examined.

When a physician functions as a clinical psychiatrist in some settings and as a forensic psychiatrist in other settings, problems may arise. The psychiatrist may not understand clearly which role to play, or may not clarify the role properly for the person being examined. Thus, one of the first rules of forensic psychiatry is to know whether one is wearing one's "forensic hat" or "clinical hat," and to share that role definition with the person being evaluated.

The following are examples of the kinds of nonclinical, nontherapeutic activities in which a forensic psychiatrist may become involved:

- evaluating whether a defendant in a criminal case is competent to stand trial
- determining if a Social Security disability claimant is truly disabled
- assessing whether a patient in a hospital who was acquitted by reason of legal insanity is likely to be dangerous if released
- determining in a divorce case which of two competing parents would be the better custodian of their child
- reconstructing the mental state of a dead person at the time the person signed a last will and testament, in order to determine the competence of the person to make the will
- reviewing records to assist the police in the development of a psychological profile of a criminal

Again, in each of these examples, the person who is the primary focus of the forensic psychiatrist's expertise is not necessarily the person being assessed or evaluated. Indeed, the person being evaluated (directly or indirectly) might have actually opposed the evaluation being done. Reflecting the fact that the primary focus of evaluation is not necessarily a patient, forensic psychiatrists tend to refer to the persons being evaluated as defendants, claimants, testators, plaintiffs, purported perpetrators, and so on. This is a way of clarifying for all parties that the psychiatrists are using their skills for forensic, not clinical, purposes.

Issues and Problems

Given its unique focus, one might question whether forensic psychiatry is compatible with psychiatry's professional ethics. The fact is that, though forensic psychiatrists do not function in a physician-patient relationship with the persons they examine, their activities and goals are not inconsistent with the ethical principles of medical practice. Indeed, in a larger context, it could be argued that many important societal tasks would be significantly impaired if psychiatric experts were constrained from assisting the legal system.

Within the profession, the practice of forensic psychiatry is clearly consistent with the code of ethics of the American Medical Association and with that code's "Annotations for psychiatrists" that were developed in conjunction with the American Psychiatric Association. As long as forensic psychiatrists are clear in their own mind as to their nontherapeutic role, and as long as they make it clear to the people they are asked to evaluate that they are not acting as their agents, they are functioning ethically—albeit outside the traditional physician role. In short, a psychiatrist may ethically use the skills acquired in the course of clinical training for ends that are not clinical, as long as all parties understand the psychiatrist's nonmedical role and objectives.

Although administrators and clinical psychiatrists in the general hospital setting are particularly concerned with the legal regulation of clinical psychiatry, they are likely, at some point, to encounter forensic psychiatrists in the courtroom. Whenever an issue in the legal regulation of psychiatric practice must be resolved by a judge, it is likely that a forensic psychiatrist will be called to testify. In such situations, if one is to make the best use of their services, it is important to understand how forensic psychiatrists analyze psychiatric legal problems. In many courtroom situations, the forensic psychiatrist may be a better witness for the administrator or clinician than a clinical psychiatrist. In some circumstances, each side in the legal contest may be represented by a forensic psychiatrist rather than a therapeutic staff psychiatrist. In general, just as one would want a clinician to deal with a clinical problem, one would want a forensic expert to deal with a legal problem.

The Psychiatric Legal Process

In general, all psychiatric legal problems can be understood in terms of a four-step analysis; this is the approach the forensic psychiatrist is most likely to utilize:

1. What is the psychiatric legal issue?
2. What are the legal criteria that will be used to decide the issue?
3. What are the relevant clinical data?
4. What is the reasoning that can apply the relevant data to the legal criteria in order to generate an opinion on the issue?

A single clinical case may involve several psychiatric legal issues. For example, if a person assaults another person, the following issues may arise:

- whether the assaultive person is a suitable candidate for involuntary psychiatric hospitalization
- whether the assaultive person may be held to be not criminally responsible for the assaultive behavior because of legal insanity
- whether the assaultive person is currently competent to stand trial

A forensic psychiatrist may be particularly useful in delineating these kinds of psychiatric legal issues. Alternatively, a more precise analysis of their implications may be obtained by consulting an attorney.

For each psychiatric-legal issue, a particular set of legal criteria must be considered. To illustrate by analogy, in a clinical psychiatric diagnosis, a specific set of psychiatric criteria must be met: If a patient has schizophrenia, the type of schizophrenia is the issue, and the criteria to be met are found in DSM-III. In a forensic psychiatric diagnosis, if the issue is whether a person is competent to stand trial, the set of criteria is to be found in the law. In such cases, the psychiatric legal issue is one that can be determined with a "yes" or "no." The legal criteria involved may be brief, lengthy, precise, vague, recent, or old; but they are the guidelines that must be used to evaluate the data. While some forensic psychiatrists are familiar with the legal criteria pertaining to particular psychiatric legal issues, it is best to obtain this information from the attorney who will represent the psychiatric administrator's or clinician's interests in the legal court hearings.

In a particular case, the *relevant* clinical data must be distinguished from all available clinical data. Relevant data are those that are germane to the legal criteria that will determine the issue. The judge or jury may be confused by all the information that the clinician possesses about the case. Or the information that the clinician has may not relate pertinently to the legal criteria that the judge or jury must use in reaching a decision on the psychiatric-legal issue. For example, in the assault case described above, the issue of criminal responsibility would require information about the assaultive person's mental condition at the time of the offense and relevant past historical data to aid in determining what in fact was going on in the person's mind. Beyond that, if further information were provided to the court, it would probably be regarded as irrelevant, and the case may well be lost as a result.

The reasoning process by which one moves from the relevant clinical data, to their application to the legal criteria, and then to an opinion regarding the specific issue at hand is the special province of forensic psychiatry. Awareness of this process will enable the administrator and clinician to make the best use of the available legal services and forensic psychiatric expertise.

The difficulties that some clinicians encounter in explaining their reasoning processes to a court may be due in part to anxiety created by the unfamiliar setting. Also it is disconcerting to have to face the challenges of the lawyer on the opposing side to the testimony the clinician is trying to present. Thus, it is particularly important that clinicians work closely with their own attorneys in order to present their testimony effectively.

Sources

As a practical matter, the general hospital psychiatric practitioner or administrator should know how to locate a forensic psychiatrist for a particular case. The best method is to write to the American Board of Forensic Psychiatry at 1211 Cathedral Street, Baltimore, Maryland 21201, to obtain a list of physicians who have been certified in the forensic subspecialty. Alternatively, one can contact the American Academy of Psychiatry and the Law, at the same address, to get a much larger list of noncertified forensic psychiatrists. At present, there are only about 150 certified forensic psychiatrists, but there are nearly 1,000 noncertified forensic psychiatrists. Another source of information is the American Academy of Forensic Sciences (AAFS), which has listings of forensic psychiatrists, forensic pathologists, forensic odontologists, forensic anthropologists, as well as specialists in criminalistics, engineering, toxicology, questioned documents, and jurisprudence. The AAFS address is 205 South Academy Boulevard, Colorado Springs, Colorado 80901. In some circumstances, a forensic psychologist may be useful; a list of these professionals may be obtained from the American Board of Forensic Psychology or from the American Psychology-Law Society (the addresses of these organizations change with the officers who are elected to lead them).

THE LAW AND PSYCHIATRY: SOME CASE STUDIES

As the technologies and conceptualizations in medicine continue to evolve, the legal framework of medical practice seems to be keeping pace. Though psychiatrists and other mental health professionals cannot be expected to remain fully up-to-date in this area of the law, they should at least understand the broad legal framework in which medicine and the mental health professions operate. In this way, they should be reasonably equipped to deal with specific cases and their derivative legal applications.

The following case studies illustrate the interface between the law and psychiatry in the general hospital setting.

Case 1: Assessment of Suicidal Risk

On a Saturday evening the psychiatric consultant received an urgent call from the emergency room. An agitated woman had brought in a comatose man. The medical intern was concerned that a suicide had been attempted and requested assistance. Upon being questioned, the woman related that she and her boyfriend had recently broken up and that she had found him in a stupor when she came by his apartment to pick up some of her belongings.

The man, responding to medical treatment, regained consciousness, but was evasive about what had happened, claiming that his state was only the result of an accident. He said that he had been having trouble sleeping and that he had taken "a couple of shots" of whiskey to relax. When the alcohol failed to help sufficiently, he took some sleeping pills. He denied a suicidal intent. The former girlfriend was terrified and guilt-ridden. She was concerned that he might try to kill himself as soon as he was released. The medical intern indicated that the man did not need admission because of his medical condition, but he insisted on obtaining "psychiatric clearance" before the man was permitted to leave the emergency room.

The psychiatric legal issue in this case was whether or not the man met the legal criteria for involuntary hospitalization. In New York State, there are two possible procedures to obtain the relevant criteria: (1) the involuntary hospitalization procedure, which requires a certification by two physicians to the effect that the patient is in need of care and treatment in a hospital *and* is suffering from a defect of judgment (due to mental illness) that prevents the patient from recognizing that need; or (2) the emergency hospitalization procedure, which requires a certification by only one physician to the effect that the patient is in need of care and treatment in a hospital because the patient is dangerous to self or others (as a result of mental illness). The psychiatric consultant attempted to collect data that would be relevant to each procedure.

In a clinical interview with the patient, the consultant first tried to establish rapport. The man was clearly not psychotic, although he was unhappy with his work and with his "failure" to satisfy his girlfriend. The consultant concluded that the patient had an adjustment disorder with depressed mood, superimposed upon a mixed personality disorder, with histrionic, dependent, and passive-aggressive features. The consultant was aware that the local courts were extremely reluctant to support the involuntary retention of nonpsychotic patients. The conclusion was that the patient was not a candidate for either involuntary or emergency psychiatric hospitalization. The girlfriend agreed to spend the weekend with the man, to ensure his safety and to assuage her guilt; and the patient was permitted to depart, with a referral to the hospital's outpatient psychiatric clinic for the following Monday morning.

Case 2: Involuntary Hospitalization

A gastroenterologist had a patient, an 87-year-old lady, who refused to take her medications and insisted on leaving the hospital. The gastroenterologist wondered if she was competent to refuse treatment and if she might be a candidate for a guardianship proceeding. The liaison psychiatrist was asked to evaluate the situation. He found the patient with her bags packed, in the presence of her niece, who explained that "Aunt Minna wants to go home."

In New York State, there are two types of guardianships. One, a conservatorship, is for persons who cannot manage their finances responsibly, although they are otherwise competent. The other, a committee, is for persons who are completely incompetent to cope with the world they live in. Did the patient fit into either of these legal categories?

The patient had been losing weight for the past two months. Her appetite was poor and she was restless and irritable. She had been chronically constipated, with nausea and vomiting, during the previous week. An initial laboratory examination included a positive guaiac test for occult blood in her stool. The gastroenterologist was concerned about a bowel obstruction, perhaps due to a malignancy. He ordered a panoply of radiological examinations, a colonoscopy, and surgical consultation. The patient would have to consent to all of these procedures. Was she competent to do so?

The patient was clearly well-oriented as to time, place, and person. She worked as a bookkeeper and read the *New York Times* daily. She did not have an organic mental syndrome. It was determined that she had adopted the cats of her neighborhood and had made it her personal mission to see that they were fed in winter. She was afraid that, if she remained in the hospital, "her" cats might starve and suffer.

With the help of the niece, arrangements were made to have the cats fed while the patient remained in the hospital. The patient agreed to stay and was concerned to get the best possible care. She wanted to be cooperative; after all, if anything happened to her, her cats would suffer. The patient was clearly not psychotic; and, if she had insisted on leaving, there would have been no legal grounds to stop her.

Case 3: Posing a Danger to Others

A middle-aged man was brought into the emergency room by his wife. The man had recently been fired from his job, and was disappointed, frustrated, and furious at his boss, whom he was threatening to kill as soon as he left the emergency room. His wife reported that her husband was excited, irritable, talkative, and filled with "plans for the future." The psychiatric consultant was called by the resident psychiatrist because of the concern that the patient might hurt his ex-boss. There was also a question regarding the hospital's duty to warn the former employer that the patient was threatening his life.

The resident was advised that in New York State there was, as yet, no clear "duty to warn" potential victims of dangerous patients. If the resident felt that the patient posed a "clear and present danger" to the boss, the patient could be offered admission to the hospital as a voluntary patient (with constant companioning by orderlies while waiting for psychotropic medications to become effective). Alternatively, if the patient refused voluntary admission, he would be an excellent candidate for emergency psychiatric hospitalization. If the patient were hospitalized, he would not be dangerous to his former employer; if the treatment was successful, the employer would also be safe. However, the consultant noted that a good after-care plan was important to minimize future risks.

SUMMARY

In each of the above cases, there is a blend of clinical and forensic considerations. Indeed, the good forensic psychiatrist is also, fundamentally, a good clinical psychiatrist. Without a solid grounding in clinical psychiatry, the tactical and logical skills of the forensic psychiatrist are of little use. On the other hand, the clinician and administrator must know how to use the skills of the forensic psychiatric consultant. In many instances, through careful clinical intervention— by taking an accurate history, making an accurate diagnosis, and treating the patient as a person rather than as a case—there may be no need to utilize the skills of a forensic psychiatrist and the reserve powers of the law. It is, nevertheless, important to know what those powers are and to be familiar with their scope and limitations, in order to decide if they are applicable in a particular case.

The legal regulation of psychiatric practice continues to evolve. The nontherapeutic psychiatric interface with the law, as represented by forensic psychiatry, encompasses a wide range of issues and variable legal criteria, with no fixed examination format or data collection model. Faced with this flux, general hospital psychiatric administrators and clinicians are better advised to understand the basic framework of legal control over psychiatry and how to utilize the services of a lawyer and a forensic psychiatrist than to learn a long list of arbitrary rules, regulations, and legal procedures. It is more important to know how to think about psychiatric legal issues, how to conceptualize the problems involved, than to be able to apply a particular legal solution.

BIBLIOGRAPHY

Allen, R.; Ferster, E.; and Rubin, J. *Readings in Law and Psychiatry,* rev. ed. (Baltimore: Johns Hopkins University Press, 1975).

Brooks, A. *Law, Psychiatry and the Mental Health System* (Boston: Little, Brown & Company, 1974).

Gutheil, T., and Appelbaum, P. *Clinical Handbook of Psychiatry and the Law* (Hightstown, N.J.: McGraw-Hill, 1982).

Rosner, R. *Critical Issues in American Psychiatry and the Law* (Springfield, Ill.: Charles Thomas, 1982).

Schwitzgebel, R.L., and Schwitzgebel, R.K. *Law and Psychological Practice* (New York: John Wiley & Sons, 1980).

Slovenko, R. *Psychiatry and Law* (Boston: Little, Brown & Company, 1973).

Chapter 18

Financing Psychiatric Services in the General Hospital

Charles Mazzone and Beatrice J. Krauss, Ph.D.

INTRODUCTION

The development and continued viability of any medical program ultimately depends on how much the service costs, who benefits from it, and who is willing to pay for it. Psychiatric services are no exception.

In the last 20 years, there have been profound changes in the sites where psychiatric services are rendered, the population to whom they are directed, the number of care providers involved, the criteria for measuring the benefits of such services, the sources of payment for the services, and, finally, the national health policies that both respond to and guide all of these factors.[1] Planning for the financial viability of general hospital mental health programs demands awareness of trends in each of these areas. It also requires, increasingly, the use of sophisticated management information systems to track local cost-benefit ratios, to determine one's unique position within the larger mental health care market, and to provide information about unmet needs to effect necessary change.[2] On the basis of the information, they can provide on these issues, financial officers have become increasingly important members of psychiatric service planning and development teams.

Site

Emphasis on health cost containment and deinstitutionalization has led to the proliferation of least-cost alternative sites and the "privatization" of sites for mental health care. For example, in 1955 outpatient settings were responsible for 23 percent of mental health episodes (cases of persons residing in or admitted to hospitals for treatment of mental disorders in one year); by 1975, outpatient settings handled 77 percent of such episodes.[3] By

367

the late 1970s, 29 percent of HMOs provided mental health services through their own full-time staffs, while 40 percent contracted such services out, and only 13 percent provided no mental health services.[4]

In the 1970s, 40 percent of psychiatric inpatients were seen in general hospitals without psychiatric wards.[5] Between 1971 and 1977, beds in dedicated psychiatric units of general hospitals increased 26 percent. The concomitant rise in new private psychiatric hospitals and community mental health centers over the last 20 years is further evidence of the national trends toward privatization and deinstitutionalization.[6] Recently, psychiatric day care has been proposed as a low-cost, effective alternative to more costly psychiatric inpatient care.[7,8]

Health Policy

In part, the growth of mental health services in the private sector is responsive to the growth in demand. However, it also reflects changes in national health policy, away from an emphasis on "accessibility" of health care by all through government programs, toward "health cost containment" through competition inherent in the private market.[9] However, the problem of accessibility to health care by the poor remains unsolved by this strategy.[10-12] Indeed, Muszynski, Brady, and Sharfstein have suggested private sector contracting of services or coverage to public institutions responsive to the indigent community.[13]

Population Served

It is estimated that, at any given time, 15 percent of the population is in need of mental health care.[14] Actual utilization, however, is lower and appears to be somewhat dependent on the strictures or incentives of third party insurance coverage for type and extent of care,[15-18] as well as complex factors leading to consistent state-by-state variations in per-capita utilization rates.[19] It is less dependent than was previously thought on the socioeconomic status of the patients,[20] other than the indigent; although sensitivity to differences in insurance coverage does appear to vary with income level for psychotherapy services.[21] Demonstrating actual low utilization rates, a recent Michigan study of 2.3 million persons covered by one comprehensive insurer noted that only 4.6 percent of the covered population made mental health claims.[22] However, because of the catastrophic nature of some mental disorders, the dollars spent on mental health care appear to be about 12 percent of all health care expenditures (as of 1977).[23] In fact, the utilization of mental health care seems to be less than, but similar in pattern to, the utilization of health care in general.[24] Moreover, despite the complexities of predicting utilization for a particular locale, several studies suggest that, for individual areas and coverage plans,[25] utilization rates tend to stabilize across the years.[26-28] As noted earlier, utilization studies also document an increased use of outpatient and other low-cost facilities. Measurement and tracking of utilization rates thus have utility for planning.

Providers

Between 1955 and 1980, the number of psychiatrists per 10,000 population doubled, while the number of psychologists and psychiatric social workers per 10,000 population trebled. Similar increases have occurred in the numbers of psychiatric nurses, counselors, and other mental health care delivery professionals.[29] The mental health care market, therefore, is now more saturated than ever with low-cost, alternative, mental health care providers.

Cost-Benefit Measurement

The difficulties inherent in demonstrating a "cure" for mental and nervous disorders have led to problems in selling psychiatric services to the public and in convincing health insurers that coverage of such services is necessary. Although a number of studies, using sophisticated methodology, seem to demonstrate the efficacy of psychiatric treatment, both physiological and psychotherapeutic,[30-32] there has been a growing trend toward selling mental health services by demonstrating the cost of *not* providing those services.

In 1977, the estimated cost to society of alcoholism, drug abuse, and mental illness was $88.1 billion. Direct care services for mental illness accounted for only $18.2 billion of this total; and "indirect" costs, including loss of productivity, morbidity, and premature mortality due to mental illness, totaled another $21.5 billion. The remaining $48.4 billion was due to the direct and indirect costs of alcoholism and drug abuse.[33]

A series of studies has suggested that psychiatric and psychotherapeutic services reduce the utilization of other modes of health care,[34-37] and also speed recovery from surgery and illness.[38-40] Since much of this mental health care involves brief psychotherapy, outpatient service, and medical liaison, the substitution tends to reduce total cost. Further research in this "cost-offset" area may provide a compelling argument to employers and health insurers to increase mental health care coverage.

Sources of Payment

Insurance coverage of mental and nervous disorders is inadequate. Even though, as of 1981, 90 percent of all insurance policies in the United States contained coverage for mental health care, coverage for mental illness almost uniformly compared unfavorably with coverage for other forms of illness.[41] Discrimination occurs in lower coverage of outpatient services, requirements for higher co-payments, and tighter caps on the number of treatments or inpatient days allowed.[42] Disparity is greatest for ambulatory care, least for in-hospital care and physicians' in-hospital visits.[43]

The major insurers remain Medicare, Medicaid, and the top nine private insurers: Blue Cross, Blue Shield, Prudential, Aetna, Travelers, the merged group Connecticut General and Insurance Company of North America (CIGNA), Equitable, Metropolitan, and the Kaiser Foundation Health Plan (the nation's largest HMO). However, self-insured employer plans are increasing.[44] In the early 1980s, self-funded employer plans served about 8 million persons. These have ceased paying health insurance premiums to traditional insurers, are providing their own segregated benefit trusts, and are putting the "management of benefit claims processing out to bid."[45]

The potential in the design of individual benefit packages for individual workplaces is immense. On the one hand, such funds emphasize cost containment. Fund managers can be approached by individual hospitals for coverage, using cost-benefit arguments and individual contracts for sites of care. On the other hand, as Goldsmith points out, such self-insured plans are likely to broker services to preferred provider organizations (PPOs) and HMOs and thus upset the previous alliance between insurers and hospitals.[46] Obviously, tracking coverage for care in the changing insurance arena will become increasingly difficult.

The most dramatic change may come from the new prospective payment system of reimbursing hospital services under Medicare, based on diagnosis-related groups (DRGs). The DRG system mandates payment for diagnosis, as opposed to fee for service or days of care. This prospective payment system shifts the responsibility for containment of cost more and more onto the health service providers, taxing their ability to work within and under payment limits.[47] Although certain psychiatric facilities were not covered by DRGs at the inception of the legislation, the exemption is scheduled for review in 1985. DRGs, as a payment concept, may spread to other insurers, as well.[48]

Thus, the financial officer of today is facing a market setting in which patients are encouraged to shop for mental health care services by the burdens of co-payment and by the availability of alternate sites and providers of care. Similarly, in the current market orientation, insurers and employers are becoming responsive to cost-benefit arguments for service coverage and contracted care. A continuing serious problem is the failure of current health policies to respond with appropriate coverage for indigent persons in need of mental health care and for the small proportion of patients whose requirements for treatment make their mental disorders financially catastrophic.[49-53]

FINANCIAL MANAGEMENT OF PSYCHIATRIC SERVICE: THE LENOX HILL EXPERIENCE

Start-Up Costs for a Psychiatric Scatter-Bed Inpatient Program

The start-up costs of a psychiatric scatter-bed program are minimal. Capital expenses are minor, because the program is based on the utilization of existing beds and space. The psychiatric patients are intermingled with the medical and surgical patients. Not having to plan, construct, and equip dedicated rooms, a floor, wing, or a building eliminates the need for large expenditures.

Modest expenses will be incurred to provide space, facilities, and materials for group therapy, conference rooms and offices for the psychiatric staff. Other costs are incurred in the areas of staffing, supplies (for example, diagnostic and therapeutic equipment, psychological tests, occupational and vocational therapy supplies, and clinical supplies), and indirect costs (for example, housekeeping, security, engineering). A budgetary listing of these types of costs is shown in Table 18–1.

The relatively low start-up costs of a psychiatric scatter-bed program remain constant after operations begin, with no significant additions as the program matures. Periodic capital expenditures may be made for the occupational/vocational therapy component. Major additions to the staffing complement may also occur, although this has not been our experience at Lenox Hill. The professional personnel changes may involve increases in nursing staff for more effective coverage of evening, night, and weekend/holiday time periods and increases in salaried, psychiatric-physician, on-site coverage of the emergency room during those time periods, thereby expanding the responsibility for effecting admission and providing the initial work-up orders and for making management decisions and acute therapeutic interventions.

Insurance Coverage for a Psychiatric Scatter-Bed Service

Insurance for psychiatric service lags behind insurance for other medical specialties. Still, more coverage is available for psychiatric services today than ever before. It is relatively rare to find that no psychiatric benefits are available under a patient's health insurance policy.

Table 18–1 Operating Costs of a Psychiatric Inpatient Scatter-Bed Program

Direct	Indirect
Professional salaries and fringe benefits	Dietary
Physicians	Heat-light-power
Psychologists	Plant maintenance repairs and
Social workers	plant operations
Nursing personnel	Medical records
Mental health nurse specialist	Housekeeping
Psychiatric staff nurse	Depreciation for bed space occu-
Mental health technicians	pied by psychiatric patients
Secretarial-clerical	Security
Medical student orderly	Malpractice insurance premiums
Teaching program—Professional and support,	Pharmacy
salaries and fringes (optional)	Ward medical-surgical nursing
Supplies and expenses	personnel
Clerical supplies	Admitting function
Occupational/activities therapy supplies	Ancillary services
ECT supplies	Radiology
Physical space cost allocations to ECT patients	Laboratory
ECT Rx room	Physical therapy
Recovery room	ECG
Equipment	EEG
Administrative space for professional/clerical sup-	
port of program	

The first step in evaluating insurance coverage for psychiatric services is to determine how each third party insurance provider classifies inpatient psychiatric patient-days. Third party insurers must be made aware that the hospital does not have a "certified," segregated inpatient unit but is planning to add short-term psychiatric inpatient services in the form of a scatter-bed program to the list of services presently provided to the general community.

Many health insurance carriers provide coverage for psychiatric inpatient services without differentiating the benefits available for these services from those available for other medical services provided by the general hospital. This could mean that a patient with a standard hospitalization plan that includes benefits for an established number of days is eligible for the same number of days for inpatient psychiatric care at the hospital. However, many health insurance carriers limit the number of days for primary psychiatric care in any setting; other carriers limit the number of days only if the patient is confined in an institution that is partly or entirely dedicated to the treatment of mental illness.

Medicaid insurance in New York State does not cover psychiatric scatter-bed services, because such services remain outside the certification process of the New York State Office of Mental Health. Such certification is required under Medicaid regulations. Other states do certify scatter-bed programs, making them eligible for Medicaid reimbursement.

In reviewing the health insurance carriers that service a particular locale, certain key questions need to be answered in regard to acute psychiatric hospitalization coverage. These are detailed in the following sections.

The Definition of a Covered Inpatient Day

Does the daily coverage include both the routine care and the use of the covered ancillary services that the mentally ill patient requires? Is there a maximum allowable charge for the combined day, routine care, or ancillary services? Are any of the covered charges limited to a percentage of the charge?

Modes of Acceptable Treatment

It is important to ascertain the specific clinical services covered under the patient's insurance plan. One must further delineate which of these services is covered only with reference to the site of the program, for example, inpatient versus outpatient, partial hospitalization versus outpatient, and so on.

Deductibles

Does the contract include a deductible that is the patient's personal responsibility? Will the insurance carrier advise if, where, and when the deductible is met? It is important to know where and for how long the patient was recently hospitalized elsewhere, especially if the other institution has not yet submitted its bill. Staff will be able to contact the other institution to determine the number of days utilized, which must then be deducted from the coverage anticipated.

What is the time frame for the deductible? Is the deductible payable for each admission, or is it payable annually? Does "annually" refer to the patient's policy enrollment date or the calendar year? Are there any circumstances in which the requirement for the deductible is waived?

Annual Usage Limitation

Is there an annual limitation of usage? Is the annual requirement based on the policy contract date or the calendar year?

Basic Coverage versus Major Medical Coverage

Most patients will at least indicate their hospitalization and medical coverage when requiring medical services. Does the insurer, especially if it is an employer or trade group, provide a major medical policy that gives additional coverage above the basic policy?

Waiting Periods

Did the patient's condition exist prior to the effective date of the patient's enrollment with the health insurance carrier? Most health insurance carriers do not provide coverage for any condition that existed before the contract enrollment date, unless a certain waiting period after the enrollment has passed, or unless this requirement is specifically waived. Many carriers include a one- to two-year waiting period after the enrollment date. This time period must elapse before they will provide any benefit related to a preexisting condition.

On occasion, a health insurance carrier may even exclude certain conditions for the patient's lifetime, if the chronic condition preexisted and was declared at the time the patient enrolled for coverage. The lifetime exclusion is usually applicable only to individual health insurance policies, and in most instances, is noted on the policy as an exclusion. Some organizations have waivers in their health insurance contracts to eliminate any waiting period.

Benefit Rejuvenation Period

Do the contracts for full-day health insurance benefits provide maximum standard benefits for a new admission or readmission to an institution only if the patient was not hospitalized within a preestablished time period since the previous hospitalization? Some health insurance contracts provide full benefits on readmission, but only for a diagnosis that is not related to the diagnosis made at previous admission.

Another term that may apply to these circumstances is "spell of illness." Benefit rejuvenation period and spell of illness have many common elements. Their particular definitions and applications may vary, however, with the organization that provides the health insurance benefits.

Special Processing Forms

Does the health insurance carrier accept and honor universal assignment and claim forms to process payments? Some organizations still insist on the notification of admission or the rendering of a bill. Some organizations accept the universal form but also request or insist upon the submission of their own forms, in addition to the universal form. Possibly as a payment delaying tactic, some organizations also insist that the patient or the enrolled member visit their offices to sign a particular type of claim or form for certification of services received. The health care institution should be able to obtain a supply of each required form for use in its admitting office.

Eligibility and Benefits Certification Authority

Has the patient's eligibility for benefits changed? Although the patient's office record may indicate the services for which the insurer reimbursed the patient in the past, it is well to view this record only as a tentative schedule of potential benefits. Another contact to verify the patient's eligibility may be in order.

For example, a local of the hospital skilled workers union may provide health insurance coverage to its members and families through a contract with a particular insurance company. The first contact is with the insurance company, and it confirms that the patient has coverage for 365 days in full for any condition without limitation. In this case, it must be determined whether the patient or the insured member of the patient's family is still a member of the union, whether the insured member has paid dues in the current month or quarter, and whether that person has worked a sufficient number of hours during the previous quarter to qualify for health care benefits. Is the patient or the insured member still employed? Has the hospital or union paid the dues or premium? All of these concerns may not be relevant in a particular case, but some or all of them can arise, usually because organizations do not record and communicate changes in their members' statuses on a current basis.

Mechanism to Reinstate Eligibility

Can lost eligibility be reinstated? The clerical staff can be trained to answer this question through periodic, detailed analysis of successful and unsuccessful cases. The analysis should be based on information available from admission records and bad-debt files. Many organizations are willing to extend assistance to their employees or members in time of need. Some help in a spirit of altruism, while others are concerned about the loss of a valued employee or dues-paying member.

Attempts to gain reinstatement of membership are likely to be more successful if the organization has a limited number of employees and the employee is personally known to the owner or major partner of the firm. On occasion, however, such requests may also be successful with a larger national or international employer. In certain circumstances, requests to reinstate eligibility may also be directed to the major health insurance provider, such as the large insurance companies, or even Blue Cross. The following three case examples of restored eligibility or discovered coverage are based on business office experience at Lenox Hill Hospital.

Case 1. A male, unemployed former employee of a small, local retail furniture establishment applied for an elective admission. In a telephone interview, it was learned that he had resigned from a 14-year job for health reasons and had been out of work for nine months. The applicant stated that he had left the job on good terms with all of his fellow employees and with the store's owner and that, in fact, he visited the store frequently just to stay in touch. With the patient's permission, the patient's former employer was contacted. The store owner's feelings towards the former employee were warm. The store owner had no idea that his loyal former employee was now without medical coverage. The result of the contact was that the store owner contacted the store's insurance agent, was able to enroll the patient retroactively in the firm's group health insurance plan, and was more than willing to pay the nine months' premium involved.

Case 2. A female patient who applied for admission had been unemployed for several years. She had been able to pay for her individual enrollment hospitalization insurance policy through Blue Cross up until six months prior to the need for hospitalization, and she had just received the cancellation policy the week before. One telephone call to Blue Cross was sufficient to learn that her cancelled contract would, in fact, be reinstated if payment were received within seven days. A subsequent conversation with the patient resulted in her borrowing the money from a relative. The premium was mailed to the carrier, and the patient's enrollment was reinstated without any adjustment to the original effective date. The relative had been more than willing to lend her the few dollars needed to ensure payment in full for a 22-day stay.

Other Cases. It is not unusual for patients to be unaware of their health insurance coverage. For example:

- Many early retirees are not aware that their former employers or trade unions maintain their hospitalization coverage. In many instances, the medical coverage is identical to that of the still-active employees. In others, the available benefits are reduced for early retirees or the disabled but remain adequate. Also, many full retirees who are enrolled in Medicare are not aware that their former employer or union continues to provide coverage for, and sometimes beyond, Medicare deductibles.
- Minors who are no longer living in their parents' homes may have health care insurance maintained by their parents' continued payments.

- Professionals may not be aware that their memberships in various trade organizations entitle them to participate in limited health insurance plans.

Coordination of Benefits

Are the benefits of several insurers complementary? Most health care insurance carriers insist on being furnished with information about other group or individual health care insurance coverage for the patient or the patient's family. With such information, it can be determined which insurance carrier is to be considered primary (first payer) and if the benefits of the first carrier are exhausted or do not cover all charges in full, which carrier is to be considered secondary (second payer). Such coordination of benefits can be seen as a multifaceted cost-containment effort. The larger insurance providers can pass along premium reductions when duplicate payments by several carriers are eliminated. Gone are the days when a patient or family member covered by two group health care plans could process a duplicate claim and retain each payment.

The determination as to which carrier is to be the primary payer can involve rather complex issues. Many households have more than one wage earner. The major breadwinner and that person's spouse are probably both covered by health care contracts that include coverage for family members. Which one is to be primary? A general rule is that the group insurance contract of the patient designates the prime payer, with the spouse's coverage considered secondary. At times, the multiple coverage may be available through the same carrier because the employers of both parties are insured through the same insurance provider or because the patient or the spouse has more than one place of business. The enrollment dates of the contracts may then be considered in order to establish the primary payment responsibility.

Another factor to consider in the coordination of benefits is how the patient was injured or how the condition developed. A condition or injury that is job-related is the determining factor for medical coverage by the workers' compensation policy of the patient's employer. All group health care is considered to be secondary to workers' compensation, as is Medicare and any other program sponsored by the federal or state governments. The same ruling applies in many states and to any federally sponsored program when the condition or injury is due to an automobile accident.

The Medicare program and the New York State Medical Assistance for Needy Persons program designate themselves as secondary carriers under certain circumstances, for example, when a third party is found to be liable for health costs because of a law suit. Several self-insured union welfare funds in New York State insist on a lien against a future award in the case of a court decision that is favorable to the patient. The lien ensures recovery of funds that were paid to the providers of care. The lien is binding in the case of a favorable award by a court or a favorable settlement without the court's decision.

Coordination of benefits requirements must be included in any survey of health care insurance providers in the service area. The business office staff's awareness of the need to coordinate benefits will facilitate payments for services that are not subject to overlapping coverage. As a carrier completes an investigation of joint coverage, an alert staff can aid in obtaining the release of covered benefits not in contention.

Admissions and Management Procedures

The financial health of a psychiatric service requires accurate record keeping. Yet, societal attitudes toward mental disorder often inhibit patients from providing information and, indeed, may result in staff assigning "less prejudicial" diagnoses. Indeed, at least one investigator has found the latter practice widespread.[54]

Hospital admissions and business office staff need the support and counsel of the psychiatric staff during training to develop knowledge about diagnoses, to learn appropriate interviewing techniques with patients, and to develop guidelines for patient confidentiality. The potential for embarrassing, costly, or serious misunderstandings is considerable if business office representatives attempt to obtain or verify data necessary for billing records or insurance forms with a spouse, family member, or workplace without adequately preparing the patient for the intrusion.

Contacts with a small place of business that has few employees are much more sensitive than contacts with a large employer, whose personnel department, remote from the job site, is likely to handle the inquiry without notifying the patient's peers or supervisor. Some patients may believe that they will lose their jobs or miss upcoming promotions if their employers should learn about their need for treatment of a mental condition. In such cases, the patients may wish to specify as a contact someone at the workplace whose discretion is particularly trusted. On rare occasions, to keep the employer from learning about the mental condition, the patient or the patient's family may elect not to use their health insurance and decide to pay for the required services themselves. Unfortunately, in many instances, the willingness to pay for such services is not always matched by the ability to do so. In such cases, a frank discussion of total costs and available coverage may be in order. In that context, a requirement for a cash deposit prior to admission that is equal to the anticipated charges for the estimated length of stay will educate the patient as to the actual costs involved and also protect the institution.

THE BILLING CYCLE

The handling and processing of a patient's account, psychiatric or nonpsychiatric, is usually divided into six primary phases:

1. preadmission
2. admission
3. interim billing
4. discharge
5. billing
6. follow-up until payment in full

With this phased process, psychiatric populations tend to be characterized by (1) extended institutional stay and outpatient treatment; (2) a potential for frequent admissions and other occasions of service; and (3) limited coverage, nonavailability of coverage, or exhaustion of benefits because of the first two conditions.

In New York City, a nonpsychiatric inpatient account that results in a bad debt is equal to losing payment for approximately nine days of service. For a psychiatric patient, this bad debt amount increases by 144 percent, amounting to a loss of payment for 22 days of service, because of the longer average length of stay. Failure to develop, implement, and adhere to policy and procedures (the preadmission through discharge phases) will result in increased bad debts at a substantially higher amount per account than would be normal for the institution.

Preadmission

The first four of the six primary phases are related. Occasionally, the first phase, preadmission, is combined with the admission phase. However, elimination of a thorough preadmission procedural routine by a hospital is equivalent to a credit-granting organization—a department store, bank, consumer finance company—granting credit to the consumer without first obtaining a credit application and acting upon it.

In the case of the credit-granting organization, there are several steps that, as a matter of sound business policy and practice, must be completed before the approval and granting of credit.

- accumulation of socioeconomic information
- review of established minimum data: name, address, employment history, credit experience, assets, liabilities, and so on
- verification of major data

- evaluation of all data
- approval or disapproval of the credit applied for
- establishment of a dollar amount limitation or a requirement for additional information, if the information submitted is inconclusive
- discussion of the approval or disapproval with the applicant

If the credit application is disapproved, the applicant is often able and willing to supply additional information or clarification in order to obtain approval.

In effect, the elimination or inadequate processing of the preadmission phase for a pending psychiatric admission is tantamount to a consumer credit-granting organization's eliminating all but the first of the above credit steps. Knowledge of the patient's financial profile prior to rendering service or incurring major expense is crucial. Business office staff verification of coverage or the patient's ability to pay for the services prior to admission and treatment ensures that losses are held to a tolerable level. An appropriately conducted preadmission phase can also benefit the patient, by reducing the patient's anxiety about finances, by reducing the waiting time on the day of admission, and by preventing delays in the start of treatment. Waiting until the day of admission or the start-of-treatment date to obtain the necessary data increases the institution's exposure to bad debts, overburdens the admitting staff, and inconveniences the patient. Thus, we strongly recommend the establishment of policies and procedures to ensure that no psychiatric admissions are completed without preadmission financial review and approval by the appropriate staff elements.

Preadmission Forms

The preadmission form must solicit sufficient data to enable the assigned staff members to readily analyze and render a sound and fair credit decision that will reduce the financial concerns of the patient, the family, and the institution. The preadmission application form and accompanying admission record that have been used successfully for several years at Lenox Hill Hospital are shown as Exhibits 18–1 and 18–2. These forms contain the basic data elements on which a sound admission decision can be based.

The Lenox Hill preadmission application form was designed to eliminate the need to contact the patient or the patient's family repeatedly about current clinical or financial conditions. In addition to the Admitting Department, several other departments are required to interact with the patient or family in order to establish financial, medical, or other records. The information on the Exhibit 18–1 preadmission application form is transcribed on the Exhibit 18–2 admission record, which is then usually distributed, in full

Exhibit 18–1 Lenox Hill Hospital Preadmission Application

LENOX HILL HOSPITAL
100 EAST 77TH STREET / NEW YORK, N. Y. 10021
Founded 1857
PRE-ADMISSION APPLICATION

REMARKS (FOR HOSPITAL USE ONLY)

▼ FOR HOSPITAL USE ONLY ▼

| ATTENDING DOCTOR | SERVICE |
| REFERRING DOCTOR | DATE OF ADMISSION |

ACCOMMODATION P ☐ S ☐ W ☐   CONFIRM ☐ ON CALL ☐   PRIVATE DUTY NURSE YES ☐ NO ☐

| LENGTH OF STAY | HISTORY NUMBER | FINANCIAL COUNSELOR |

PRINT OR TYPE   PLEASE COMPLETE AND RETURN THIS APPLICATION IMMEDIATELY

FILL IN ALL SPACES, INCLUDING SHADED AREAS, COMPLETELY

If you have any questions, please call (212) 794-4218

PATIENT DATA

PATIENT'S NAME (LAST NAME FIRST) · BIRTH DATE · BIRTH PLACE · AGE · MARITAL STATUS (SINGLE / WIDOWED / MARRIED / SEPARATED / DIVORCED) · SEX · RELIGION · SOCIAL SECURITY NO.

STREET ADDRESS · APT. NO./IN CARE OF · CITY AND STATE · ZIP CODE · HOME PHONE NO. · YRS AT THIS ADDRESS · NO. OF OTHER

OCCUPATION · EMPLOYER'S NAME · EMPLOYER'S ADDRESS (STREET) · CITY AND STATE · ZIP CODE · BUSINESS PHONE

YEARS EMPLOYED · ANNUAL INCOME IN THOUSANDS OF $ (☐ 2-5 ☐ 10-15 ☐ OVER ☐ 5-10 ☐ 15-20 ☐ 20) · HAVE YOU EVER BEEN HOSPITALIZED · WHEN? · WHERE? · HOW LONG? · IS HOSPITALIZATION RESULT OF ACCIDENT? YES ☐ NO ☐ · WAS ACCIDENT AT WORK? YES ☐ NO ☐

HAVE YOU BEEN PREVIOUSLY ADMITTED TO THIS HOSPITAL? YES ☐ NO ☐ INPATIENT ☐ OUTPATIENT ☐ YEAR 19 __ · IF CLAIMING BLOOD CREDITS GIVE NAME OF ORGANIZATION? · ARE YOU A VETERAN? YES ☐ NO ☐

ANY OTHER FAMILY MEMBERS HOSPITALIZED WITHIN PAST TWO YEARS? (NAME, DATE, HOSPITAL, HOW LONG?)

FINANCIAL MISC.

NEAREST RELATIVE OR FRIEND · RELATIONSHIP · ADDRESS · HOME PHONE · BUSINESS PHONE

FATHER'S NAME · BIRTH PLACE · LIVING YES ☐ NO ☐ · MOTHER'S MAIDEN NAME · BIRTH PLACE · LIVING YES ☐ NO ☐

RESPONSIBLE PARTY'S NAME · RELATIONSHIP · HOME PHONE · BUSINESS PHONE · ANNUAL INCOME (IN THOUSANDS OF $) ☐ 3-5 ☐ 10-15 ☐ Over 20 ☐ 5-10 ☐ 15-20

RESPONSIBLE PARTY'S ADDRESS (STREET) · (APT. NO.) · (CITY AND STATE) · ZIP CODE · OCCUPATION · YEARS NO. OF EMPLOYED

EMPLOYER OF RESPONSIBLE PARTY · EMPLOYER'S ADDRESS (STREET) · (CITY AND STATE) · (ZIP CODE)

SPOUSE'S NAME · AGE · BIRTH PLACE · OCCUPATION · YEARS EMPLOYED · BUSINESS PHONE · ANNUAL INCOME IN (THOUSANDS OF $) ☐ 3-5 ☐ 10-15 ☐ Over 20 ☐ 5-10 ☐ 15-20

SPOUSE'S EMPLOYER · EMPLOYER'S ADDRESS (STREET) · (CITY AND STATE) · (ZIP CODE)

INSURANCE

CERTIFICATE OR GROUP NO. · SUFFIX · EFFECTIVE DATE · SUBSCRIBER'S NAME (AS IT APPEARS ON CARD) · ADDRESS

RELATIONSHIP · SOCIAL SECURITY NO. · NAME OF GROUP · ADDRESS · BLUE SHIELD YES ☐ NO ☐

POLICY NUMBER · INSURANCE COMPANY NAME · ADDRESS · TELEPHONE NUMBER

GROUP ☐ INDIV ☐ IF UNION LOCAL IF GROUP GROUP NAME · NAME OF POLICY HOLDER · SOCIAL SECURITY NO.

UNION ☐ EMPLOYER ☐ UNION ☐ · ADDRESS · TELEPHONE NUMBER TO CONFIRM BENEFITS

M A NUMBER · SUFFIX · TYPE OF ASSISTANCE · EXPIRATION DATE · CASE NAME (NAME ON CARD)

TYPE OF SERVICE · ADULTS · CHILDREN · WELFARE CENTER AND NUMBER

M C NUMBER · SUFFIX · EFFECTIVE DATE PART A · EFFECTIVE DATE PART B · NAME ON CARD

SENIOR CARE NUMBER · SUFFIX · EFFECTIVE DATE

WCS NUMBER · EMPLOYER AT TIME OF INJURY · ADDRESS · PHONE NUMBER

CARRIER · ADDRESS · DATE OF INJURY

DELAY IN ADMISSION WILL RESULT UNLESS ALL NECESSARY INSURANCE IDENTIFICATION AND CLAIM FORMS ARE PRESENTED AT TIME OF ADMISSION.

Form No. F159 Rev. 7/73

Source: Courtesy of Lenox Hill Hospital, New York City.

Exhibit 18–2 Lenox Hill Hospital Admission Record

LENOX HILL HOSPITAL

ADMISSION RECORD

100 EAST 77TH STREET / NEW YORK, N.Y. 10021

CHART COPY

HISTORY NUMBER	ADMIT DATE	ROOM NO.	BED NO.	ROOM TEL. NO.	ACC. TYPE	TRANS. ROOM NO.	BED NO.	ROOM TEL. NO.	ACC. TYPE	JO. NO.	FIN. CL.	# PLANS	ADMITTING DR. NO.

P

PATIENT NAME (LAST NAME FIRST)		ADDRESS: STREET	CITY		COUNTY	STATE	ZIP CODE	APT. NO.	IN CARE OF

HOME TELEPHONE NO.	BIRTH DATE	BIRTH PLACE		AGE	SEX	MAR. ST.	MA	RELIGION	RACE	SOCIAL SECURITY NO.

DISCHARGE DATE	DISCHARGE TIME	OCCUPATION	ADMISSION CODES	PAI

UBF-1   DDA

EMPLOYER'S NAME	EMPLOYER'S ADDRESS: STREET	CITY & STATE	ZIP CODE	BUSINESS PHONE	YEARS EMPLOYED

REFERRING DOCTOR	REF. DR. NO.	ATTENDING DOCTOR	ATTEND. DR. NO.	HOSP. SERV.

SPOUSE'S NAME	AGE	SPOUSE'S BIRTHPLACE	SAI	OCCUPATION	SPOUSE'S EMPLOYER

SPOUSE'S EMPLOYER'S ADDRESS	PATIENT'S NEXT OF KIN	RELATIONSHIP

NEXT OF KIN'S ADDRESS: STREET	CITY & STATE	ZIP CODE	HOME TELEPHONE NO.	BUSINESS TELEPHONE NO.

FATHER'S NAME & BIRTHPLACE	LIVING?	MOTHER'S MAIDEN NAME & BIRTH PLACE	LIVING?

PRIOR HOSPITALIZATION - NAME	DATE FROM	DATE THRU	IN P	OUT P

IS HOSPITALIZATION RESULT OF ACCIDENT?	WAS ACCIDENT AT WORK?	OCCUPATIONAL INJURY OR ILLNESS	MOTOR VEHICLE RELATED	OTHER	ARE YOU CLAIMING BLOOD CREDITS?	NAME OF THE ORGANIZATION RELEASING THE BLOOD CREDITS

ADMITTING DIAGNOSIS (PRIMARY)	ADMITTING DIAGNOSIS CODE	EST. NO. OF DAYS

ADMITTING DIAGNOSIS (SECONDARY)	SECONDARY CODE

INFECTIOUS PROCESS	INFECTIOUS PROCESS CODE

GUARANTOR'S NAME	ADDRESS: STREET	CITY & STATE	ZIP CODE

GUARANTOR'S TELEPHONE NO.	GUARANTOR'S OCCUPATION	GAI	NAME & ADDRESS OF GUARANTOR'S EMPLOYER

INSURED'S MAILING ADDRESS: STREET	CITY	COUNTY	STATE	ZIP CODE

CERTIFICATE OR GROUP NO.	SUFFIX	DATE EFFECTIVE	SUBSCRIBER (AS NAME APPEARS ON CARD)	BLUE SHIELD

NAME & ADDRESS OF GROUP

MEDICARE NUMBER	SUFFIX	PART A: EFFECT. DATE	PART B: EFFECT. DATE	NAME ON CARD	SENIOR CARE: NO/SUFFIX	EFFECT. DATE

INSURANCE POLICY NO.	NAME OF POLICY HOLDER	POLICYHOLDER'S SOCIAL SECURITY NO.

INSURANCE COMPANY'S NAME & ADDRESS	INS. CO. TEL. NO.

MEDICAID NUMBER	NAME ON CARD

TYPE OF ASSISTANCE	TYPE SERVICE	COVERAGE		WELFARE CENTER NO.	EFFECTIVE DATE	EXPIRATION DATE
		ADULT	CHILDREN			

WORKMAN'S COMP. WCB. NO.	EMPLOYER AT TIME OF INJURY	ADDRESS	EMPLOYER'S TELEPHONE NO.

CARRIER	ADDRESS	DATE OF INJURY

ATTORNEY'S INFORMATION	ADMITTED BY	ADMIT TIME

REMARKS (IF ACCIDENT GIVE DATE. TIME. PRECINCT & BADGE NO.)	VALUABLES ENVELOPE NO.

189 1/FF (6/80)

Source: Courtesy of Lenox Hill Hospital, New York City.

or in part, to a number of service departments that will interact prior to, during, and often after the patient's stay. Most of the preadmission application forms for elective admissions to Lenox Hill Hospital are completed by the patient or the patient's family at home. Some are completed by business office staff when the patient visits the office or is scheduled for admission as an inpatient from the outpatient department (clinic).

The institution's preadmission application form can be made available to the patient separately or as part of a more complete information package available to the patient in the physician's office or by mail when the admission date is first booked. Alternatively, a business or admitting office representative can contact the patient or family by telephone, explain the reason for the requested information, and proceed to complete the form.

Key Features

Key features of the Exhibit 18-1 preadmission application form—indicated by element numbers I through XI superimposed on the form—and their relation to psychiatric admissions are detailed in the following paragraphs.

Element I, the remarks section at the top of the form, is completed by the representative who conducts the financial review, evaluation, and approval process. Element II identifies the attending physician, the referring physician, the service, and the tentative date of admission. It also notifies the financial reviewer if a private room accommodation has been requested.

In Element III, in addition to the traditional identifying features (name, address, and so on), the patient's Social Security number is requested to facilitate identification. "Apartment number" and "in-care-of" data are requested to minimize the possibility of mail returns.

Element IV, the patient's occupation, is an indirect verification of income. Quite often, the patient's occupation can lead to additional insurance information, through membership in a trade union or other professional organization. For example, physicians usually maintain their own individual health insurance plans, but they may have additional coverage through the local or national medical organizations of which they are members.

In Element V, the employer's name, address, and telephone number are requested. This information may be of assistance in developing additional coverage and in enhancing the ability, when necessary, to contact the patient to collect final payments.

Elements VI and VII, the years employed and income, may be indicators of stability and the ability to pay for services not covered by a third party insurance provider. In the Lenox Hill experience, the request for income information has not been a problem. Though, in general, people with better-than-average incomes are not comfortable indicating their exact incomes, the income "block" indicators create little resistance. The "over-$20,000" block creates no problems, since the average patient at Lenox Hill does not have an income over $20,000 and may indeed derive a certain amount of satisfaction from being grouped with individuals in a substantially higher income bracket. The same is true of the other four income blocks; at least half of the patients in each block will fall into the bottom half of the indicated income bracket and thus may experience some satisfaction in being grouped with individuals earning a higher income.

Most institutions request the Element VIII information about prior admissions at their hospitals. The section regarding "any other family members hospitalized within the past two years" often leads to additional third party insurance coverage.

Element IX information on other responsible parties is important in a credit environment. The other responsible party's home address, business, and telephone number are needed to ensure that the guarantor has sufficient stability and income to repay the debt. With regard to Element X, in addition to the spouse's name, it is important to obtain information on the spouse's occupation, employer, and income. Every opportunity to uncover additional health insurance is worth investigating.

Element XI, the insurance section, has subsections relating to the major types of health insurance providers. The pertinent information is that relating to the patient's or the spouse's health insurance providers. The separate sections for each major coverage ensures that the information needed to identify and qualify the patient for eligibility and benefits for each type of insurance is obtained. Because of cost-containment measures established by federal, state, and local governments and by individual insurers, it is important to coordinate multiple benefits to make certain that the primary insurance provider is billed and pays for the service rendered to its member. Often, the patient is not aware of multiple coverage and may be anxious, or prepared, to pay the remaining balance after the primary insurer payment is calculated. If second or third insurance coverage is discovered, it can provide additional benefits after the initial benefits from the primary insurer have been exhausted, thus obviating payment by the patient.

Medical Transfers

With the development of more active psychiatric consultation-liaison services in many general hospitals, an important, but often neglected, issue has emerged. This concerns the status of the medical patient for whom primary psychiatric care is clinically indicated at some point in the hospitalization. In such cases, it is advisable that the psychiatric professional staff treat the patient on a consulting basis pending the business office's financial review, evaluation, and approval.

Admission

Essential Procedures

The admission of the patient involves much more than a nonmedical registration. Admitting office staff who pride themselves on getting new elective-admission patients in their assigned rooms within 15 minutes of their arrival may be doing the institution, and probably the patient, a grave financial disservice.

A "new" patient is one who either has not previously been admitted to the institution or who has not been processed during the preadmission phase. In either case, a financial review and evaluation, however brief, is necessary. This does not present a problem if the general hospital has a combined admitting-business office arrangement, or if the admitting clerical staff have been trained to make financial reviews, and evaluations of patients' admission data. If no such arrangement exists, it is advisable for the patient to be referred to the business office for the financial review and evaluation. If referral is inconvenient for the patient or staff, a business office representative may be sent to the admitting office to undertake the financial review and evaluation.

A quick admission without a relevant financial review sometimes leads to a financial liability for the hospital, patient, or family. The requisite accumulation, verification, and evaluation of the key data elements are best accomplished in a controlled environment. An early preadmission phase will allow sufficient time to address concerns arising from incomplete or inaccurate information. The additional time spent in the preadmission phase will reduce the element of risk for both the hospital and the patient by giving the reviewer more verified factors on which to base judgment. The admitting office staff can further reduce the element of financial risk by photocopying all documents that the patient brings in.

Signatures authorizing the release of information regarding assignment of insurance benefits should be obtained prior to the admission. Various consent forms should also be signed prior to the admission. It is often advisable to have such forms signed by the patient's family member who is responsible or who, in the case of an insurance claim, is the insured party.

Emergency or acute admissions present the greatest financial risk. All available socioeconomic information about the psychiatric patient who has been admitted, or is about to be admitted, from the emergency room must be conveyed to the business office staff as soon as possible so that the financial review process can be started. If the patient is unable or unwilling to communicate, an escort (a family member, employer, coworker), can often supply sufficient data to establish a working file.

If socioeconomic information on an acutely ill patient is incomplete or inadequate, that fact should be made known to the admitting psychiatrist, who can then obtain the required information when the patient is able or willing to communicate. Members of the floor nursing staff and the social service staff should also be alerted to the fact that further information is required. They may then either try to obtain the required information directly or refer the patient's visitors to the business office to be interviewed.

Miscellaneous Charges

The patient may clinically require, or the family may request, services that are not included as covered services by the insurance provider. The two highest-cost items in this category are private rooms and private duty nurses. If, because of the patient's special condition, it is determined by the admitting physician that such a service is required, the health insurance carrier may allow, or may pay for, such services. However, in many cases, such coverage is doubtful. A patient should not be admitted under the auspices of a psychiatric scatter-bed program if the patient's condition warrants a higher level of care than can be provided under the program's protocol. In such cases, serious consideration should be given to transferring the patient to a segregated inpatient psychiatric unit.

Interim Billing

Some institutions do not render interim bills to the patient, family, or third party health insurer while the patient is still in-house. Yet, interim billing has many advantages, whether or not the patient is insured. As a matter of sound business practice, we recommend interim billing, even if it is not required by the third party insurer.

The major advantages of interim billing are that it makes it possible to:

- accelerate cash flow
- verify the third party insurer's benefits
- verify the patient's ability to pay, as judged by the business office staff during the preadmission phase
- reduce the need for the hospital to borrow operating cash, thereby reducing interest costs
- to apprise the hospital of the patient's potential need for financial assistance in the event the interim bill is not paid by the patient or family

- limit loss exposure and control the amount lost at the earliest possible point
- monitor admission procedures to ensure that benefits have not been exhausted

If the patient needs financial assistance (for example, Medicaid), the relevant application usually requires considerably more information than was required by the admitting institution. Copies of documents (birth certificates, bank books, rent receipts, proof of income, and so on) may have to be submitted to the qualifying agency, along with the application for assistance. The patient and the family are usually better motivated to assist with the additional information and documentation while the patient is still undergoing treatment. A determination after discharge that the patient, the family, or the third party will not or cannot pay the bill can easily lead to a bad debt.

It is recommended that, as a matter of policy, uninsured patients or patients responsible for a portion of the expense be billed at 7-day intervals. Third party insurers should be interim-billed at 21-day intervals, unless the insurer mandates otherwise.

Discharge

The discharge phase provides the last opportunity for the business office staff to review and obtain additional information or signatures before the patient leaves the hospital. Unfortunately, the patient's willingness to provide additional information or documentation progressively decreases after the crisis is ended. In essence, the review in the discharge phase is similar to that of the preadmission phase, but it must be performed in a relatively shorter time. As indicated earlier, a full review in an earlier phase is much more desirable and effective, for both the business office and the patient.

All patients should be accompanied to the business office for discharge unless previously cleared for discharge by the business office staff. An appropriate procedure for this, involving the nursing department and the business office, should be established. The advantages of such a procedure will be obvious to both the nursing and the business office staff.

Billing

To be effective and provide adequate cash flow, billing must be prepared and submitted within a few days of the discharge. The bill should be complete and accurate and should contain any attachments previously identified as necessary to support the charges. The bill should be directed to the appropriate third party or individual payer, as identified and verified during an earlier phase. Consideration should be given to (1) the primacy of responsibility for payment; (2) the completeness of the mailing address, including the name of someone who may be able to expedite payment; (3) the number of required copies; (4) required attachments, including:

- specified claim or assignment forms
- record of partial payments
- formal confirmation of benefits, as supplied by the patient's employer or insurance carrier
- rejection or partial-payment documentation from the primary insurance carrier
- copies of the required portion of the patient's medical record to certify the treatment and final diagnosis

The required attachments should be identified before the billing phase. Other documentation required to support the bill may be determined as a result of the business office staff's follow-up with the insurance carrier. The business office should anticipate any extraordinary requirements, in order to ensure immediate processing of the bill, and to avoid any delay in cash flow.

Follow-up

A follow-up effort with an insurer to collect for psychiatric services is virtually identical to that required to collect for nonpsychiatric services; both are based on data identified in the billing phase. The normal billing cycle that is utilized for other services should be used for follow-up. The waiting period prior to written or telephone contact with the carrier is likely to vary with the institution's experience with that carrier, or with the period designated by the carrier.

Any extraordinary delay in payment patterns should be formally addressed by the institution's financial managers. The difficulty may lie with the quality of the billing or attachments, or it may be due to the failure of the hospital, physician, or patient to respond in a timely fashion to the insurer. The development of a delayed payment pattern must be analyzed and attended to. The hospital's billing policy and procedures should be examined before any contact is made with management personnel of the insurer. The hospital's self-examination should then form the basis for an evaluation of the insurer's processing policy and procedures in order to identify the problem and expedite both the outstanding claim and any future claims.

The nature and extent of the follow-up effort will be determined by the quality and effectiveness of the business office staff's work during the earlier phases of the billing cycle. The individual's ability and willingness to pay should have been established before the final bill was prepared after discharge. The individual should have been made aware of the approximate cost and responsibility for payment. Other than rejection by an insurer for unanticipated reasons, the balance due from the individual should be for the period from the last interim billing to the patient's discharge.

An unanticipated insurer rejection should be explored, upon receipt, with the patient, the insured party, or the insurer before a bill is rendered. An error in a minor item, such as an omitted or incorrect digit in an identification number, can be quickly adjusted to avoid any additional anxiety to the patient and ensure payment without further delay.

A special dunning cycle is not necessary for a patient treated for a mental illness. The standard bill and statements in use for other patients are. adequate. The time between discharge and billing and the type, number, and timing of the dunning statements are matters to be determined by policy. However, we recommend billing the patient within 5 days of discharge, with two or three follow-up dunning statements at 15-day intervals. To effect payment, each statement should contain a progressively stronger legend, as indicated in the following formats:

Format	Legend
Bill:	"Payment due upon receipt of bill."
First statement (optional):	"Perhaps you overlooked our bill."
Second statement:	"Past due. Please pay immediately."
Third (final) statement:	"Final notice. Nonpayment within ten days will result in referral to our attorney for legal action."

Telephone or special letter contact may also be implemented, depending on institutional policies, past experience, policy, the amount due, and so on.

As with any other kind of patient, the socioeconomic condition of a mentally ill patient may not return to normal immediately after discharge. The patient's ability to function at business or in the home environment may be impaired, temporarily or permanently. In these situations, sound judgment must be exercised, based upon facts supplied by the individual, the family, and the physician or therapist. The payment arrangements, including delay or waiver of payments, must be based strictly on the individual's ability to pay, not merely on a promise that cannot be substantiated by the individual's socioeconomic condition.

FINANCING AND MARKETING OUTPATIENT SERVICES AND ALTERNATIVE MODES OF CARE

Most acute care general hospitals have (or want to have) outpatient psychiatric services, in addition to inpatient psychiatric scatter-bed services or a segregated inpatient unit. Health insurance providers cover, in varying degrees and without standardization, all modes of outpatient treatment. Among third party health insurance providers, there is no common key or identifier to determine if a particular mode of psychiatric outpatient service is covered, and if so, to what extent. Thus, for a particular clientele or region, it is necessary first to document the relevant coverage in a careful survey of insurance providers that service that clientele and region. The resulting information can be then utilized by the business office staff to develop an overview of available psychiatric coverage. The determination of benefits available in the target area will provide direction for marketing both scatter-bed programs and outpatient services. The existing psychiatric coverage in the area may dictate which programs to offer initially.

The survey data can also provide the foundation for a long-range plan. An inquiry about uncovered services may create in the group or employer being interviewed an interest in considering coverage. Because of the current trend toward cost containment, enquiries about less expensive modes of treatment, such as those provided on an outpatient basis, may lead to their promotion as alternatives to more expensive inpatient services. In the case of insurance provided by employers, an additional selling point is the fact that inpatient service results in greater loss of productivity at the individual's workplace and home, compared to outpatient service.

Program features that are supported but not accepted currently by governing bodies, employers, self-insured groups, or the general service population may become the seeds of future expansion to meet the growing needs of the community. In this way, the documentation of service trends can help the institution anticipate and plan growth and encourage coverage.

The survey and resulting interviews may cover, but need not be limited to, the following services. We suggest input from each member of the psychiatric service development team to modify or expand the list prior to the initiation of the community survey.

- day care
- night care

- vocational rehabilitation
- recreational rehabilitation
- teen or young adult programs
- parent educational programs
- child psychiatry services
- clinic visits; individual or group therapy
- day or evening outpatient clinics
- pain treatment programs: inpatient and outpatient
- counselling programs for cancer patients: coping with terminal care
- alcohol and drug-abuse programs
- weight-loss and smoke-ending groups

REFERENCES

1. A. Biegel and S. Sharfstein, "Mental Health Care Providers: Not the Only Cause or Only Cure for Rising Costs," *American Journal of Psychiatry* 141 (1984): 668–672.

2. S. Muszynski, J. Brady, and S. Sharfstein, "Paying for Psychiatric Care," *Psychiatric Annals* 14 (1984): 861–869.

3. C. Kiesler, "Mental Hospitals and Alternative Care: Noninstitutionalization as Potential Public Policy for Mental Patients," *American Psychologist* 37 (1983): 349–360.

4. B. Levin and J. Glasser, "Mental Health Coverage within Prepaid Health Plans," *Administration in Mental Health* 7 (1980): 271–281.

5. National Institute of Mental Health, *The Financing, Utilization and Quality of Mental Health Care in the United States* (Rockville, Md.: Prather, 1976).

6. Biegel and Sharfstein, "Mental Health Care Providers," 668–672.

7. W. Guillette et al., "Day Hospitalization Care: A Pilot Study," *Hospital and Community Psychiatry* 29 (1975): 525–527.

8. S. Washburn et al., "A Controlled Companion of Psychiatric Day Treatment and Inpatient Hospitalization," *Journal of Consulting and Clinical Psychology* 44 (1976): 665–675.

9. J. Goldsmith, "Death of a Paradigm: The Challenge of Competition," *Health Affairs* 3 (1984): 5–19.

10. Muszynski, Brady, and Sharfstein, "Paying," 861–869.

11. J.K. Inglehart, "Hospitals, Public Policy and the Future: An Interview with John Alexander McMahon," *Health Affairs* 3 (1984): 20–34.

12. R. Mollica and F. Redlich, "Equity and Changing Patient Characteristics—1950–1975," *Archives of General Psychiatry* 37 (1980): 1257–1263.

13. Muszynski, Brady, and Sharfstein, "Paying," 861–869.

14. *Report from the Presidents' Commission on Mental Health* (Washington, D.C.: U.S. Government Printing Office, 1978).

15. K.B. Wells et al., *Cost-Sharing and the Demand for Ambulatory Mental Health Service*, Contract No. 278-81-0045(DB) (Rockville, Md.: Department of Health and Human Services, National Institute of Mental Health, 1982).

16. J. Hankin, D. Steinwachs, and E. Chapmian, "The Impact of Utilization of a Copayment Increase for Ambulatory Psychiatric Care," *Medical Care* 18 (1980): 807–815.

17. R. Frank and T. McGuire, *Progress Report on the Demand and Utilization of Specialty Mental Health Services* (Washington, D.C.: American Psychiatric Association, 1983).

18. Edwin C. Hustead, *The Hay Associates Model for Determining Costs of Mental and Nervous Care Insurance* (Washington, D.C.: Hay Higgins Group, 1983).

19. John Krizay, "Federal Employees' Experience as a Guide to the Cost of Insuring Psychiatric Services in Various States," *American Journal of Psychiatry* 139 (1982): 866–871.

20. Washington Psychiatric Society, *Report on Utilization Characteristics of the FEHBP Mental Health Benefits* (Washington, D.C.: Washington Psychiatric Society, 1980).

21. T. McGuire *Financing Psychotherapy: Costs Effects and Public Policy* (Cambridge, Mass.: Ballinger, 1981).

22. B. Liptzin, "The Effects of National Health Insurance on Canadian Psychiatry. The Ontario Experience," *American Journal of Psychiatry* 134 (1977): 248–252.

23. *Report of the Research Triangle Institute, The Cost to Society of Alcohol, Drug Abuse and Mental Illness,* Contract 283-79-001 (Rockville, Md.: Alcohol, Drug Abuse, and Mental Health Administration, 1980).

24. Wells et al., *Cost-Sharing.*

25. Krizay, "Federal Employees' Experience," 866–871.

26. Liptzin, "Effects," 248–252.

27. E. Hustead, *Utilization of Mental Illness Benefits under the Federal Employees Health Benefits Program* (Washington, D.C.: United States Civil Service Commission, 1977).

28. S. Sharfstein and H. Magnas, "Insuring Intensive Psychotherapy," *American Journal of Psychiatry* 132 (1975): 1252–1256.

29. Biegel and Sharfstein, "Mental Health Care Providers," 668–672.

30. A. Reifman and R. Wyatt, "Lithium: A Brake in the Rising Cost of Mental Illness," *Archives of General Psychiatry* 37 (1980): 385–388.

31. M. Smith, G. Glass and T. Miller, *The Benefits of Psychotherapy* (Baltimore, Md.: Johns Hopkins University Press, 1980).

32. U.S. Congress, Office of Technology Assessment, "The Efficacy and Cost Effectiveness of Psychotherapy," in *The Implications of Cost-effectiveness Analysis of Medical Technology,* Background paper no. 3 of the OTA study (Washington, DC: Government Printing Office, 1980).

33. A. Cruze et al., *Final Report: Economic Costs to Society of Alcohol, Drug Abuse and Mental Illness—1977,* Alcohol, Drug Abuse and Mental Health Administration Contract No. 283-79-001 (Rockville, Md.: National Institute of Mental Health, 1981).

34. R. Anderson et al., "Psychologically Related Illness and Health Service Utilization," *Medical Care* suppl. 15 (1977): 59–73.

35. I. Goldberg, G. Krantz, and B. Locke, "Effect of a Short-Term Outpatient Psychiatry Therapy Benefit on the Utilization of Medical Services in a Prepaid Group Practice Medical Program," *Medical Care* 8 (1970): 419–428.

36. J. Jameson, L. Schuman, and W. Young, *The Effect of Outpatient Psychiatric Utilization on the Costs of Providing Third-Party Coverage,* Research Services 18 (Blue Cross of Western Pennsylvania 1970).

37. E. Mumford, H. Schlesinger, and G. Glass, *A Critical Review of the Literature up to*

1978 of the Effects of Psychotherapy on Medical Utilization, part I of the final report, NIMH Contract 278-77-0049 (Rockville, Md.: National Institute of Mental Health, 1984).

38. Ibid.

39. E. Mumford, H. Schlesinger, and G. Glass, "The Effects of Psychological Intervention on Recovery from Surgery and Heart Attacks: An Analysis of the Literature," *American Journal of Public Health* 72 (1982): 141–151.

40. S. Levitan, and D. Kornfeld, "Clinical and Cost Benefits of Liaison Psychiatry," *American Journal of Psychiatry* 138 (1981): 790–793.

41. Muszynski, Brady, and Sharfstein, "Paying," 861–869.

42. S. Sharfstein, S. Muszynski, and A. Gattozzi, *Maintaining and Improving Psychiatric Insurance Coverage: An Annotated Bibliography* (Washington, D.C.: American Psychiatric Association, 1983).

43. Muszynski, Brady, and Sharfstein, "Paying," 861–869.

44. Ibid.

45. Goldsmith, "Death of a Paradigm," 5–14.

46. Ibid.

47. Ibid.

48. Muszynski, Brady, and Sharfstein, "Paying," 861–869.

49. Biegel and Sharfstein, "Mental Health Care Providers," 668–672.

50. Muszynski, Brady, and Sharfstein, "Paying," 861–869.

51. Goldsmith, "Death of a Paradigm," 5–19.

52. Inglehart, "Hospitals," 20–34.

53. Sharfstein, Muszynski, and Gattozzi, *Maintaining and Improving.*

54. O. Towery, S. Sharfstein, and I. Goldberg, "The Mental and Nervous Disorder Utilization and Cost Survey (MANDUCS): An Analysis of Insurance for Mental Disorders," *American Journal of Psychiatry* 137 (1980): 1065–1070.

Chapter 19

Marketing Mental Health Services

Roger Barker and Herbert H. Krauss

INTRODUCTION

Marketing is seen as a peripheral enterprise by most members of the mental health professions. There are many reasons for this attitude: the mistaken belief that marketing is synonymous with advertisement; the justified, long-standing, fundamental proscriptions in the ethical canons of medicine, psychology, and social work against certain forms of advertising and self-promotion; the view that laymen are insufficiently prepared to evaluate the public claims of the professions; and, finally, the widely held opinion of professionals that the hurly-burly of the marketplace is beneath them.

The fact that some advertising and promotional material is misleading or false has fueled professional disdain for marketing activities. Historically, we are in fact not far removed in time from the medicine show and its panaceas. Too often, advertising overstates, pushes, intrudes, and demands attention, like a bad child. Indeed, for most mental health professionals, advertising is still regarded as little more than hucksterism. These professionals have been taught throughout their careers that ideas and practices are best reviewed and evaluated by peers, that their practices must be based on scientific merit alone. As long as these perceptions persist, mental health professionals will resist engaging in marketing activities.

Given these circumstances, it is not surprising that, until recently, there has been relatively little effective and sophisticated marketing of mental health services. Much of the marketing of such services has been limited to public information slots on local radio and television stations and to an occasional laudatory newspaper article describing a hospital's mental health services. Unfortunately, the avoidance of mental health marketing activities by professionals has deprived many potential beneficiaries of needed services, simply because they did not know that help was available. In many instances, the lack of a sophisticated marketing strategy—one that links consumer need and institutional responses—has retarded the development of desirable, cost-effective mental health services.

In recent years, however, the recognition has grown that the marketing of mental health services is an essential component of the hospital's commitment to the effective care of its patients and to the community.[1] Several factors have contributed to this more accepting attitude toward marketing:

- more sophisticated view of the nature of the marketing enterprise, including an awareness that marketing is an orientation and process designed to study, plan, and manage exchange relationships between service consumers and service providers in a systematic manner[2-4]
- changes in the attitudes of professional associations toward promotional activities
- the decision of the federal government to "reprivatize" health care and foster competition among health service providers
- the growing penetration of the health care sector by institutions with a business orientation toward marketing practices[5-7]
- government pressure on health care providers to offer consumer-oriented, cost-effective services[8]
- an attempt on the part of all third party providers (both government and private insurers) to shift a greater portion of their costs, especially mental health costs, back upon the consumers of these services, thereby increasing consumer reservations about seeking such services and making those who need them more selective about their options

Taken together, these factors suggest that, in the coming years, marketing will play an increasingly important role in determining the success—perhaps survival—of health care institutions in a more intensely competitive marketplace. If this is true for health care services in general, it is likely to be doubly true for mental health services, which have long been the neglected step-children of the health care establishment.

MARKET ORIENTATION AND PLANNING

Apart from the many functions it performs, the hospital exists as a business. And "the purpose of business," as Levitt points out, "is to get and keep a customer."[9] Thus, without a reasonable proportion of solvent customers, there will be no business. If the hospital cannot produce and deliver services that its potential clients want, at prices and under conditions that are attractive when compared with those of its competitors, the hospital will fail, regardless of the quality of care it offers.

To continue to function, the hospital must reliably produce revenues in excess of, or in some reasonable balance to, costs. This cannot be accomplished by accident or instinct; it requires strategic and tactical business planning. A plan for marketing is an essential component of the total business strategy. A modern marketing orientation is not simply to "sell" available services to a reluctant customer. Rather, marketing plans require that:

- external factors that will significantly influence the service market be evaluated
- the internal strengths and weaknesses of the service provider be analyzed
- opportunities to offer specific services to the community be identified
- promotional strategies for each offered service be developed and the likelihood of their success be assessed[10]

By external factors, the marketer means the configuration of economic, demographic, technical, and governmental factors that significantly influence the health care provider in the arena in which he must compete. Such external factors include rates of inflation, taxation, and unemployment; the institution's cost of doing business and its likely cost trajectory; the rate structure for services in the community; the income, age, employment, and ethnic mix of the community; the community's acceptance of the institution; and the availability, reliability, and cost of needed technology (computers, biofeedback equipment, and so on).

The internal strength of the hospital resides, not only in its client base, technical facilities, financial resources, and equipment, but also in the perceived quality of its management, services, and personnel. In "high-contact" service businesses, the quality of the service is inseparable from the quality of the service provider and the patient's perception of that quality.[11]

To a marketer, the key to developing a service spectrum is the subdivision of the market into relatively homogeneous groups of potential clients, that is, into market segments. For each market segment, certain questions are asked. Steps are taken to provide objective answers to the questions: What are the health care needs of potential consumers? Does the institution possess the ability to offer or develop such services? What factors will influence consumers' decisions to seek such services? How can needed services be offered in a readily available, cost-effective manner? To what extent will health-care users be able to afford the proffered services? How will regulatory factors influence the services to be offered? How will the services be promoted? How successfully will they compete in the marketplace with those offered by other providers? What is the long-range future of these services? To what extent will the institution be committed to provide them or similar services?

For any potential service, the strategic marketing plan describes the service to be offered, specifies how it is to be priced, details the plans for its promotion, assigns it a place and priority in the overall package of services to be offered to clients by the institution, and develops criteria to assess whether the provided service is likely to be successful in the marketplace. Such a plan is best subdivided into three segments, depicting the tactics to be employed (1) when the service is first offered, (2) when the acceptance of the service by consumers has been achieved, and (3) when the service has matured, that is, when it has achieved its greatest impact upon its targeted market segment.[12]

For each service the following questions are asked:

- What is the nature of the service?
- What type of relationship does the service organization have with its customers?
- How much room is there for customization and judgment on the part of the service provider?
- What is the nature of the demand for the service?
- How is the service delivered?
- What are the attributes of the service product?

ORGANIZATIONAL STRUCTURE: THE MARKETING COMMITTEE

The successful implementation of a modern marketing plan for mental health services in the general hospital requires more than just a change of attitude toward marketing by professionals. It requires that marketing professionals and mental health professionals act as a team. The marketing plan must be developed and implemented by trained personnel who are allocated sufficient resources and responsibilities by the hospital to enable them to function successfully. Investing in marketing competence requires the same commitment to excellence as investing in clinical departments.

In developing an organizational structure for marketing operations, however, one has to be realistic. It may not be possible to recruit a quality marketing professional because of cost constraints or the inherent difficulty of attracting such a person to a health care facility. But the hospital can still establish an effective marketing division. It can choose either to avail itself of marketing consultants or to develop its own internal resources for marketing its services.

Each path has its advantages and disadvantages. The use of marketing consultants provides direct access to high-level outside experts with marketing skills. Yet these consultants may not be sufficiently aware of the hospital's unique marketing position, its personnel, or its internal capacity to formulate a workable and effective marketing plan. Marketing plans require repeated modification and fine tuning. Thus, the cost in money, time, and lost efficiency from using consultative services may well make it more expensive than originally anticipated.

On the other hand, every general hospital has on its staff a number of individuals who have excellent communication, business, and research skills, who already have the requisite knowledge of the hospital and its capacities, and who have intimate contacts with the community. Such individuals, given appropriate institutional support and perhaps additional training, could form the cadre necessary to formulate a marketing strategy.

This cadre could, in effect, become a "marketing committee" that would be responsible for the entire range of marketing hospital services. Its membership would include representatives from:

- the clinical departments
- the department of public relations
- the department of resources development
- the department of community relations
- the department of quality assurance
- the business office
- the administration
- the department of planning
- a marketing staff professional or consultant

The leadership of the committee should be determined by the particular strengths of the hospital's staff relative to the marketing area. It may be necessary to entrust the marketing staff professional or consultant with the chairmanship.

The committee's tasks would be to:

- ensure that the hospital maintains an ongoing marketing orientation and program

- coordinate the clinical services and financial and other support divisions of the hospital to ensure that economic returns are maximized and quality services are provided to the community
- plan, review, and promote the service program initiatives of the hospital
- determine the adequacy of both the mix of clinical services being offered and their delivery systems
- recommend modification in either the mix or the delivery of clinical services

Whatever the organizational structure that is developed, effective marketing will require that an accurate, reliable, and effective communication network be established between the hospital's administrative and clinical service departments and the clients who are to be served. This network must be open continuously to mutually informative dialogue.

Obviously, the development of an effective marketing committee will take time and effort, but its value will surely become apparent as the hospital aggressively searches for new ways to accomplish its mission.

TARGETING MENTAL HEALTH SERVICES

Community Needs

The general hospital must begin its mental health marketing activities by ascertaining the mental health needs of the community. Epidemiological studies; surveys by federal, state and local governments; reports by health systems agencies, and analyses of community utilization of the mental health services the hospital already offers—all are useful in determining patterns of need.

Unfortunately, there is no necessary correlation between understanding community needs and translating that understanding into a workable mental health delivery system. As in the industrial sector, determining that a consumer need exists does not guarantee development of a product that will meet that need. Nor does it ensure that, if the product is created, it will meet with consumer acceptance and be profitable. In fact, the most creative and demanding of all mental health marketing challenges is to determine which service, if developed, will, at one and the same time, meet the professional standards of those who deliver the service, be desired by those for whom the service is intended, and contribute to the fiscal well-being of the provider institution.

The Service Review

Before establishing any new mental health services, the hospital's mental health division should of course evaluate the quality, accessibility, and acceptability of existing services. For most hospitals, the list of offered mental health services will encompass a broad range of activities and programs that have been developed as a result of government mandate, staff interest, community pressure, or experienced need. In many instances, the services may be provided throughout the hospital under the joint auspices of several clinical divisions. Thus, mental health professionals may be attached to pediatrics, neurology, oncology and cardiology, as well as psychiatry. This wide complexity makes the development of a comprehensive, coordinated mental health program an arduous task, but one that is clearly essential if the hospital is to develop an effective marketing program.

The following are examples of existing mental health services that should be reviewed and evaluated before embarking on a major marketing effort:

- psychiatric consultation-liaison services
- psychiatric emergency services
- acute care psychiatric hospitalization services
- psychiatric outpatient services
- preventive mental health services
- health education services (for example, parent education workshops)
- occupational and vocational therapy
- inpatient and outpatient rehabilitation
- behavioral medicine or health psychology
- psychological evaluation
- pain management

In reviewing these existing services, the overall positioning of the hospital's mental health services in the community must be noted. For better or worse, as hospitals move increasingly toward the provision of prepaid service plans,[13-15] their fiscal solvency will depend to an ever-greater extent upon the nature of the market segments they serve.[16] For example, the provision of long-term psychotherapy, especially if a large percentage of those being treated are chronically or characterologically disturbed, may prove to be financially embarrassing to the hospital,[17,18] even though society's long-range interest requires that such services be made available.[19]

In conducting the service review, it should be kept in mind that the utilization of services by one segment of the hospital's potential service community may preclude their utilization by another. As Berry has pointed out, when high-contact services are offered (that is, those that require intense consumer-provider interaction), it is rarely the intrinsic quality of the generic service or its price that determines its viability in the market-place. Rather, it is the complex of associations that the product evokes in the mind of the consumer. The perceived quality of the service, the reputation of the service provider, and the perceived quality of the clientele that purchases it are key elements in determining the product's success.[20] For example, a hospital that is known as a provider of drug-abuse services to lower socioeconomic elements is unlikely to be successful in marketing those services, regardless of their quality, cost, or accessibility, to middle- and upper-level corporate executives.

Thus, the evaluation of existing services must take into account the target consumer's view. Are the price, accessibility, and style with which the services are offered likely to appeal to the particular segment of the consumer market that the hospital wants to attract? Bearing in mind that the relationship between a buyer and seller does not end when the service is purchased,[21] every attempt should be made to ensure that, not only the providers of the services, but also the hospital's support component (billing, housekeeping, scheduling, and recordkeeping) operate with the consumer's interest in mind and that these components demonstrate this concern in their daily transactions with the service consumers.

Hospitals operate in a dynamic external environment. Services that were once needed, were effectively provided, and were fiscally sound may no longer be wanted. Similarly, services offered successfully today may prove problematic tomorrow. On the other hand, advances in technology or changes in reimbursement policies may make the creation of new services both possible and desirable. Thus, the service review should aim at both improving the quality and internal marketing of existing services and evaluating the hospital's total mental health service mix. It should also provide the hospital with an assessment of the appropriateness of the market segments its services are reaching in terms of its marketing objectives.

For each service in the total service mix, these questions should be asked:

- Is the service of acceptable quality?
- Under what circumstances can it be offered to ensure its economic viability?
- Is appropriate news of its availability reaching its intended market segment?
- Has it achieved sufficient acceptance with its targeted audience?

If the answer to any of these questions is no, corrective action should be taken. Even if a service passes all these tests, a decision to modify or eliminate it may still be made if its impact upon the total array of services is negative and too difficult to correct.

Changing the Service Mix

Obviously, in those instances in which a mental health service is deemed deficient, the chief of the service, in conjunction with other interested parties, should initiate improvements. In certain circumstances, improvement may not be possible; the relevant specialist may not be available or may be too costly, or the necessary reallocation of departmental resources might weaken services of higher priority. In such circumstances, consideration should be given to eliminating the service.

It is always difficult for a hospital to make changes that will, in effect, deprive patients of existing services. Yet, marginal services not only require the commitment of scarce resources out of proportion to the benefits they generate, they also weaken the ability of the hospital to respond effectively to consumer needs of greater importance. Thus, the paring down of services must be as much a part of service planning and marketing as the creation of new services.[22,23]

In many ways, the process of creating new mental health services parallels that involved in assessing existing ones. It, too, is a protracted task that requires continual interactive dialogue between the hospital and the community. It requires evaluations of community needs and the hospital's willingness and capacity to meet those needs at reasonable cost. It demands a strategic assessment of how the proposed new programs will articulate and complement the hospital's present mental health service mix.

Ideally, the new service will:

- supplement existing programs
- aid the hospital in further penetrating the market segments it intends to serve
- build upon existing programmatic strengths in personnel and technology
- potentially produce financial gains
- stimulate professional growth and morale
- portray the hospital as forward-looking and as a positive agent for change in the community

Using these criteria, it would be feasible, for example, to add chronic pain management and cognitive rehabilitation programs to rehabilitation units, to supplement cardiology and internal medicine services with biofeedback and stress management programs, or to add parent effectiveness training to existing well-baby pediatric programs. In any event, even more than in the case of existing services, new programs need to be presented and promoted effectively to the market segment to which they are targeted.

Promotional Activities

Broadly defined, marketing and promotion are roughly synonymous. However, by custom, promotion refers to activities designed to produce sales, for example, advertising, public relations, and salesmanship. Often, for convenience, promotional activities are divided into two classes: direct and indirect. For the hospital, direct promotional activities are those in which there is face-to-face contact between the hospital's representative and the potential consumer. In indirect promotion,[24] the hospital's message is communicated to potential consumers via intermediary media, for example, radio, television, or print.

On the whole, mental health professionals prefer direct promotion, particularly when attempting to sell a service that requires extensive explanation and is purchased infrequently.[25] This preference, though not firmly based in research, undoubtedly reflects the professionals' suspicion that media advertisements are inherently incomplete or deceptive. It probably also is due to the professionals' inclination to approach potential consumers and referral agents directly, in the belief that direct communication ensures accurate communication, and in the hope that such an approach will have a more effective impact on the potential consumer. Even if these suppositions were supported by evidence, however, direct promotional activities need to be supplemented by indirect methods. In short, a well-thought-out promotional campaign must rely upon a mix of direct and indirect approaches, the exact mix to be determined by the marketing committee and available resources.

Goals

A program designed to promote a hospital-based, mental health service must have multiple aims. It must motivate appropriate potential consumers to seek the service, effectively convey a range of information about the service, and begin to educate the consumers about how they are expected to act if they are to benefit from the service. The program must reach these goals as best it can within the constraints of time, space, and cost. And it must do so without violating professional ethics.

Unlike those who purchase tangible products, the consumers of services operate at a disadvantage.[26,27] They have, in general, little direct experience with the service until they engage in it. They recognize that the quality of the service frequently depends upon the particular characteristics of the service provider and that providers consistently vary in quality, even when evidence of professional competency is required. They recognize that, to a significant extent, they are buying a service whose success cannot be guaranteed. In sum, they recognize that they are at risk.

In addition to these complexities, promoters of mental health services are faced with a special challenge: they must overcome the consumer's natural hesitancy to admit publicly (even if the admission is held in confidence) that the consumer needs outside assistance to cope effectively with some aspect of living. The degree to which the potential consumer's fear of seeking a mental health service is replaced by a realistic hope about the gains the consumer may achieve with that service will determine the success of the promotional campaign.

Reaching the Goals

In any given situation, the choice of means to achieve the promotional goal is crucial.[28] Promotion is more art than science. Thus, the success of the promotional effort will depend upon the effectiveness with which it translates the intangible qualities of the offered service into concrete images, metaphors, and similes that touch the hopes and aspirations of the targeted audience. Exactly how this is done will, of course, depend upon the unique characteristics of the audience—age, educational accomplishments, ethnic identification, and so on.

In addition to the subtle use of images of a better future or institutional reliability, the promotional program can reduce uncertainty on the part of potential consumers by providing concrete information about the service:

- the exact nature of the service
- the quality of the service and of the institution that offers it
- the ease with which the service may be obtained
- the cost of the service
- the gains a client may reasonably expect from the service
- the risks faced by the client who uses the service
- the service's potential users
- advantages of seeking this particular service at this particular hospital

The marketing committee should keep in mind that, while the goal of promotion is to communicate with potential users of mental health services in a manner that will persuade them to buy the services, only a fraction of the promotional dollar should be aimed directly at those consumers. Referral sources must also be convinced that it is worthwhile to direct their clients to the hospital's services. Thus, considerable promotional activity, probably differing from that employed for more general audiences,[29] must be directed toward those who are now, or will be, in contact with potential clients, for example, other mental health and social service agencies, fellow professionals, employee assistance programs, and corporate personnel departments. This is particularly important when the hospital wishes to attract to its services individuals who may benefit from treatment but are unlikely to self-refer. An example of such a situation is that of corporate executives who are in need of alcoholism services but who deny being alcoholics.[30]

The marketing committee should assume responsibility for monitoring the effectiveness of the hospital's promotional efforts. It should also be able to redirect them when it is necessary to do so. In such efforts, it should be aided by systematically conducted surveys that are designed specifically to assess the impact of the hospital's promotional campaigns on the targeted audiences and to determine the patterns of referral to, and the utilization of, the promoted services.

REFERENCES

1. R.W. Gibson, "Strategic Planning and Marketing of Mental Health Services," *Psychiatric Annals* 14 (1984): 846–850.

2. C.H. Lovelock, *Services Marketing* (Englewood Cliffs, N.J.: Prentice-Hall, 1984).

3. T. Levitt, *The Marketing Imagination* (New York: Free Press, 1983).

4. E.R. Corey, *Industrial Marketing: Cases and Concepts,* 3rd ed (Englewood Cliffs, N.J.: Prentice-Hall, 1984).

5. Lovelock, *Services Marketing*.

6. P. Starr, *The Social Transformation of American Medicine* (New York: Basic Books, 1983).

7. "Trends in the Number of Psychiatric Hospitals, Services, Costs, Staff Uncovered by NIMH Survey," *Psychiatric News* (3 February 1984): 24–25.

8. Lovelock, *Services Marketing*.

9. Levitt, *Marketing Imagination*.

10. Corey, *Industrial Marketing*.

11. R.B. Chase, "Where Does the Customer Fit in a Service Operation?" *Harvard Business Review* 516 (1978): 137–142.

12. Corey, *Industrial Marketing*.

13. Gibson, "Strategic Planning."

14. Starr, *Social Transformation*.

15. "Trends."

16. T.E. Bittker, "The Industrialization of American Psychiatry," *American Journal of Psychiatry* 142 (1985): 149–154.

17. "Trends."

18. P. Solomon, J. Davis, and B. Condon, "Discharged State Hospital Patients' Characteristics and the Use of Aftercare: Effect on Community Tenure," *American Journal of Psychiatry* 141 (1984): 1566–1570.

19. Ibid.

20. L.L. Berry, "Service Marketing Is Different," *Business* 30 (1980), 25.

21. Levitt, *Marketing Imagination*.

22. S.H. Rewoldt, J.D. Scott, and M.R. Warschaw, *Introduction to Marketing Management: Text and Cases* (Homewood, Ill.: Irwin, 1982).

23. P. Kotler, *Marketing for Nonprofit Organizations* (Englewood Cliffs, N.J.: Prentice Hall, 1982).

24. Ibid.

25. Ibid.

26. Levitt, *Marketing Imagination*.

27. Berry, "Service Marketing."

28. J. Rohlman et al., *Marketing Human Service Innovations* (Beverly Hills, Calif.: Sage, 1983).

29. Kotler, *Marketing*.

30. Gibson, "Strategic Planning."

Chapter 20

The Future of Mental Health Services in the General Hospital

Herbert H. Krauss and Allen H. Collins

HISTORICAL PERSPECTIVE

The destinies of medicine, the general hospital, and mental health services are—and will be for the foreseeable future—intricately interwoven. This has not always been the case. "Before the Civil War," Paul Starr reminds us, "an American doctor might contentedly spend an entire career in practice without setting foot on a hospital ward."[1] Similarly, from the early years of the nineteenth century until the psychopharmacological revolution of the mid-twentieth, the evolution of treatment for the mentally ill proceeded upon a path that diverged significantly from that followed by "normal" medicine. Today, however, there are signs of increasing rapprochement between general medicine and the psychiatric treatment of mental illness.

The reconciliation, partial though it may prove to be, is the result of the transformation of medicine, mental health services, and the general hospital. "Few institutions," Starr has demonstrated, "have undergone as radical a metamorphosis as have hospitals in their modern history."[2] The same may be said of medicine and mental health treatment delivery systems.

At one time, hospitals were pest holes, far removed from the center of medical practice. Run by religious or charitable organizations, hospitals provided long-term custodial care to the unwashed and unwanted of society—care that the relatives of these unfortunates could not or would not provide for them.

Today, hospitals serve patients from all walks of life, providing rich and poor alike with equivalent care, if not equivalent consideration. The modern hospital is now a well-scrubbed center of high medical specialization and engineering technology. In organization and ethos, it increasingly resembles the modern corporation. Although the sick are still tended in hospitals, it is for ever-shorter periods. Long-term care has been superseded as the hospital's primary task by a new priority: the provision of focused biomedical interventions designed to cure, or at least ameliorate, organic dysfunction. No longer places of asylum, hospitals have become bastions of therapeutic hope.

Medicine has undergone a remarkable parallel evolution. Lewis Thomas, in describing his medical education at Harvard in the 1930s, wrote:

> My medical education was, in principle, much like that of my father. The details had changed a lot since his time . . . but the *purpose* of the curriculum was, if anything, even more conservative than thirty years earlier. It was to teach the recognition of disease entities, their classification, their signs, symptoms, and laboratory manifestations, and how to make an accurate diagnosis. The treatment of disease was the most minor part of the curriculum, almost left out altogether.[3]

Needless to say, a revolution has since transformed medicine. Clearly, there has been exponential progress in the treatment of bacterial infections, the prevention of many viral diseases, and the development of surgical techniques. Any remaining doubts about medicine's progress are now confined to relatively few issues. Two such issues are (1) the fear that medical technology has surpassed medical wisdom, and (2) that the physician-patient relationship has deteriorated. In part, these are related concerns, both of which we examine more closely later in the chapter.

The history and treatment of mental disorders are distinct from those of the more obviously physical dysfunctions. There are many reasons for this. For one, until quite recently, the development of psychiatry was associated with the rise of the mental asylum, not the general hospital. Physically isolated from their medical colleagues, electing or given largely social control and custodial functions, psychiatrists came to resemble in role and action administrators more than physicians.[4] This trend was, no doubt, magnified by the tendency to transfer to the ministrations of "normal" medicine all patients for whom a definitive cure could be effected. To cite but one example, at one time, the wards of insane asylums were filled with psychotic patients who suffered from general paresis. Today, the treatment of syphilis is the concern of the internist, not the alienist, as the psychiatrist was once called.

In the early to mid-twentieth century, psychoanalysis made the private practice of certain aspects of psychiatry both rational and possible. But it also widened the gap between psychiatry and the rest of medicine. Psychoanalysis remained mentalistic as "normal" medicine became increasingly physicalistic. Also, the psychoanalytic regimen required long-term, intensive interpersonal contact with a rather select group of patients, while medicine was becoming more technical, favoring short-term objective encounters with a more varied population of patients. In 1930, the average general physician in private practice treated 50 patients a week; by 1950, the number was about 100, and by 1980, 117.[5]

Further, despite protestations to the contrary by American psychiatrists, there appeared to be little that was "medical" about psychoanalysis. Freud himself strongly argued against the medical exclusivity of his clinical creation, an argument that has been firmly resisted by the American psychoanalytic establishment for over four decades. It is only in recent years that "lay" analysts have come close to being grudgingly accepted by their psychiatric colleagues, even as psychoanalysis itself has come under more severe attack from many quarters.

The mental health professions—psychiatry, psychology, and to some extent social work—gained credibility throughout the 1940s and early 1950s. In part this was attributable to the public's growing romance with psychotherapy. Of course, psychiatry had developed a number of other promising therapeutic procedures. Psychosurgery, electroconvulsive therapy (ECT), and insulin coma therapy were but a few. But, promising as psychotherapy was believed to be, and despite the overblown claims for the few somatic interventions available, it was clear that the vast majority of psychotic patients housed in state hospitals would remain there unless more effective therapies were discovered.

It is debatable whether the introduction of the antipsychotic drugs in the early 1950s, the antidepressants in the late 1950s, and lithium in 1970 would have, in themselves, provoked the far-reaching changes that occurred in the mental health system, or whether the particular sociopolitical background of the times was a necessary condition for the revolution that ensued. But a transformation of the mental health system did indeed take place.[6,7] One consequence of that revolution has been the opportunity afforded for the "re-medicalization of psychiatry." Another was the return of great numbers of state mental hospital residents to the society-at-large. Thus, to a greater extent than previously considered possible, the general medical hospital has become the center of society's mental health delivery network.

The transmutation of the general hospital, medicine, and mental health practice has many causes. So, too, does their reassociation. The advance of biomedical science is one important factor; others are admixtures of social, economic, and political changes, making it possible to assess more accurately the cost-benefit considerations of mental health treatment. The complex action of these forces is illustrated by the changing pattern of authority in American general hospitals over the years:

Authority in American hospitals, Charles Perrow argues, has passed successively from the trustees to the physicians and finally to the administrators, a development he explains as resulting from the changing technology and needs of hospitals. The domination of the trustees was rooted in the need for capital investment and community acceptance. Doctors then assumed control because of the increasing complexity and importance of their skills. Finally, there has been a trend toward administrative domination because of the complexity of internal organization and relations with outside agencies. This argument suggests virtually an imminent process of change in organizations, depending entirely on their functional needs. Yet, as we have seen, the changing structure of authority was related to specific historical conditions. The growing power of physicians at the turn of the century rested in large part on their new ability to bring in revenue because of the increasing use of hospitals by paying patients; the rising influence of hospital administrators depended in part on the resistance to both centralized coordination of the hospital system and full-time responsibilities for physicians practicing in hospitals. These were the results, not of functional necessities, but of a particular configuration of interests.[8]

CURRENT TRENDS

Identifying and predicting the action of a "particular configuration of interests" operating at a given time is more successfully accomplished with hindsight. Still, even at this point, a number of variables indicate that the development of mental health services in the general hospital is far from complete. The most obvious of these is the determination on the part of both the government and nonhealth-related corporations to reduce the cost of health care in general, and mental health services in particular.

In 1965, when Medicare and Medicaid were enacted, the total cost of health in the United States was estimated to be 39 billion dollars. This came to 6 percent of the gross national product (GNP), or approximately 181 dollars per capita. Of this amount, patients paid 45 percent, insurers 25 percent, and the federal government 11 percent. By 1981, the bill for health care had risen to 287 billion dollars, 9.8 percent of the GNP, and 862 (inflation-corrected) dollars per capita. Insurers paid 28 percent of these costs, the federal government 30 percent, while the patients' out-of-pocket share had decreased to 27 percent. Hospital costs alone were more than 5.5 times higher in 1982 than in 1965. The proportion of GNP devoted to health care reached 10.3 percent in 1982, and was still climbing.[9] By 1990, Inglehart estimates, it will be 12.3 percent of GNP.[10]

The cost of mental health services has followed a similar trajectory. In 1955, 1.2 billion dollars was spent on mental health services. This was approximately 6 percent of the total of all health care costs. By 1977, 19.6 billion dollars, or about 12 percent of all health costs, was spent on mental health services. Of this amount, the federal government contributed 25 percent, state and local governments 28 percent, insurers 13 percent, and the remainder was paid directly by the patient. Undoubtedly, the monies spent on mental health services at that point would have been even larger if the insurance coverage available for them more closely approximated that for other medical care.

The rising cost of medical care, however, was but one precipitant of the shift in health care policy that is now under way. Starr argues that, "like American politics more generally, the politics of health care passed through three phases in the 1970s:

1. "A period of agitation and reform in the first half of the decade, when broader entitlements to social welfare and stricter regulation of industry gained ground in public opinion and law.
2. "A prolonged stalemate, beginning around 1975, when the preoccupation increasingly became coping with inflation, doubts arose about the value of medical care, and initiatives such as national health insurance were set aside.
3. "A growing reaction against liberalism and government culminating in the election of President Reagan in 1980 [and his reelection in 1984] and the reversal of many earlier redistributive and regulatory programs."[11]

Today, the consumer, the insurance industry, employers, and the government are arrayed in a coalition that is determined at least to hold down, and at best to reduce, the cost of medical care. The strategy of the government is clear: (1) competition among health care providers will be encouraged; (2) incentives will be provided for reducing health care costs; (3) patients will pay a higher proportion of their medical bills out-of-pocket; (4) the government will become less involved in the direct delivery of health care services, that is, the health delivery system will be "reprivatized;" (5) the government will take additional steps toward further control of health costs, whenever it deems it necessary to do so.

The growing penetration of for-profit corporations in the health care field is having, and will continue to have, an enormous impact upon the health care service delivery system. By the early 1980s, over 30 percent of all hospital beds were controlled by multiinstitutional corporations. The total was lowest for New England (10 percent) and highest in the West (40 percent).[12] These facts (taken together with the high frequency with which physicians are entering into other than fee-for-service relationships with their patients) seem to guarantee that "reprivatization" will not return health care to the private practitioner model of times past.

Mental health practitioners will be affected more by some particular trends in privatization. For example, comprehensive plans for diagnosis related groups (DRG) reimbursement in the area of mental health are under discussion, but they are not as yet ready for implementation. It is hoped that the particular difficulties involved in applying such a policy to mental disorders will be duly considered and mastered. Two of the problem areas are (1) the lack of a sharp delineation between normal and abnormal behavior,[13,14] and (2) the poor correlation between diagnosis and length of treatment.

On the other hand, the growing number of for-profit, prospective payment plans will undoubtedly accentuate the "re-medicalization" of psychiatry and increase the number of nonmedical practitioners rendering psychotherapeutic services to patients. This will occur, if for no other reason, because psychotherapy is less expensive when an adequate supply of substitute personnel is readily available.[15]

Against this background of change, the pressing need for an effective, comprehensive delivery system for mental health services must be considered.

> The true prevalence of mental disorders as measured in western countries since WWII is unlikely to average less than 15% at any given time. One of the most important findings from these studies is that only a small percentage of the persons judged to be suffering from these disorders have ever been treated by mental health professionals. For all disorders combined, an average of almost three fourths of the cases appear to be untreated. Even for schizophrenia, probably the most severe disorder, the median community rate of untreated cases is 20%, increasing to 40% for all psychoses.[16]

Not only does a significant portion of our population suffer from serious emotional and cognitive disorders, many of which are untreated, but, for many of those who come to treatment, the response of the mental health system has been far from adequate. This is nowhere more obvious than in New York City, where a stroll down any of the major thoroughfares—Madison, Park, Fifth, Lexington, or Broadway—will provide the pedestrian with stark evidence of the failure of the deinstitutionalization crusades of the 1960s and 1970s. Confused individuals are seen sleeping on the streets and rummaging in the trash. Especially vulnerable to therapeutic abandonment are the poor or those who will become poor because of their emotional condition and society's response to it.[17,18]

If we add to the number of individuals who suffer from primarily psychiatric disorders those individuals who develop emotional or behaviorial dysfunction in reaction to physical injury, disease or substance abuse, those who experience adjustment failure in the face of adversity, and those who could profit from preventive programs with mental health components (cardiac patients, those suffering from chronic pain syndromes, the overweight, smokers, hypertensives), the proportion of potential mental health clients in the general population would be enormously larger. This is not to say that all those at risk should seek, or would profit from, mental health interventions. Rather, it argues that the appropriate provision of these services is a public health and economic necessity. To cite but one example of many available:

> Retrospective analysis of health insurance claims data and meta-analyses of time-series studies and prospective controlled experimental studies converge to provide evidence of a general cost-offset effect following out-patient psychotherapy. The widespread and persistent evidence of reduced rate of increase of medical expense following mental health treatment argues for the inseparability of mind and body in health care and it also argues specifically for the likelihood that mental health treatment may improve patients' ability to stay healthy enough to avoid hospital admission for physical illness.[19]

THE FUTURE

Clearly, the general medical hospital will play an increasingly central role in the delivery of mental health services. The manner in which this role will be performed will depend in part upon the nature of the hospital (voluntary, municipal, proprietary) and its defined mission. However, some general predictions can be made on the basis of current trends.

Psychiatric Inpatient Services

Psychiatric inpatient services, units, and nonsegregated facilities will become "hyperacutely" oriented. They will increasingly concentrate upon local, crisis-oriented, short-term interventions designed to arrest fulminating psychiatric emergencies. These services will become primarily, if not exclusively, located in general hospital settings because of the increasing availability of more powerful psychiatric technologies—imaging techniques, blood tests, and so on—that can be utilized in fast, accurate diagnostic work-ups. In these settings, the psychiatrist, acting within the medical model, will employ an increasing armamentarium of somatic therapies.

The remarkable development of clinically effective psychoactive agents will continue; new drugs will be available that will be both more disease-specific and more applicable to a wider group of disorders. For example, the availability of antidepressants that have a considerably faster onset of action, more effective blocking agents for the treatment of opiate addiction and abuse, antipsychotic drugs that have far fewer side effects, and psychoactive agents for the treatment of some "personality disorders" will make hospital-based psychiatric treatment both necessary and more desirable. These types of somatic treatments will have major effects in decreasing lengths of stay for psychiatric illnesses, thereby making health insurance coverage for these treatments indistinguishable from those for "medical" conditions.

Once the patient's care has stabilized, psychotherapeutic and social interventions, as well as aftercare coordination, are likely to be managed more frequently by nonmedically trained mental health specialists. In some instances, the inpatient psychiatrist will assume total responsibility for the patient's care. In others, the psychiatrist will function as a consultant to other professionals upon whom patient care will devolve—primary care physicians, psychologists, social workers, psychiatric nurse specialists, drug treatment counselors, and so on.

Cost Containment

The impact of peer review organizations (PROs) and their cost-containment successors will be substantial in reducing hospitalization lengths of stay and the number of clinical problems for which patients are treated in the hospital setting. Prospective payment reimbursement systems (for example, DRGs) and other government- and third party payer-mandated mechanisms will force hospitals to wield greater control over attending physicians and other mental health care providers who admit patients. The inherent difficulties between hospitals and their affiliated private practitioners to cooperate within the cost-containment guidelines may lead hospitals to employ professionals directly so that more effective control over clinical care can be exerted.

Hospital Privileges

Hospital admitting, treatment, and discharge privileges will be broadened to encompass a wider range of mental health professionals, most notably clinical psychologists, psychiatric nurse specialists, and psychiatric social workers. Such privileges will be limited by functional considerations consistent with the developments described above. The utilization of nonphysician professionals will accelerate because of cost efficiency and legal considerations. This will be especially true in proprietary institutions that have a history of responding to fiscal changes by modifying services and professional providers.

Consultation Services

Mental health professionals will be more frequently requested to consult and assist in the treatment of general medical patients. Psychiatric consultation-liaison services provide an organizational format for such interdisciplinary collaboration. Other formats may be found in semiautonomous or autonomous departments of behavioral medicine and health psychology. Consultation-liaison programs are likely to remain inpatient-focused, while behavioral medicine and health psychology programs are likely to remain outpatient-based.

The Mental Health Delivery System

More so than ever before, the general hospital is likely to serve as the hub of a complex mental health delivery system. Attached to its core inpatient facilities, either by affiliation agreement or intrainstitutional development, will be an increasingly large array of services—outpatient clinics, partial hospitalization units, preventive outreach programs, long-term custodial care centers (nursing homes), and so on. Many of these will depend on changes in third party reimbursement policies that to date have emphasized inpatient care. As these other services come to be appreciated for their cost-containment potential, they will be more appropriately funded and will serve as alternatives to hospitalization whenever clinically possible.

Service Marketing

Mental health services will be increasingly marketed. The marketing programs will be professionally orchestrated and directed toward that mix of potential patients who are, at any given time, likely to generate the greatest net income. Once again, the indigent will largely fall to the tender mercies of underfunded public facilities and programs. The pressures on such local public mental health services might become so great that state mental hospitals will once again open their doors and expand their roles in the care of these patients.

Planning and Coordination

Because of the "reprivatization" of health care—the reinvigoration of competition and the profit motive—and a failure in will on the part of the government, mental health planning and coordination of mental health services will prove even more difficult than they are now. This is not to suggest that there will be an end to regulation. Indeed, regulation will increase as health centers and government continue to debate the feasibility of diagnosis-related groupings (and whatever successor reimbursement systems are formulated) and the real costs of "doing business." Extensive and expensive data-retrieval systems will be necessary to monitor a growing variety of variables, including treatment effectiveness and costs, patient progress, hospital costs, and practitioner incomes.

Specific Changes

Significant modifications will be made in the health delivery system of which general hospitals are a part. These will stem from the following developments:

- An increasing share of payment for health care will fall on consumers.
- The health care provided to those who cannot pay for it will deteriorate.
- The number of corporation-controlled health care facilities will increase, restricting the number to whom they provide services and the nature of those services.
- The autonomy of the individual health care service provider will be reduced.

CONCLUSION

It is clear that major changes in many areas will profoundly affect the provision of mental health care services in the general hospital setting. The technology, professional personnel, and perhaps even the disease processes themselves, are all assuming unfamiliar appearances. It is likely that many general hospitals will not be capable of adapting to the stress of all these changes and will not survive.

Yet, it is equally clear that the very nature of the complexities that increasingly characterize our appreciation of medical and psychiatric disorders, the progressively more powerful therapeutic armamentaria that we possess to ameliorate or cure disease processes, and the increasingly closer relationships that have evolved between the biological and psychosocial approaches to human disorder—all make general hospitals more important than ever in the provision of patient care services.

REFERENCES

1. P. Starr, *The Social Transformation of American Medicine* (New York: Basic Books, 1982), 146.

2. Ibid.

3. Lewis Thomas, *The Youngest Science* (New York: Viking Press, 1983).

4. Starr, *Social Transformation,* 27.

5. Thomas, *Youngest Science.*

6. M.L. Zaphiropoulos, "On Remedicalizing Psychiatry and Demedicalizing Psychoanalysis," *Academic Forum* 28 (1984): 6–8.

7. A.H. Calobeisi, "General Hospital Psychiatry Update," *Psychiatric Annals* 13 (1983): 598–601.

8. Starr, *Social Transformation,* 178–179.

9. S.S. Sharfstein and A. Beigel, "Less Is More? Today's Economics and Its Challenge to Psychiatry," *American Journal of Psychiatry* 141 (1984): 1403–1408.

10. J.K. Inglehart, "Fixed-Fee Medicine for Medicare: An Introduction," *Science and Technology* 1 (1984): 94–100.

11. Starr, *Social Transformation,* 880.

12. Ibid.

13. B.S. Dohrenwend et al., "Social Functioning of Psychiatric Patients in Contrast with Community Cases in the General Population" *Archives of General Psychiatry* 40 (1983): 1174–1182.

14. D. Eddy, "Variations in Physician Practice: Role of Uncertainty," *Health Affairs* 3 (1984): 74–89.

15. A. Beigel and S.S. Sharfstein, "Mental Health Care Providers: Not the Only Cause or Only Cure for Rising Costs," *American Journal of Psychiatry* 141 (1984): 668–672.

16. Dohrenwend et al. "Social Functioning," 1174.

17. C.E. Flemister and J.A. Talbott, *Alternative Futures for Mental Health Services in New York: 2000 and Beyond,* Report of the New York State Health Planning Commission (Albany, NY: New York State Health Planning Commission, 1984).

18. L.R. Marcos and R.M. Gil, "Psychiatric Catchment Areas in an Urban Center: A Policy in Disarray," *American Journal of Psychiatry* 141 (1984): 875–881.

19. E. Mumford et al., "A New Look at Evidence about the Reduced Cost of Medical Utilization Following Mental Health Treatment," *American Journal of Psychiatry* 141 (1984): 1145–1158.

Index